The Neurology of Olfaction

The Neurology of Olfaction

Christopher H. Hawkes

Richard L. Doty

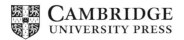

CAMBRIDGE
UNIVERSITY PRESS

CAMBRIDGE UNIVERSITY PRESS
Cambridge, New York, Melbourne, Madrid, Cape Town, Singapore, São Paulo, Delhi

Cambridge University Press
The Edinburgh Building, Cambridge CB2 8RU, UK

Published in the United States of America by Cambridge University Press, New York

www.cambridge.org
Information on this title: www.cambridge.org/9780521682169

First published 2009

Printed in the United Kingdom at the University Press, Cambridge

A catalogue record for this publication is available from the British Library

Library of Congress Cataloguing in Publication data
Hawkes, Christopher H.
    The neurology of olfaction / Christopher H. Hawkes, Richard L. Doty.
        p. ; cm.
    Includes bibliographical references and index.
    ISBN 978-0-521-68216-9 (pbk.)
    1. Smell disorders.   2. Smell.   3. Nose–Innervation.   I. Doty, Richard L.   II. Title.
    [DNLM: 1. Olfaction Disorders.   2. Neurodegenerative Diseases–complications.
    3. Olfactory Pathways–anatomy & histology.   4. Olfactory Pathways–physiology.
    5. Olfactory Pathways–physiopathology.   6. Smell–physiology.   WV 301 H392n 2009]
    RF341.H387 2009
    616.8′ 56–dc22   2008045143

ISBN 978-0-521-68216-9 paperback

Contents

The plates are to be found between pages 82 and 83

Foreword

As a 20-year-old I stepped outdoors and in an instant was taken back in time to my grandmother's garden, the aroma of baking bread from her kitchen reawakening in me visual memories, feelings, and experiences of clarity and intense familiarity. I looked about me and saw a bakery nearby.

At the age of 45 my mother lost her sense of smell, and at the age of 65 she developed Parkinson's disease.

When I was a medical student as part of a course in public health our class visited a building on Manhattan's lower east side where coffee was roasted commercially. On entering the building the fragrance of roasting coffee was deliriously wonderful. A workman by the door said: "After 20 minutes you won't be able to stand the smell." He was right.

When playing soccer in school I suffered a hard knock on the head colliding with an opposing player and in that instant smelled an odor as peculiar as it was intense.

The olfactory system is, paradoxically, primitive yet complex and sophisticated, not following many of the rules pertaining to other sensory systems, intimately and immediately connected to deep and important brain structures. It declines with age, and its loss may foretell serious and progressive degenerative disease of the brain. Despite the obvious importance of this vital sensory system, olfaction has largely been neglected by neurologists.

Where have the neurologists been all this time and why have they neglected this important modality? The nose is the "eye" for most nonprimates and just because other sensory modalities have proven critical in human evolution does not make the sense of smell unimportant to human beings. Indeed, this sense plays a critical role in safety and nutrition, and recent studies suggest its understanding may help to unravel the mysteries of certain neurologic diseases.

The *Neurology of Olfaction* connects olfactory science to human neurology for the first time. Jointly authored by Professor Christopher Hawkes, a leading clinical neurologist with a special interest in olfaction, and Professor Richard L. Doty, a world-renowned specialist in smell and taste, this monograph provides an engaging overview of the sense of smell and its importance in human neurological disease. The book is replete with compelling experimental findings and fascinating clinical case studies, and each time I picked it up I found myself spending much more time with it than I had planned. It will serve as a valuable reference source for neurologists and others truly interested in the newly developing world of the chemical senses. Every neurologist should have this book in their library.

Thomas R. Swift, MD FAAN
Professor Emeritus and Former Chair
Department of Neurology
Medical College of Georgia
President
American Academy of Neurology, 2005–2007
Past President
American Association of Electromyography and Electrodiagnosis
Past President
Society of Clinical Neurologists

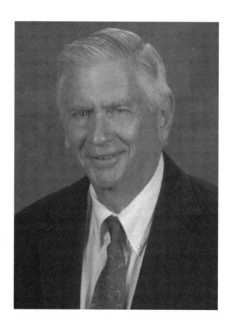

Preface

Olfaction evolved at least 550 million years ago and, in conjunction with the ability to move, eat, and reproduce, detecting chemicals by specialized receptors was about all that invertebrates could do. Today the sense of smell is commonly viewed as a somewhat more primitive modality than its sister sense of taste, in that it does not rely upon the thalamus for cortical transmission. Vision and hearing are even more recent phylogenetically, employing the thalamus in their projections to cortical regions. They have received major attention because of their perceived biological importance in humans. However, the significance of the olfactory system for everyday life is rarely appreciated until dysfunction occurs, and this primary sensory modality is far from immune to disease – in fact it is *more* vulnerable than any other sensory system. This is largely because of its virtually unprotected contact with the external environment in the nose and its close neural connections with temporal lobe and limbic brain regions associated with memory and emotion. As we describe, this anatomy provides access for neurotropic agents and facilitates their spread to regions associated with developmental and degenerative diseases. Clearly, the studious avoidance and trivialization of smell testing by clinicians is unwarranted, but until recently the excuse was always that the sense of smell is not important, and that it provides information of minimal diagnostic value. All this is in the process of change as we try to show here. For example, many studies demonstrate the consistency and probable premotor development of decreased smell function in degenerative disorders, notably Parkinson's and Alzheimer's diseases. This is clearly important: if a simple smell test can assist with a diagnosis, it might replace more complex procedures and, more importantly, it may help to identify those family members at risk of future illness.

This book provides a resumé of the anatomy and physiology of the olfactory pathways and how the sense of smell may be measured. We elaborate those diseases where smell loss is a notable feature that may assist the clinician in making a diagnosis. Approaches are detailed for diagnosing, investigating, and treating a number of olfactory disorders and for counseling patients how to cope best with impairment of olfactory function. Finally, we describe strategies that help to minimize food poisoning and avoid dangerous situations, such as leaking natural gas.

We hope this book will stimulate others to take up a clinical and research interest in olfaction and give this ancient modality the full attention it richly deserves.

CHH

RLD

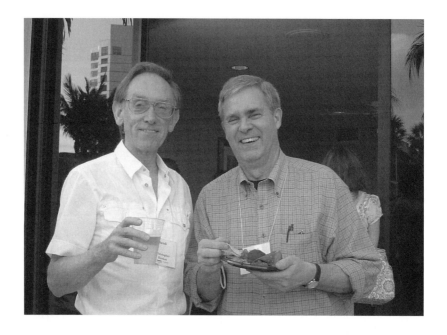

Acknowledgments

The authors wish to express their thanks to the following colleagues who provided invaluable assistance in writing this book. Their names are presented alphabetically and not in order of their contribution.

Professor Kailash Bhatia, Institute of Neurology, London, UK

Dr. David Bowsher, Pain Research Institute, University Hospital Aintree, Liverpool, UK

Professor Heiko Braak, JW Goethe University, Frankfurt, Germany

Dr. Sanjiv Chawda, Queen's Hospital, Romford, UK

Dr. Jacquie Deeb, Queen's Hospital, Romford, UK

Dr. Kelly del Tredici, JW Goethe University, Frankfurt, Germany

Professor Jay Gottfried, Northwestern University Feinberg School of Medicine, Chicago, USA

Dr. Ranjan Gunasekara, Queen's Hospital, Romford, UK

Professor Thomas Hummel, University of Dresden, Germany

Professor Tim Jacob, University of Cardiff, UK

Professor Paul Moberg, University of Pennsylvania School of Medicine, Philadelphia, USA

Dr. Nizar Muhammed, Queen's Hospital, Romford, UK

Professor Krishna Persaud, UMIST, Manchester, UK

Dr. Paola Piccini, MRC Clinical Sciences Centre, Imperial College, London, UK

Dr. Muss Shah, Queen's Hospital, Romford, UK

Dr. Greg Smutzer, Department of Biology, Temple University, Philadelphia, USA

Dr. Sarah Tabrizi, Institute of Neurology, London, UK

Anatomy and physiology

The sense of smell, viewed as the sentinel of the brain by Macdonald Critchley (Critchley, 1986), largely determines the flavor of foods and beverages, and provides an early warning system for the detection of such hazards as fire, leaking natural gas, and spoiled food. Aside from playing a critical role in safety, nutrition, and quality of life, this important sense provides an index of the health of sectors of the brain not discernible by other means. Thus, decreased smell function can signify the early development of neuropathology within limbic structures associated with Alzheimer's disease and idiopathic Parkinson's disease – neuropathology that can occur several years before the onset of other clinical signs (see Chapter 4). Before undergoing the ravages of old age and associated neural dysfunction, humans are exquisitely sensitive to odors, detecting some substances, such as mercaptans added to odorize natural gas, in the parts-per-billion range.

Despite such importance, olfaction has been neglected by most neurologists, with the majority failing even to test its function. Fortunately this has been changing in recent years, in part because of (1) the development and proliferation of practical quantitative smell tests, (2) a better understanding of its association with neurodegenerative diseases, (3) the elucidation of its transduction mechanisms, and (4) a broader appreciation of its general importance to human health and well-being.

In this chapter we describe the anatomy and physiology of the olfactory system, as well as a number of factors which influence its normal function. Emphasis is placed on the system's complex and dynamic nature, including its unique regenerative properties and critical associations with brain structures related to emotion and memory. The influences of diseases on olfactory function are discussed in Chapters 3 and 4.

The nasal cavity

For odorant molecules to reach the olfactory receptors, they must first pass through the upper recesses of the nasal cavity, the first part of the respiratory passages. This highly vascularized cavity is separated into two chambers by a partition, the nasal septum. Three or, more rarely, four structures, termed nasal turbinates, project from the lateral wall of each side of the nose into the cavity. These structures receive their blood supply from branches of the sphenopalatine artery, the end artery of the internal maxillary branch of the external carotid artery (Lee et al., 2002). The lymphatic system of the nasal mucosa drains into the superficial cervical lymph nodes, which drain into the posterior cervical lymph nodes. Medial to each turbinate is a cleft or meatus. It is the most superior of these clefts, the olfactory cleft, through which air passes to reach the olfactory receptor region. These features and parts of the olfactory forebrain are displayed in Figure 1.1.

The nasal turbinates, particularly the inferior and middle, are richly endowed with a network of tortuous veins that can rapidly swell with blood. Such engorgement dramatically alters nasal passage volume, influencing the amount of air that reaches the olfactory cleft and respiratory processes in general. When the turbinates are moderately distended, more air is delivered to the olfactory cleft than when they are markedly engorged or disengorged (Schneider & Wolf, 1960). In the human, 5–15 percent of the inhaled air-stream is diverted to the receptor region, depending upon such engorgement, the strength of sniffing, idiosyncratic aspects of nasal cavity anatomy, the thickness of the mucus, and the size and shape of the nasal valve (Keyhani et al., 1995). Exercise, hypercapnia, and increased sympathetic tone are among the factors that constrict turbinate engorgement, whereas cold air, irritants, hypocapnia, and increased parasympathetic tone are among those that increase such engorgement (Jones, 2001). Short repetitive sniffs appear to be less efficient than long sustained sniffs in optimizing olfactory sensitivity and the delivery of odorants into the human olfactory cleft (Laing, 1983; Mainland & Sobel, 2006; Zhao et al., 2004, 2006). High flow rates favor absorption of hydrophilic compounds, whereas low flow rates favor absorption of hydrophobic substances (Mozell et al., 1991).

It is now known that most people experience changes in the relative engorgement of each side of the nose over time (Haight & Cole, 1984). In some individuals, such changes are coordinated, resulting in periodic shifts of relative left–right airflow. These side-to-side fluctuations have been reported to have period lengths ranging from one to five hours in adults and to be absent in children. Although this "nasal cycle" has been said to be present in up to 80 percent of adults, recent studies suggest that this may be an over-estimate (Flanagan & Eccles, 1997). Thus, if one accepts the commonly held definition of cycle (regular periodicity) and assumes that 180° phase differences are required for the left–right engorgement periods, very few humans have a true nasal cycle. In one study using autocorrelation analysis, for example, only 9 (15 percent) of 60 subjects exhibited the classical nasal cycle, 28.3 percent exhibited parallel cycles (i.e., left–right engorgement changes

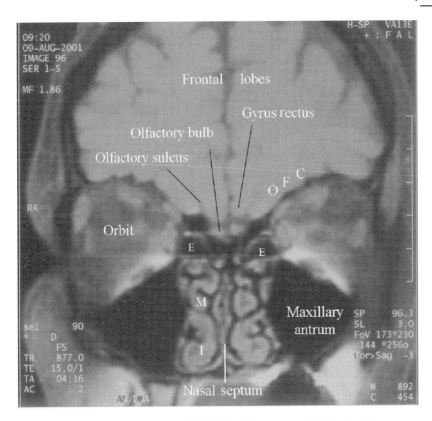

Figure 1.1 MRI scan (coronal, T1 weighted) in healthy 45-year-old lady showing frontal lobes; orbits; olfactory bulbs, olfactory sulcus and gyrus rectus. OFC is the orbitofrontal cortex. Letter "E" indicates part of the ethmoid sinuses, which are frequently honeycomb structures. Letter "I" is the right inferior turbinate; "M" is the right middle turbinate. The superior turbinate and infundibulum are not clearly shown due to the posterior coronal section. (Reproduced with permission from Hawkes, 2002. Copyright © 2002, Elsevier.)

that are in phase), 23.3 percent exhibited hemicycles (i.e., only one side showing engorgement fluctuations over time), and 33.3 percent were acyclic (Mirza et al., 1997). Another study, also based upon statistical criteria, found a classic nasal cycle in only 2 of 16 (13 percent) adults evaluated. Hemicycles were observed in seven (44 percent) (Gilbert & Rosenwasser, 1987).

Regardless of its periodicity, left–right fluctuations in nasal engorgement are claimed to be an overall index of autonomic tone (Werntz et al., 1983). When the left nasal chamber is more congested than the right, general sympathetic activity predominates over parasympathetic activity. When the

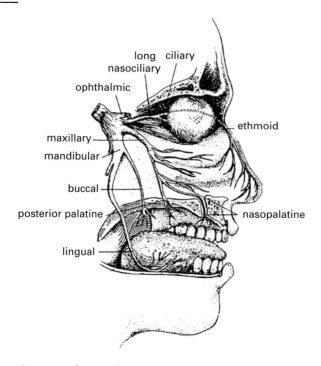

Figure 1.2 Schematic diagram of the branches of the trigeminal nerve that innervate the nasal, oral, and ocular epithelia. (From Bryant and Silver, 2000. Copyright © 2000, Wiley–Liss. Reprinted with permission of Wiley–Liss, Inc., a subsidiary of John Wiley & Sons, Inc.)

right nasal chamber is more engorged than the left, the opposite is the case. Importantly, the relative degree of left–right engorgement correlates with such measures as: (1) the relative electroencephalographic (EEG) activity of the two cerebral hemispheres (Werntz *et al.*, 1983); (2) rapid eye movement (REM) and non-REM sleep activity patterns (Goldstein *et al.*, 1972); (3) verbal and spatial cognitive processing (Klein *et al.*, 1986); and (4) asymmetrical activity in paired body organs, including the release of hormones from paired glands such as the adrenal glands (Shannahoff-Khalsa *et al.*, 1996). Olfactory thresholds tend to be lower on both sides of the nose during the heightened sympathetic component of engorgement, that is, when the left nasal chamber is more occluded (Frye & Doty, 1992). Interestingly, when subjects sniff a two-odor mixture composed of a hydrophobic and a hydrophilic odor, the hydrophobic element of the mixture is better perceived through the low-flow nostril and the hydrophilic element through the high-flow nostril (Sobel *et al.*, 1999a).

The general somatic nerve supply to the nose derives from branches of the trigeminal nerve (Doty & Cometto-Muniz, 2003), whereas the autonomic

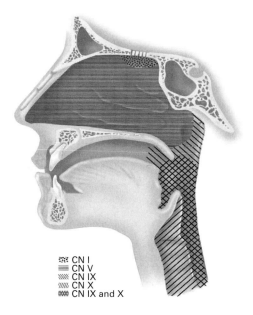

CN I
CN V
CN IX
CN X
CN IX and X

Figure 1.3 A schematic of the regions within the nasal and oral cavities innervated by several cranial nerves that can be stimulated by some odorants and irritants. CN I, olfactory nerve; CN V, trigeminal nerve; CN IX, glossopharyngeal nerve; CN X, vagus; CN VII innervates the taste buds in the anterior tongue and is not shown in this diagram. The cross-hatched regions represent areas of overlap between CN IX and CN X. CN V also innervates the region innervated by CN I. CN I may extend farther down onto the middle turbinate than depicted here. (Copyright © 2002, Richard L. Doty.)

supply to the nose comes from the sphenopalatine ganglion. The anterior and posterior ethmoid nerves, which are branches of the nasociliary nerve (ophthalmic division of V), supply the upper part of the nasal cavity (Figure 1.2). The posterior part of the nasal cavity is fed by the nasopalatine nerve, a branch of the maxillary nerve. The autonomic supply to the nose comes from the sphenopalatine ganglion.

Some airborne odorants and other chemicals are capable of stimulating trigeminal free nerve endings distributed throughout the nasal mucosa, as well as trigeminal and other sensory nerve endings dispersed in other regions of the throat and mouth (Figure 1.3). Examples of sensations resulting from such stimulation are warmth, coolness, and sharpness (Doty *et al.*, 1978). These somatosensory sensations should not be confused with odors, although they can contribute to the overall appreciation of an odor.

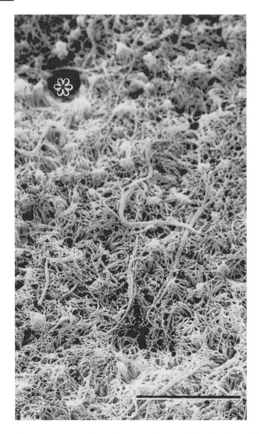

Figure 1.4 Scanning electron micrograph of surface of human olfactory epithelium showing where thin parts of olfactory cilia form a blanket covering the epithelial surface. Asterisk indicates opening into duct of a Bowman's gland. Bar, 10 μm. (From Menco and Morrison, 2003. With permission.)

The olfactory epithelium

In the human nose, there are an estimated six million specialized olfactory receptor cells per nostril (Moran *et al.*, 1982). The receptor cells are embedded in a matrix of supporting cells within a pseudostratified columnar epithelium located high in the nasal chamber (Figure 1.4, Figure 1.5, Figure 1.6). This neuroepithelium covers the cribriform plate and lines sectors of the superior septum, superior turbinate, and, to a lesser extent, the anterior portion of the middle turbinate. The existence of some olfactory receptor cells (ORC) on the middle turbinate (Leopold *et al.*, 2000) is a useful aspect of applied anatomy for those wishing to biopsy ORC for culture, histology, or patch clamp studies, as it is more accessible and less risky to

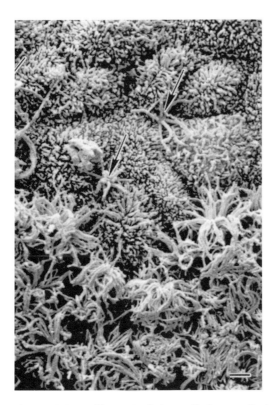

Figure 1.5 A transition region between the human olfactory (bottom half) and respiratory (top half) epithelia. Arrows signify two examples of olfactory receptor cell dendritic endings with cilia. (From Menco and Morrison, 2003. With permission.)

sample than the main olfactory area. Whilst most of the bony and cartila-ginous structures within the nasal cavity, including the turbinates, are covered with a mucus-secreting respiratory epithelium, the olfactory region is covered with a distinctly different epithelium whose mucus is mainly derived from specialized glands, termed "Bowman's glands" (for review, see Menco & Morrison, 2003).

The bipolar olfactory receptor cells serve as the first-order neurons of the system, and their central limbs project directly from the nasal cavity to the olfactory bulb without synapse, making them a major conduit for central nervous system (CNS) viral and xenobiotic invasion, as described in Chapter 4. These receptor cells form tight junctions with adjacent non-neural cells. The apical end of each cell has a knob-like protrusion from which receptor-containing cilia project into the mucus (Figure 1.7). Embryologically, these cells are derived from the olfactory placode and are thus of CNS origin (Chuah *et al.*, 2003). Their somata are found at all levels within the

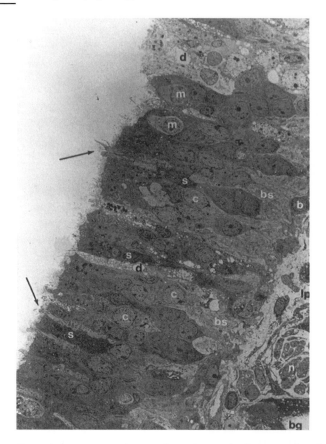

Figure 1.6 Low-power electron photomicrograph of cross-section of the human olfactory neuroepithelium depicting the four major types of cells: bipolar receptor cells (arrows point to cilia at dendritic knob; c, cell body), microvillar cells (m), sustentacular cells (s), and basal cells (b); bg, Bowman's gland; lp, lamina propria; n, collection of axons within an ensheathing cell; d, degenerating cells; bs, basal cell undergoing mitosis. (Photo courtesy of Dr. David Moran, Longmont, Colorado.)

epithelium, with the somata of the older cells being closer to the mucosal surface than those of more recently differentiated cells. The axons of the bipolar olfactory cells are extremely small (~0.2 μm in diameter), making them among the thinnest and slowest conducting (~1 m/s) axons in the nervous system. In humans, the cilia number, on average, ~25 per cell, whereas in other species, such as the dog, this can number in the hundreds. Although the olfactory cilia contain the familiar 9+2 arrangement of microtubules, i.e., two central microtubules surrounded by nine outer doublet microtubules, they lack the muscle-like dynein arms required for

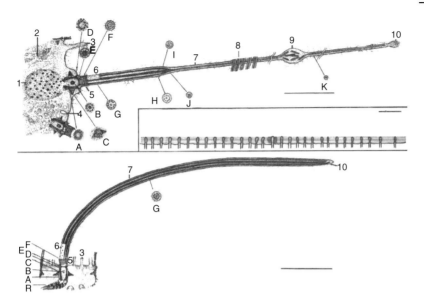

Figure 1.7 Diagram of mammalian olfactory (top) and respiratory (bottom) cilia. Features of the two diagrams have been drawn to scale. The olfactory cilium is interrupted at two places, indicating that the cilia are actually much longer. A–E, basal body cross-sections; F–H, cross-sections through proximal regions of olfactory cilia (top) and homologous regions of respiratory cilia (bottom); I–K, cross-sections through distal parts of olfactory cilia; R, striated rootlet of respiratory cilium; 1, fibrogranular microtubule pool (cilium precursor pool); 2, microtubules inside dendritic endings; 3, microvilli of dendritic endings (sparse) and of ciliated respiratory cells; 4, coated vesicles; 5, ciliary necklaces (seven strands for olfactory cilia, five strands for respiratory cilia); 6, ciliary membranes studded with membrane particles reflecting proteins which are more numerous in olfactory than respiratory cilia; 7, nearby glycocalix; 8, bundle of tapers of other, nearby, cilia; 9, vesiculated expansion along distal part of cilium; 10, ciliary tips which in the case of olfactory cilia terminate in a small vesicle. The inset demonstrates that the cilia of one receptor cell dendrite can extend over about 15 other endings. Top and bottom bars = 1 μm; center bar = 10 μm. (From Menco and Morrison, 2003. With permission.)

motility (Figure 1.7; Menco & Morrison, 2003). Hence, they do not beat synchronously, unlike the cilia of the respiratory epithelium, and simply waft in the mucus.

The supporting cells, also termed "sustentacular cells," are predominant within the olfactory epithelium. These relatively large cells insulate the receptor cells from one another, regulate mucus microcomposition, deactivate odorants, and protect the epithelium from foreign agents. Although these cells lack cilia, they project many microvillae into the mucus.

In addition to the olfactory receptor and supporting cells, the olfactory epithelium harbors cells which line the glands and ducts of the Bowman's glands, microvillar cells, and two types of basal cells (namely, horizontal and globose basal cells), as well as other cellular elements (Figure 1.6). The microvillar cells, whose function remains poorly understood, resemble so-called brush cells of the upper and lower airways of many species. They are located at the epithelial surface and, like the supporting cells, extend micro-villae from their apical surfaces into the olfactory mucus (Moran et al., 1982). In the human, they occur in about a 1:10 ratio with the bipolar receptor cells, numbering around 600 000 in an intact epithelium. The horizontal (dark) and globose (light) basal cells are located near the basement membrane and are stem cells from which other classes of cells arise (Figure 1.6).

In addition to odorants, numerous volatile compounds, as well as nonvolatile ones that adsorb from small particles in the air, are readily taken up by the nasal mucosa (Schlesinger, 1985; Stott et al., 1986). For example, herbicides such as dioxins (Gillner et al., 1987) and chlorthiamid (Brittebo et al., 1991) are selectively absorbed by the olfactory epithelium, causing damage to the cells. Compounds absorbed by the nasal mucosa are actively metabolized in situ. In some cases they are detoxified, but in other cases they are transformed into metabolites of greater toxicity or carcinogenicity (Bond, 1986; Dahl, 1986). Whilst the high concentration of P450 in hepatic microsomes is well known, microsomes in the olfactory epithelium also have high levels of P450 mono-oxygenases, as shown, for example, in the rat (Hext & Lock, 1992) and rabbit (Ding & Coon, 1990). Supporting cells, as well as the acinar and duct cells of Bowman's glands, are particularly endowed with such xenobiotic metabolizing enzymes (Ding & Dahl, 2003), serving to metabolize agents that become absorbed in the olfactory mucus. More than 10 different P450s have been identified in mammalian olfactory mucosa, including members of the CYP1A, 2A, 2B, 2C, 2E, 2G, 2J, 3A, and 4B subfamilies (Ding & Dahl, 2003). Several P450s are preferentially expressed in this mucosa, including CYP2G1. The P450 levels are sometimes in excess of those in the liver, depending on the particular subtype. Compounds that have been shown to be metabolized in vitro by the nasal P450 dependent mono-oxygenase system include nasal decongestants, essences, anesthetics, alcohols, nicotine, cocaine, and many nasal carcinogens (Dahl, 1988).

When the olfactory epithelium is damaged, the same type of basal cell, most likely a globose cell, gives rise to both neural and non-neural cells, allowing for the replacement of damaged receptors (Huard et al., 1998). Although at one time it was believed that the sensory neurons of the olfactory epithelium are automatically and continuously replaced by the differentiating basal cells over the course of a month or so, we now know this is not true. Thus, long-lived receptor cells have been observed in rats (Hinds et al., 1984), and regulatory mechanisms have been identified that alter the timing and extent of neurogenesis from the basal cell population (Mackay-Sim, 2003). Unfortunately, receptor restoration following damage is often incomplete in both humans and animals.

The unmyelinated receptor cell axons coalesce within the lamina propria into bundles containing approximately 200 axons, each surrounded by glial cells that have features in common with astrocytes and Schwann cell mesaxons. Metabolic and electrical interactions may occur among the axons of these bundles, which are virtually in direct (~100 Å or 10 nm) contact with one another (Gesteland, 1986). These bundles further coalesce into the ~50 olfactory fila that project from the nasal cavity into the brain through the cribriform plate of the ethmoid bone. These olfactory ensheathing cells play a significant role in axon guidance and have been harvested and used experimentally to promote axon regeneration after traumatic insult. For example, transplantation of cultured olfactory ensheathing cells into an injured spinal cord of animals induces regeneration and remyelination of severed spinal nerve fibers, and facilitates functional recovery (Ibrahim *et al.*, 2006).

The olfactory receptors

The olfactory receptor proteins located on the olfactory receptor cells are members of a large G-protein-coupled receptor superfamily that comprises the largest multigene family in the mammalian genome. About 1000 genes express such receptors in mammals, although a considerable number of such genes are pseudogenes, i.e., gene copies that do not produce full-length functional proteins. For this reason, the number of functional receptor genes is probably fewer than 400 in humans (Gilad *et al.*, 2005). Interestingly, recent data suggest that pseudogenes may play an important role in gene regulation, such as governing mRNA stability of homologous coding genes, making the situation more complex than originally envisioned (Hirotsune *et al.*, 2003; Yano *et al.*, 2004). The human olfactory receptor gene family is distributed over all but two chromosomes, with the majority on chromosome 11 and most of the remainder on chromosomes 1, 6, and 9 (Glusman *et al.*, 2001).

In a 1991 landmark study that led to the 2004 Nobel Prize for Physiology or Medicine, Linda Buck and Richard Axel identified the first 18 members of the olfactory receptor gene family using a degenerate polymerase chain reaction (PCR) strategy (Buck & Axel, 1991). Like other G-protein-coupled receptors, olfactory receptor proteins have seven transmembrane domains with a stereotyped topology (Figure 1.8). The internal transmembrane domains, which are hypervariable in evolution, are believed to interact with odorants in a manner analogous to the α_2 adrenergic receptor-ligand interaction (Buck & Axel, 1991).

In mammals, each receptor cell expresses only one type of olfactory receptor, although such cells also express other types of receptors, thereby

(a)

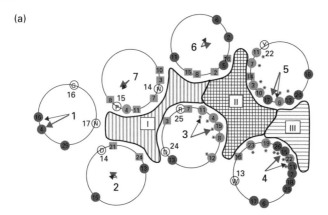

Figure 1.8 (See also Figure 1.8 in the color plate section, p. 82–3.) Presumed odorant-binding pockets of an odor receptor protein. (a) Schematic drawing depicting an overhead view of the seven transmembrane-spanning barrels of an odor receptor protein modeled against the rhodopsin G-protein coupled receptor (GPCR). Residues that are conserved among all GPCRs are shown in opencircles. Colored squares and circles represent positions of conserved and variable residues, respectively, in olfactory receptor (OR) proteins. Residues that align with ligand contact residues in other GPCRs are colored green and residues that do not align with such residues are colored red. The residues in each helix are numbered separately, according to the predicted transmembrane boundaries. Hypervariable residues (putative odorant-binding residues) are indicated by asterisks. Area II denotes a hypervariable pocket that corresponds to the ligand-binding pocket in other GPCRs. (Reproduced from Pilpel and Lancet, 1999.)

facilitating the modulation of their activity by hormones and neurotransmitters (Hague *et al.*, 2004). Those cells expressing the same olfactory receptor project to the same glomeruli, globe-like structures within the olfactory bulb where the first synapses occur (Mombaerts *et al.*, 1996; Serizawa *et al.*, 2003). Thus, the molecular features to which a given receptor type is sensitive (e.g., chain length, functional group configurations) are in effect mapped to circumscribed regions of the olfactory bulb (Figure 1.9). At least in the mouse, a receptor cell carrying a given type of olfactory receptor is more or less randomly distributed within one of four largely non-overlapping strip-like zones of the olfactory neuroepithelium that roughly parallel the dorsal–ventral axis of the cribriform plate (Breer, 2003). Thus, a "functional topography" exists in this system from the epithelium to the olfactory bulb.

The primary second messenger for mammalian odor transduction is cAMP (Breer & Boekhoff, 1992), whose essential function is to amplify the incoming signal from odorant receptors and ultimately facilitate release of glutamate, the primary neurotransmitter of the olfactory receptor cells. The opening of a cyclic-nucleotide-gated channel (CNG) causes movement of Na^+ and Ca^{2+}

(b)

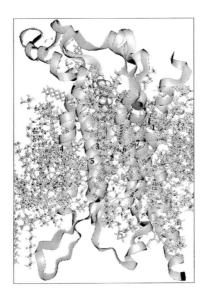

Figure 1.8(b) (See also Figure 1.8 in the color plate section, p. 82–3.) Predicted structure for mouse olfactory receptor (OR) S25. Model depicts the putative binding pocket for the hexanol ligand (purple) to the receptor protein (side view). Each transmembrane and inter-transmembrane loop is labeled. The membrane is represented in yellow. This computed model of the S25 odorant receptor protein atoms successfully predicts the relative affinities to a panel of odorants, including hexanol, which is predicted to interact with residues in transmembranes 3, 5, and 6. (From Floriano *et al.*, 2000. With permission.)

into the cell (Figure 1.10). As Ca^{2+} enters the cytoplasm of the cilium through this channel, a secondary depolarizing receptor current is activated that mediates an outward Cl^- movement in the receptor neuron. Due to the high Cl^- concentration within this neuron, an elevated reversal potential for Cl^- is induced. This increases the outward movement of Cl^- across the membrane and the induction of depolarization. Both *N*-methyl-D-aspartate (NMDA) and non-NMDA receptors are subsequently activated by glutamate on the dendrites of the second-order neurons. The former are unique in being both ligand- and voltage-dependent (Lane *et al.*, 2005).

Most odorant receptor cells express the enzyme adenylyl cyclase, which contains 12 transmembrane domains (Ronnett & Snyder, 1992). When activated, this enzyme catalyzes the breakdown of cytosolic adenosine tri-phosphate (ATP) into the second messenger $3',5'$-cyclic adenosine mono-phosphate (cAMP) and pyrophosphate. Odorants increase the activation of adenylyl cyclase within the cilia (Sklar *et al.*, 1986). Indeed, the ability of an odorant to activate adenylyl cyclase correlates with its perceived odor intensity to humans, as well as the magnitude of the summated electrical

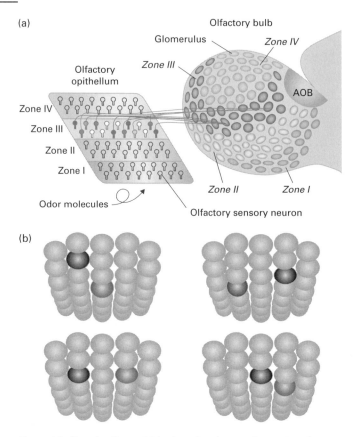

Figure 1.9 (See also Figure 1.9 in the color plate section, p. 82–3.) Patterns of connectivity between olfactory epithelium and olfactory bulb. (a) The olfactory epithelium of mouse and rat can be subdivided in four zones of equal surface area. A given olfactory receptor (OR) gene is expressed in olfactory sensory neurons (OSNs) whose cell bodies are restricted to a zone. Their axons converge on to one or a few glomeruli in each of the two half-bulbs. Shown here is the medial face of the right bulb; AOB, accessory olfactory bulb. Epithelial zones correspond to equivalent domains in the bulb, although the precise boundaries of the bulbar domains remain to be defined. (b) Glomeruli for a given OR do not occupy stereotyped positions in the bulb, but exhibit local permutations. Their position has a degree of uncertainty, both in absolute and relative terms. Shown are glomeruli for three different ORs, occupying a variety of positions within an area of ~30 glomeruli. (From Mombaerts, 2001. Reproduced with permission from Macmillan Publishers Ltd.)

response it produces in frog epithelia (Doty *et al.*, 1990). This presumably reflects the relation between the numbers of cells activated and perceived odor intensity – a relationship that is highly conserved across a wide range of mammalian forms.

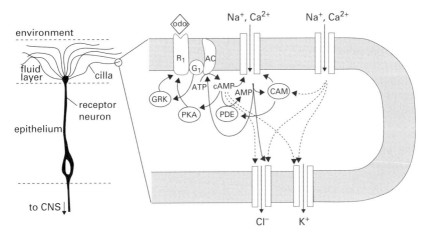

Figure 1.10 Schematic diagram summarizing the intracellular signaling pathways implicated in mammalian olfactory transduction. The major signaling pathway involves a receptor protein (R_1), a GTP-binding protein (G_1, likely G_{olf}), an adenylyl cyclase (AC) that produces adenosine 3′,5′-cyclic monophosphate (cAMP), and a cation channel that is gated directly by cAMP. ATP, adenosine triphosphate; CAM, calcium calmodulin; GRK, G-protein-coupled receptor kinase; PDE, phosphodiesterase; PKA, phosphokinase A. This signaling pathway can target secondary ion channels that carry some, and possibly most, of the transduction current. Solid lines represent better established pathways. Dashed lines represent proposed pathways. (Modified from Ache and Restrepo, 2000. With permission of Wiley–Liss, Inc., a subsidiary of John Wiley & Sons, Inc.)

Some olfactory receptor neurons do not express adenylyl cyclase, and utilize other transduction enzymes, such as guanylyl cyclase or the cyclic-glucose-monophosphate- (cGMP-) stimulated phosphodiesterase 2 (PDE2), an enzyme that leads to the breakdown of cGMP to GMP (Bruch, 1990). Neurons that express PDE2 and membrane-bound guanylyl cyclase D (an olfactory-specific cyclase) are thought to project, at least in rodents, to distinct regions within the posterior olfactory bulb. Thus, selective compartmentalization of different phosphodiesterases and cyclases may regulate odorant signal transduction in olfactory neurons, thereby modulating the sensitivity of subpopulations of sensory neurons to specific odorants. Although the second messenger inositol 1,4,5-trisphosphate (IP_3) has been implicated in both invertebrate and vertebrate olfactory transduction, it does not appear to be involved in the initial steps of mammalian olfactory signal transduction (Gold, 1999).

Both cAMP and cGMP produce distinctly different Ca^{2+} signaling kinetics and different cytosolic concentrations for CNG channel activation. Thus, when activated, cGMP reaches significantly lower levels in olfactory receptor neurons than does cAMP (Kaupp and Seifert, 2002). These differences influence the rate and amount of cation influx into the cytosol. This influx may occur through a common CNG or through functionally similar CNG channels with different subunit compositions. The second messenger signal is longer lasting or persistent for cGMP than for cAMP. It is likely that cGMP participates in long-term cellular events in vertebrate olfactory receptor neurons such as desensitization, sensory adaptation, or neuronal activity-dependent transcription (Anholt, 1989).

The vomeronasal organ

Many vertebrates, including the majority of mammals, possess a vomeronasal organ (VNO), also known as "Jacobson's organ." The VNO is a tube-like structure located at the base of the septum which functions in a number of activities, including those related to mating. In humans, this structure is rudimentary and vestigial (Bhatnagar *et al.*, 2002; Smith *et al.*, 2002). Although this remnant often connects to the nasal cavity through a small opening, it lacks the full complement of cells thought necessary for function. Moreover, there appears to be no neural connection to this organ, and the primary central brain structure to which vomeronasal nerves ordinarily project (accessory olfactory bulb) is absent in humans (Meisami *et al.*, 1998) and key elements of the VNO probably disappear by the 28th week of intrauterine life (Nakashima *et al.*, 1984). Human VNO receptor genes are pseudogenes, most of which are presumed to have no function (Liman *et al.*, 1999). Also lacking is the VNO-specific TRP2, a non-selective cation channel critical for VNO function in lower mammals (Leypold *et al.*, 2002; Tirindelli *et al.*, 1998).

The olfactory bulb

The paired ovoid-shaped olfactory bulbs, each of which measures approximately 50 mm^3 in a healthy adult, are laminate-like structures located under the ventral surface of the frontal lobes immediately above the cribriform plate (Figure 1.11; see also Figure 1.15). Contrary to some textbook descriptions, the olfactory bulb is not a simple relay station within the olfactory pathway, but a complex centre where sensory input is filtered and modified by neural elements intrinsic and extrinsic to the bulb (Kratskin & Belluzzi, 2003). A convergence rate of around 1000 receptor cell axons for every second-order neuron occurs in this structure, at least in the rabbit, resulting in a tremendous summation, i.e., amplification, of information. The general anatomy of the distinctly layered bulb is shown in Figure 1.12 and Figure 1.13, along with a listing of some of its 20 or more known neurotransmitters and neuromodulators.

The most superficial layer of the bulb, termed the *olfactory nerve layer*, is made up of bundles of unmyelinated olfactory receptor cell axons that

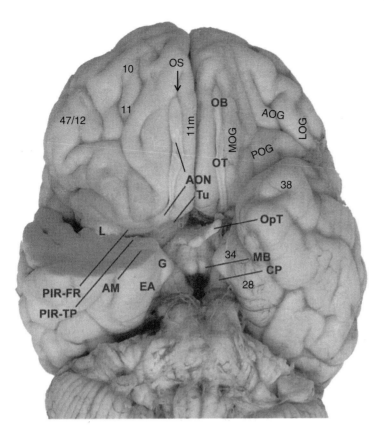

Figure 1.11 (See also Figure 1.11 in the color plate section, p. 82–3.) Base of human brain showing the ventral forebrain and medial temporal lobes. The blue oval area represents the monkey olfactory region, whereas the pink oval represents the probable site of the human olfactory region as identified by functional imaging studies. (Modified from Gottfried *et al.*, 2006, with permission). Key: numbers refer to approximate position of Brodmann areas as follows: 10, fronto-polar area; 11/11m, orbitofrontal/gyrus rectus region; 28, posterior entorhinal cortex; 34, anterior entorhinal cortex; 38, temporal pole; 47/12, ventrolateral frontal area; AM, amygdale; AOG/POG/LOG/MOG, anterior, posterior, lateral, medial orbital gyri; AON, anterior olfactory nucleus scattered throughout the olfactory tract and bulb; CP, cerebral peduncle; EA entorhinal area; G, gyrus ambiens; L, limen insule; MB, mamillary body; PIR-FR, frontal piriform cortex; PIR-TP, temporal piriform cortex; OpT, optic tract; OS, olfactory sulcus; OT, olfactory tract; Tu, olfactory tubercle.

interweave across its surface. The next layer, the *glomerular layer*, contains the aforementioned olfactory glomeruli. Although younger people have thousands of these structures arranged in single or double layers, these decrease in number with age and are nearly absent in people over the age of 80 years (Smith, 1942).

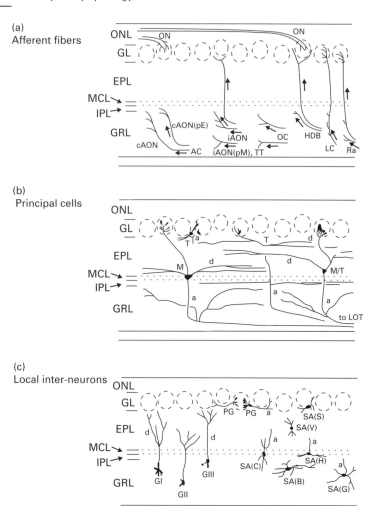

Figure 1.12 Schematic representation of afferent fibers, principal cells, and local interneurons in the olfactory bulb. ONL, olfactory nerve layer; GL, glomerular cell layer, EPL, external plexiform layer; MCL, mitral cell layer; IPL, internal plexiform layer; GRL, granule cell layer. (a) ON(m) and ON(l), medial and lateral groups of olfactory axons. Centrifugal fibers originate in the ipsilateral and contralateral anterior olfactory nucleus (iAON and cAON), tenia teca (TT), olfactory cortex (OC), nucleus of the horizontal limb of the diagonal band (HDB), locus coeruleus (LC), and raphe nucleus (Ra); pE, pars externa of the AON; pM, pars medialis of the AON. (b) The axons (a), axon collaterals, and dendrites (d) of a mitral cell (M), displaced mitral or internal tufted cell M_d/T_i, middle tufted cell T_m, and external tufted cell T_e; LOT, lateral olfactory tract. (c) GI, GII, and GIII designate three types of granule cells; PG, periglomerular cell. Various short axon cells are shown: SA(B), Blanes's cell; SA(C), Cajal's cell; SA(G), Golgi cell; SA(H), Hensen's cell; SA(S), Schwann cell; SA(V), van Gehuchten cell. (From Shepherd, 2004, with permission.)

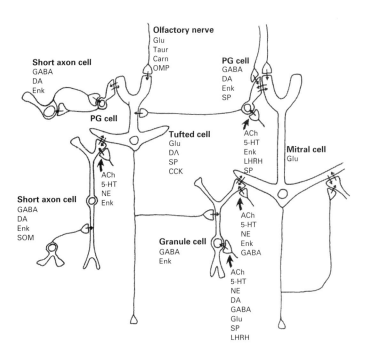

Olfactory nerve
Glu
Taur
Carn
OMP

Short axon cell
GABA
DA
Enk

PG cell
GABA
DA
Enk
SP

PG cell

Tufted cell
Glu
DA
SP
CCK

ACh
5-HT
Enk
LHRH
SP

Mitral cell
Glu

ACh
5-HT
NE
Enk

Short axon cell
GABA
DA
Enk
SOM

ACh
5-HT
NE
DA
GABA
Glu
SP
LHRH

Granule cell
GABA
Enk

ACh
5-HT
NE
Enk
GABA

Figure 1.13 Neurotransmitters and neuromodulators in the olfactory bulb. ACh, acetylcholine; Carn, carnosine; CCK, cholecystokinin; DA, dopamine; Enk, enkephalin; GABA, γ-aminobutyric acid; Glu, glutmate; 5-HT, serotonin; LHRH, luteinizing hormone releasing hormone; NE, norepinephrine; OMP, olfactory marker protein; PG cell, periglomerular cell; SOM, somatostatin; SP, substance P; Taur, taurine. Small arrows show the direction of synaptic transmission; solid arrows indicate centrifugal projections to the bulb. (Adapted from Halasz and Shepherd, 1983. With permission from Elsevier.)

These structures are dependent upon trophic influences from the receptor cells which undergo age-related damage, either from environmental xenobiotics (Nakashima *et al.*, 1984) or from the pinching of their axons by oppositional bone growth within the cribriform plate (Kalmey *et al.*, 1998).

The glomeruli encompass the initial synapses between the axons of the olfactory receptors and the dendrites of the bulb's primary projection neurons, the mitral and tufted cells. The glomeruli also receive processes from local interneurons, such as the juxtaglomerular or periglomerular cells. While each olfactory axon innervates a single glomerulus, and the primary dendrites of a given mitral or tufted cell are similarly confined to a single glomerulus, this is not the case with interneurons. For example, the spine-laden dendrites of periglomerular cells ramify within multiple glomeruli (usually two), and their axonal processes extend across several glomeruli (up to six), making contacts with other local interneurons. The periglomerular cells are heterogeneous in their morphology, neurochemistry, and physiology, and about 10 percent lack synapses with olfactory axons (Kratskin & Belluzi, 2003).

Deep to the bulb's glomerular layer is the *external plexiform layer*. This layer, which contains very few cell bodies, is formed largely by dendrites of granule cells and numerous secondary dendrites of mitral or tufted cells. Granule cells, the most numerous cells within the olfactory bulb, are relatively small axonless cells whose somata are located in the middle-most layer of the bulb (the *granule cell layer*). The processes of these cells traverse several layers of the bulb, having as their primary neurotransmitter γ-aminobutyric acid (GABA). About 80 percent of the synaptic contacts between the granule cells and the mitral or tufted cells are organized as reciprocal pairs, so that the mitral-to tufted-to-granule synapse is excitatory and the granule-to-mitral or tufted synapse is inhibitory (Kratskin & Belluzi, 2003). Since the latter is the only type of contact between the granule cells and the mitral or tufted cells, activation of granule cells inhibits mitral and tufted cell activity. It is noteworthy that there are between 50 and 100 granule cells for each mitral cell, and that each granule cell has at least 50 gemmules, short thorn-like extensions that are reciprocally connected to mitral or tufted cell dendrites. This arrangement provides a rich substrate for strong interactions between these cells. The cell bodies of the mitral cells (so-called because of their resemblance to a bishop's headdress) are found within the *mitral cell layer*, which is adjacent and medial to the external plexiform layer.

The olfactory bulb receives a large number of centrifugal fibers from the primary olfactory cortex (see below), as well as from central structures outside of this cortex (Zaborszky *et al.*, 1986). While most centrifugal fibers terminate within the granule cell layer, a number also end within the external plexiform, internal plexiform, and glomerular layers. The *internal plexiform layer* is largely composed of myelinated axons from the mitral and tufted cells. These axons exit from the olfactory bulb as the olfactory tract, although before leaving the bulb they send off collaterals that terminate within the bulb's deeper regions. In the mouse, about 75 percent of the centrifugal fibers originates from structures within the olfactory cortex (e.g., anterior olfactory nucleus and piriform cortex). The major share of centrifugal fibers that arise from ipsilateral non-olfactory structures come from the nucleus of the horizontal limb of the diagonal band via the medial forebrain bundle, the ventral part of the nucleus of the vertical limb of the diagonal band, the substantia innominata, the ventral pallidum, the subthalamic zona incerta, and regions of the medial hypothalamus. Bilateral centrifugal projections to the bulb come from the dorsal and medial raphe nuclei and the locus coeruleus. As discussed in Chapter 4, these routes may be used by various pathogens to access the brainstem – a point of possible relevance to the etiology of encephalitis and Parkinson's disease.

Like the olfactory neuroepithelium, some cell populations within the olfactory bulb undergo replacement over time (Altman, 1969), in some cases facilitated by odorant stimulation (Rochefort *et al.*, 2002). The stem cells responsible for such replacement are found within the anterior subventricular zone of the brain, a remnant of the lateral ganglionic eminence (Gheusi *et al.*, 2000). These astrocyte-like cells generate large numbers of neuroblasts, a subpopulation of which undergoes restricted chain migration along a path known as the rostral migratory stream (Lois *et al.*, 1996; Rousselot *et al.*, 1994). This migration terminates in the core of the olfactory bulb and occurs without guidance from radial glia or astrocytes. The migrating neuroblasts express the neuronal marker, neuron-specific class III β-tubulin (TUJ1), and the highly polysialated neural cell adhesion molecule (NCAM) that aids their migration (Rousselot *et al.*, 1994). After their release, the differentiating neuroblasts migrate outward along glial processes, terminating within the periglomerular and granular layers of the bulb. Some of these new neurons repopulate the granule cells, whereas others mature into periglomerular cells, a sizable number of which synthesize both dopamine and GABA (Kratskin & Belluzzi, 2003). Odorant exposure stimulates the expression of tyrosine hydroxylase, the initial and rate-limiting enzyme of dopamine biosynthesis, within the periglomerular cells. The precursor cell proliferation is markedly decreased by experimental depletions of dopamine, as occurs in Parkinson's disease (Höglinger *et al.*, 2004).

The migrating stem cells, which only recently have received widespread attention, indicate that the plasticity of the olfactory system is not confined to the olfactory neurocpithelium. What role such regeneration plays in odor perception is not clear, although reducing the number of interneurons generated by this process impairs odor discrimination performance in rodents (Gheusi *et al.*, 2000). Clearly, such regeneration is an integral component of the olfactory process.

The olfactory cortex

The olfactory system is unique among sensory systems in communicating directly with the cerebral cortex without first relaying in the thalamus, although reciprocal relays do exist via the dorsomedial nucleus of the thalamus between primary and secondary olfactory cortical structures. Those areas receiving fibers directly from the olfactory bulb (OB) are known as the "primary olfactory cortex" (Figure 1.14), which consists of the following six structures: (1) anterior olfactory nucleus (AON) located in the posterior parts of the OB and olfactory tract near the trigone; (2) olfactory tubercle (poorly developed in humans); (3) piriform cortex – the major recipient of OB output; (4) anterior cortical nucleus of the amygdala; (5) periamygdaloid complex; and (6) the rostral entorhinal cortex. The majority of mitral and

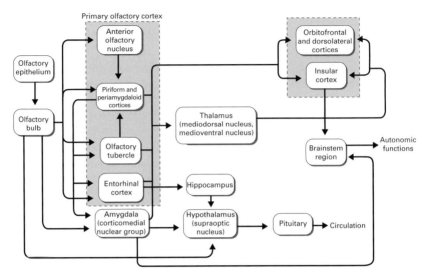

Figure 1.14 Schematic diagram of the central olfactory projections of the olfactory system. Note: the connection between the olfactory bulb and the hypothalamus is not established in humans and most other mammals. (Modified from Doty and Bromley, 2000. With permission.)

tufted cell axons exit the OB and enter the olfactory tract. This tract, which is relatively flat, extends backward from the OB on the undersurface of the frontal lobe to a point called the olfactory trigone just in front of the anterior perforated substance. Here the tract splits into three – the medial, intermediate, and lateral olfactory strie (see Figure 1.11 and Figure 1.15). Contrary to traditional teaching, in humans all fibers from the OB pass through the lateral olfactory strie and the other two strie in humans are merely vestiges (Price, 2004). Unlike other major sensory pathways, the main cortical projection of the bulb is ipsilateral.

It should be noted that even though sectors of the AON are outside the brain, it is a CNS structure that receives fibers from the bulb. This poorly defined cortical structure contains pyramidal cells whose dendrites receive synapses from mitral and tufted cells, as well as from the contralateral AON, via the anterior commissure and numerous central brain structures. The pyramidal cell axons project to ipsilateral bulb neurons (mainly granule cells), the contralateral AON, the OB, and the rostral entorhinal cortex.

All structures of the primary olfactory cortex have rich and reciprocal relations with one another and with other central brain structures, including the hippocampus. Indeed, the olfactory system is unique in that it has the most direct access to the hippocampus of all other sensory systems in terms of synaptic connections.

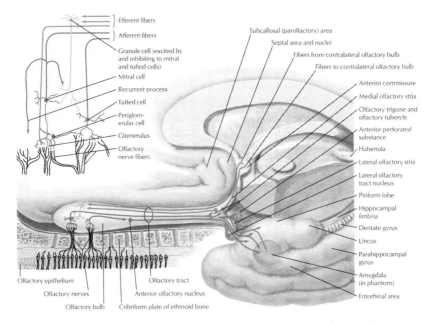

Figure 1.15 (See also Figure 1.15 in the color plate section, p. 82–3.) Schematic diagram to show anatomy of the olfactory bulb, tract, and connections in the temporal lobe. (Reproduced with permission from Felton and Jozefowicz, 2003. © Elsevier.)

Early clinical studies, including a classic study of "H.M." – whose temporal lobes were resected bilaterally – suggested that lesions of the medial temporal lobe interfered with odor identification and discrimination, but not detection (Eichenbaum *et al.*, 1983; Eskenazi *et al.*, 1986). Such observations led to the oversimplified concept that detection is performed by the bulb and that all other tasks, such as identification, discrimination, and memory, are performed by the temporal lobe. We now know, however, that such functions are also altered by lesions to the frontal cortex, and that in some instances lesions beyond the bulb affect odor detection. The removal of either frontal lobe can produce ipsilateral olfactory impairment; removal of the right lobe may influence discrimination ability bilaterally. Functional imaging studies have reported greater right than left odor-induced frontal lobe activity (Zatorre *et al.*, 1992), suggesting the right orbito-frontal cortex may be more dominant than the left in higher-order analysis of odors (Zatorre *et al.*, 1992; see, however, Royet *et al.*, 2001).

Piriform cortex

The piriform cortex (PC), literally meaning "pear-shaped," is a three-layer structure located in the anteromedial temporal lobe that receives input from most of the fibers in the lateral olfactory tract (Figure 1.15). Although there are anterior (frontal) and posterior (temporal) regions defined anatomically in humans, little is known about any differences in their function. In the rat, the response of the posterior regions to odorants may be more plastic than the anterior parts (Chabaud et al., 2000). The main region, layer II, contains tightly packed cell bodies of pyramidal cells (Haberly & Price, 1978). Layer III also contains cell bodies of these cells, but they are less numerous and packed less densely. Dendrites of the pyramidal cells extend into layer I, where they receive axonal terminals from the mitral and tufted cells of the lateral olfactory tract. The more proximal dendritic regions of the pyramidal cells receive associational and commissural input from the other components of the olfactory cortex. Inhibitory interneurons, most of which express GABA, are found within layers I and III of the PC.

Initial studies on the PC suggested that it was simply a relay station for olfactory information, but it is now known to have a far more complex function. The PC responds to sniffing odorless air (Sobel et al., 1998), implying that sniffing primes it for optimal reception of an odor – a concept proposed over 60 years ago by Adrian (1942). It rapidly habituates in the continuous presence of odor (Poellinger et al., 2001; Sobel et al., 1999b). It is responsive to odor pleasantness ("valence;" Gottfried et al., 2002), odor reward value (Gottfried & Dolan, 2003), and attention to odor (Zelano et al., 2005). It is involved in odor recognition memory and familiarity judgment (Dade et al., 2002; Plailly et al., 2005), and probably stores olfactory traces of multisensory episodic memories (Gottfried et al., 2004). Recent data suggest that the PC supports olfactory perceptual learning (Li et al., 2006); functional magnetic resonance imaging (fMRI) experiments demonstrate that the PC becomes conditioned to the sight of food and that satiety results in reduced activity. The PC is concerned also with high-order representation of odor quality or identity. According to Gottfried et al. (2006), there is a "double dissociation" in PC whereby posterior piriform regions encode quality but not odor structure (chemical class), and anterior regions encode structure but not the identity of smell. The presence of structure-based codes suggests that fidelity of sensory information arises from the olfactory bulb and that quality-based codes are independent of any simple structural configuration, implying that synthetic mechanisms underlie our experience of smell. In other words, we perceive most odors (which usually consist of multiple odorous molecules) as a single unified percept. This synthesis underlies our perception of a smell and probably how the brain interprets smell information.

Amygdala

Human evoked-potential recordings demonstrate that the amygdala (literally meaning almond) is unequivocally concerned with olfactory processing, although the precise nature of this has yet to be elucidated (Hudry et al.,

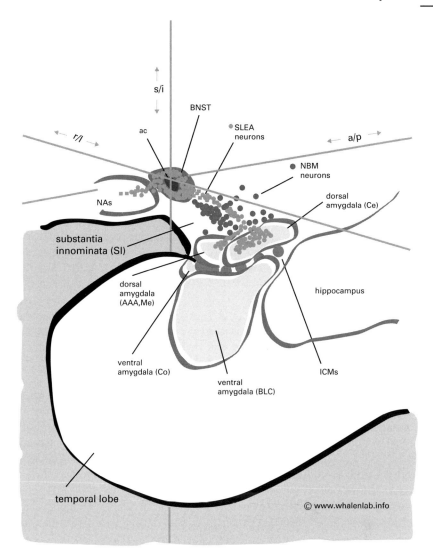

Figure 1.16 (See also Figure 1.16 in the color plate section, p. 82–3.) Schematic diagram of the nuclear complexes in the left amygdala. Abbreviations: ac anterior commissure; r/l, right/left plane; s/l, superior/inferior plane; a/p, antero-posterior plane; BNST, bed nucleus of stria terminalis; SLEA, sublenticular extended amygdala neurons; NBM, nucleus basalis of Meynert; Ce, central nucleus of amygdala; AAA, anterior amygdala area; Me, medial nucleus of amygdala; Co, cortical nucleus of amygdala; BLC, basolateral complex of amygdala; NAs, nucleus accumbens shell division; ICMs, intercalated cell masses. (Reproduced with permission from Paul Whalen, available at: www.whalenlab.info/About%20Amygdala.html.)

2001). This anteriorly located temporal lobe structure is usually divided into four anatomical regions, as shown in Figure 1.16: (1) corticomedial nuclei that receive most of the output from the OB, which includes the peri-amygdaloid area, anterior, and posterior cortical nuclei, nucleus of the lateral olfactory tract, and medial nucleus; (2) lateral nucleus; (3) basolateral nuclei; and (4) central nuclei. Apart from strong two-way connections to and from the olfactory bulb, the amygdala has connections from the corticomedial nuclei to its lateral, basolateral, and central nuclei, as well as to the basal ganglia, thalamus, hypothalamus, and orbitofrontal cortex.

It has been suggested that the amygdala is activated chiefly in accord with the pleasantness ("valence") element of an odor (Zald & Pardo, 1997), but the situation is not clear: some experiments suggest a prime role in intensity and not valence. For example, in an fMRI study by Anderson et al. (2003), intensity and valence were dissociated by presenting one pleasant odor (citral; lemon), and one unpleasant odor (valeric acid; sweaty socks), each at low and high intensity. It was found that amygdala activation was related only to intensity and not valence. This concept was addressed in further experiments using neutral odors of varying intensity, in addition to pleasant and unpleasant odors (Winston et al., 2005). Contrary to earlier work, neutral odors did not result in amygdala activation, only high-intensity pleasant or unpleasant odors did so, suggesting that the amygdala is concerned with an integrated combination of intensity and valence that reflects the overall behavioral salience of an odor.

The contribution of the amygdala to odor memory has received scant attention until recently. Buchanan et al. (2003) assessed olfactory memory in 20 patients with unilateral amygdala damage related to temporal lobe resection and one patient with selective bilateral amygdala lesions. Fifteen odors from the University of Pennsylvania Smell Identification Test (UPSIT) were presented without response alternatives, followed one hour later by an odor–name matching test and an odor–odor recognition test. Both unilateral groups were impaired in their memory for matching odors with names, but not for odor–odor recognition. The patient with bilateral amygdala damage displayed severe impairment in both odor–name matching, as well as in odor–odor recognition memory. Importantly, none of the patients were impaired on an auditory verbal learning task, suggesting a specific impairment in olfactory memory, not merely a more general memory deficit.

In common with the PC, the amygdala is probably concerned with associative learning between olfactory and visual signals. It has been proposed that the amygdala is involved with new associations but not their long-term storage (Buchel et al., 1998; Gottfried et al., 2004), a function more likely reserved for the orbitofrontal cortex as described below. The amygdala is probably concerned with emotional aspects of odor memory and these aspects may be more important than non-olfactory signals, reflecting the strong connections between the amygdala and other elements of the limbic system (Herz, 2004).

In summary, the corticomedial nucleus of the amygdala and PC have major input from the olfactory bulb and then connect to multiple regions, in particular the basal ganglia, thalamus, hypothalamus, and orbitofrontal cortex. Functional imaging studies have made it clear that the earlier concept of the PC as a simple relay within the olfactory pathway is incorrect. Both the amygdala and PC respond to intensity, valence, and memory components of smell to produce an olfactory percept for analysis by tertiary centers, most notably the orbitofrontal cortex (OFC), which in turn governs behavioral responses to a given odor.

Orbitofrontal cortex

The OFC is an area of prefrontal cortex commonly defined as that region in receipt of projections from the medial part of the dorsomedial thalamic nucleus. It is located above the roof of the orbit in the basal surface of the caudal frontal lobes, which includes the gyrus rectus medially and the agranular insula laterally. The putative human olfactory OFC is several centimeters more rostral than the primate counterpart, as based on an imaging meta-analysis (Figure 1.11, Gottfried & Zald, 2005), implying that there may have been anterior migration of function between monkeys and humans, or that the functions of monkey and human OFC are fundamentally different. Its location above the orbit makes it vulnerable to lesions within the orbit and to frontal pole disorder, typically resulting from head injury, tumor, vascular and neurodegenerative processes. It has two-way connections with the olfactory tubercle, PC, amygdala, and entorhinal cortex. There are other diverse connections which allow integration of sensory signals from visual, tactile, gustatory and visceral (hypothalamic) areas, as depicted in Figure 1.17 (Rolls, 2004). The OFC has a lateral zone which receives taste input from the frontal operculum and constitutes a secondary taste cortex in which the reward value of taste is represented (Baylis *et al.*, 1995). There is probably a hierarchical arrangement within OFC, in that the postero-medial OFC, which receives olfactory signals from the amyagdala and PC, is concerned with passive smelling and odor detection, and transfers this information to more rostral zones of the OFC (Gottfried, 2006). The rostral zones are thought to be concerned with higher-order processing, including associative learning, working memory, and odor recognition memory. It is proposed that there exists a medial–lateral specialization, whereby pleasant odors evoke activity in the medial and ventromedial areas of the OFC and unpleasant ones in the lateral part (Gottfried, 2006). Thus the OFC contains secondary and tertiary olfactory regions in which information about the identity and reward value of odors is represented. The diverse inputs from inferior temporal visual cortex,

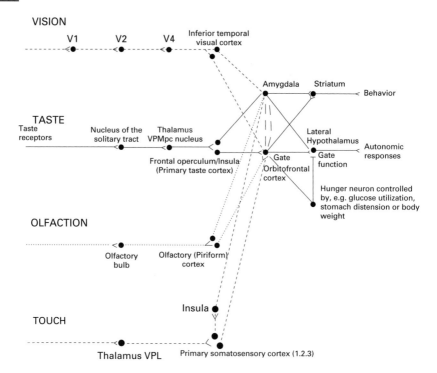

Figure 1.17 Schematic diagram showing some of the gustatory, olfactory, visual, and somatosensory pathways to the orbitofrontal cortex (OFC) and some of the outputs of OFC in primates. The secondary taste cortex and the secondary olfactory cortex are within the OFC. V1, primary visual cortex; V4, visual cortical area V4. *Abbreviations*: VPMpc, thalamic ventroposterior medialis nucleus pars compacta (taste relay); VPL, thalamic ventroposterior lateralis nucleus (somatosensory relay). (Modified from Rolls, 2004. With permission from Elsevier.)

primary somatosensory cortex, and hypothalamus allow the OFC to learn, and, if need be, suppress sensory signals to which the cells would normally respond (Figure 1.17; Rolls, 2004). Initial imaging studies (Zatorre *et al.*, 1992) suggested that the right OFC is dominant for olfaction, but this concept is probably only partially correct. Regional blood flow studies imply that the right OFC is concerned with appraisal of the presence, intensity, hedonicity, familiarity, or potential edibility of different odorants, but it is most active when making familiarity judgments of odor (probably relying on input from the PC) and least active during detection tasks (Royet *et al.*, 2001). The left OFC is thought to be more active when making hedonic assessments but it would appear that both OFCs have a medio-lateral specialization for hedonic variables, with pleasant odors being more represented medially within OFC.

These observations, although intriguing, nonetheless should be regarded as preliminary and in need of replication. Finally, a model of parallel processing has been proposed in which the level of activity in both OFCs depends on whether the evaluation involves recognition or emotion (Royet *et al.*, 2001). Therefore a lesion of OFC has the potential to interfere with identification and discrimination of smell and taste signals but, contrary to earlier concepts, the damage probably has to be bilateral.

Cerebellum

The cerebellum plays a key role in modulating the act of sniffing. Aside from serving to direct pulses of air into the olfactory region, as well as modulating sniff size in relation to the intensity or pleasantness of odorants, sniffing can result in independent neural activation of brain regions intimately associated with odor perception, such as the piriform and orbitofrontal cortices (Sobel *et al.*, 1998). Moreover, regions of the cerebellum are activated by odorants independent of sniffing activity, suggesting the cerebellum plays a critical role in the coordination of sensory and motor function. There is evidence that the cerebellum may be concerned with smell identification (Sobel *et al.*, 1998). As described in detail in Chapter 4, several cerebellar ataxias are associated with olfactory dysfunction, although it is not known whether the cerebellum, per se, contributes to such dysfunction.

Odor processing and CNS coding mechanisms

Odorants are typically small (<300 Da) hydrophobic and lipophilic molecules with binding affinities in the micromolar range. Before reaching and activating receptors on the olfactory receptor cilia, they must traverse the largely aqueous mucus barrier of the olfactory mucosa, being assisted in some cases by soluble proteins, termed odorant-binding proteins (Pelosi *et al.*, 1990). Such proteins can also serve to "filter" the amount of odorant reaching receptors. Contrary to popular belief, the human nose can detect most chemicals at extremely low concentrations. For example, the fishy-smelling substance trimethylamine can be detected by some people at less than one part per billion, whereas β-ionone, a violet-smelling substance, can be detected at levels less than 10 parts per trillion (Buttery *et al.*, 1990).

How the olfactory system decodes molecular information to ultimately produce an odor percept is complex. Odor quality is not accounted for by simple analytical chemistry, as structurally similar molecules, even stereo-isomers, can have quite different odors, and structurally dissimilar molecules

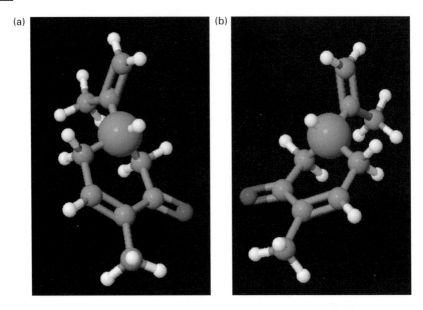

Figure 1.18 (See also Figure 1.18 in the color plate section, p. 82–3.) The enantiomers of carvone. (a) S–(+) carvone smells like caraway; (b) R–(–) carvone smells like spearmint. Red is oxygen, white is hydrogen, and gray is carbon. The large grey carbon atom is the chiral centre of the molecule. (Reproduced with permission from Steve Cook, available at: www.steve.gb.com/science/biochemical_nomenclature.html.)

can have very similar odors (Figure 1.18). Odorants are typically recognized by more than one type of receptor, and a single receptor can recognize a variety of structurally diverse stimuli, often exhibiting different thresholds to various odorants. Thus, a unique combination of activated olfactory receptors appears to encode information related to the physiochemical structures of a given odorant – a combination that is mapped to specific bulbar glomeruli.

Odorant mixtures produce mixture-specific patterns of glomerular activations analogous to patterns induced by single odorants, reflecting interglomerular neural processes that selectively establish the activated pattern of neural activity of the second-order neurons. Importantly, elements of such mixtures can act as agonists or antagonists at the receptor level, facilitating or depressing membrane depolarization. This was clearly demonstrated for a derivative of isoeugenol (spicy clove-like odor), which acts as a potent competitive antagonist for receptors responsive to eugenol (Oka *et al.*, 2004).

Like other sensory systems, the olfactory system has means of enhancing the signal:noise ratio, and much of the olfactory bulb circuitry seems to be devoted to this process. In effect, this system filters out or adapts background odors to make foreground odors more salient. The amount and pattern of output concerning both olfactory receptor cells and the second-order neurons, i.e., the mitral and tufted cells, are modulated by intrinsic and extrinsic factors. For example, GABA or dopamine release from juxtaglomerular cells can, via presynaptic receptors, inhibit glutamate release by the olfactory receptor cells, as well as modulate mitral and tufted cell activity (Davila *et al.*, 2003; Sassoe-Pognetto & Ottersen, 2000). D_2 dopamine receptor activation reduces the size of odor-evoked glomerular spatial patterns (Sallaz & Jourdan, 1992), whereas reducing bulbar dopamine content does the opposite (Wilson & Sullivan, 1995), suggesting that dopamine may serve as a volume control to mitigate olfactory nerve activity during periods of marked odorant stimulation. Importantly, the activity of a broad array of cells within the bulb is influenced by context, previous learning, and bodily state. For example, if young rats are continuously exposed to an odorant, when they reach adult life they show enhanced focal glomerular 2-deoxyglucose uptake specific to that odorant (Coopersmith *et al.*, 1986). The responses of mitral or tufted cells to food odors or odors associated with food are larger in food-deprived than food-satiated rats, emphasizing the role of bodily state in altering bulbar activity. When the centrifugal input to the bulb is lesioned, this deprivation-induced modulation is eliminated (Pager *et al.*, 1972).

Combinations of odorants produce unique perceptual wholes – termed "odor objects" by Wilson and Stevenson (2003) – that cannot be predicted from perceptual or physiochemical properties of the constituents. The PC plays a significant role in this process. Thus, this cortical region combines, in a global fashion, odorant molecular features into odor percepts. Whilst a mitral or tufted cell responds to a set of odorants based upon the presence of a common feature that dominates its receptor input, a cortical pyramidal cell responds to multiple odorant features derived from spatially dispersed mitral or tufted cells and other sources. This gestalt is, in turn, matched to existing cortical memory stores or templates for recognition. Evidence for this "coincidence detection system" comes from numerous sources. For example, cells within the PC do not exhibit as much cross-habituation to the same set of closely related odorants as olfactory bulb mitral or tufted cells, implying that these are tuned to a broader array of molecular features (Wilson, 2000).

In contrast to rodents (Rajan *et al.*, 2006), humans cannot localize to which side of the nose an odorant is presented unless the trigeminal system is activated (Kobal *et al.*, 1989; von Skramlik, 1925). This most likely explains why the major flavor sensations of foods are perceived globally during eating and are not localized to the region of the olfactory receptors. During chewing and swallowing, the olfactory receptors are stimulated by molecules passing from inside the mouth through the nasal pharynx, so-called retronasal olfaction (Burdach & Doty, 1987).

Perception of odor hedonics

As discussed above, both the amygdala and PC are thought to be concerned with valence and intensity appreciation. However, it has been suggested that pleasant and unpleasant odors differentially stimulate the left and right sides of the brain. For example, Kobal *et al.* (1992) reported that event-related evoked responses to two "unpleasant" odors, menthol and hydrogen sulphide, were shorter and of smaller amplitude when presented to the left than to the night nostril. The reverse was the case for two "pleasant" odors (vanillin and phenyl ethyl alcohol). These authors claimed that their observations could not be explained on the basis of simple differences in perceived intensity. More research with additional odors is needed, however, before the generality of this observation can be determined.

People who are able to smell the steroid androstenone describe it variously as pleasant or unpleasant – like body odor. In one study, all subjects gave androsterone an equal intensity rating, but those who classed androstenone as body odor-like showed a larger amplitude N1-P2 component ("P3") of the OERP than those who found the smell to be pleasant (Lundstrom *et al.*, 2006). There was no difference in amplitude between those finding androstenone unpleasant and their responses to hydrogen sulphide. From this it was deduced that "P3" was a measure of odor pleasantness.

Odor adaptation

In keeping with other sensory systems, repeated presentation of the same stimulus at a high enough intensity can produce a temporary decrement in an individual's ability to perceive that specific odorant (adaptation) or other odorants (cross-adaptation), as reviewed by Cometto-Muniz and Cain (1995). The rate and degree of adaptation, as well as the rate and degree of recovery, depends upon the duration and concentration of the adapting stimulus, as well as the attention level of the subject. Interestingly, adaptation of one nasal chamber produces adaptation in the other nasal chamber, a phenomenon likely mediated via fibers within the anterior olfactory nucleus and anterior commissure. For intense odorants, adaptation can be relatively rapid. Thus, continuous exposure to lemon or orange oil vapors results in more or less complete loss of olfactory sensations, on average, in three minutes (Aronsohn, 1886). Cross-adaptation is most commonly asymmetrical. For example, while exposure to odorant A decreases the perceived intensity of odorant B, exposure to odorant B may not decrease the intensity of odorant A to the same degree. In general, the sensitivity to a given odorant is reduced more by the exposure to that odorant than to any other odorant, although, in rare instances, the opposite may occur. It is noteworthy that odorants that strongly self-adapt tend to be reduced markedly by other odorants, and that adaptation to complex odorants (i.e., odorants made up of more than one chemical) is generally less than adaptation to single-component odorants.

Odor memory

Humans have an uncanny ability to remember smells, and from an early age odors quickly become associated with environmental objects, such as food. Evidence that smell can evoke memories from the distant past is well described in the lay literature. This is exemplified by the famous passage from Marcus Proust's novel *Remembrance of Things Past.* Whenever Proust was offered a *petit madeleine* (sponge cake), this immediately brought forth vivid childhood memories of an old gray house where his Aunt Leonie used to give him a *madeleine*, dipping it first in her own cup of tea. In a similar vain, Emile Zola, the French novelist, noted that the smell of olives would invariably conjure up scenes of Provence where he spent his childhood (Zola, 1928).

Although some studies suggest that odors are not forgotten to the same extent as other sensory experiences (Engen & Ross, 1973), this not generally the case (Davis, 1977), and the novelty of the stimulus and its emotional and semantic associations are critical in establishing its salience (Herz, 1998). The vividness of odor recall associated with emotional experiences can be quite marked as, for example, in some Vietnam War veterans who suffer severe flashbacks when exposed to smells reminiscent of tent mould, jet fuel, or burning flesh (Pain, 2001). As described earlier, one possible reason for these observations is the strong anatomical connections between the olfactory pathways in the medial temporal lobes (amygdala, PC) and the limbic system regions which are concerned with memory and emotion. Hence memory, emotion, and smell frequently seem to be interrelated. Conditioning fragrances, such as lavender and jasmine, with relaxation in massage or bathing is one explanation of the efficacy of aromatherapy, and odors are known to alter sleep patterns. Thus, lavender fragrance significantly increases the percentage of deep or slow-wave sleep (Goel *et al.*, 2005). However, it is possible that such effects are caused by systemic absorption of the odorous agent. For example, phyto-estrogens in lavender oil used in personal care products can pass into the bloodstream transdermally, producing gynecomastia in prepubescent boys (Henley *et al.*, 2007).

In common with most other memories, women rely more than men on semantic processes (typically left temporal lobe) in remembering odors (Larsson *et al.*, 2003; Oberg *et al.*, 2002). This may explain why women perform better than men on the left than on the right side of the nose on a standardized odor memory test (Doty & Kerr, 2005). The sex difference is most marked at the 10-s delay interval, where verbal rehearsal was least affected by counting backwards.

Human pheromones

In 1932, the entomologist Bethe distinguished, in insects, between hormones secreted within the body ("endohormones") and hormones excreted outside of the body ("ectohormones"), dividing the latter into those with intraspecific, and those with interspecific, effects (termed "homoiohormones" and "alloiohormones," respectively) (Bethe, 1932). In 1959, Karlson and Lüscher replaced the term *homoiohormone* with the term *pheromone*, defining pheromones as "substances which are secreted to the outside by an individual and received by a second individual of the same species, in which they release a specific reaction, for example, a definite behaviour or a developmental process" (Karlson & Lüscher, 1959). Soon thereafter a number of insect pheromones were identified, most notably the primary sex attractant of the female silkworm moth, *Bombyx mori* (for a history of the pheromone concept, see Doty, 2003).

In the 1960s, several prominent zoologists, including the entomologist E. O. Wilson, suggested that pheromones are also present in mammals, mediating, for example, sexual attraction, responses to territorial odors, and alterations in endocrine state. Although hundreds of studies have since appeared in the mammalian literature claiming their effects are mediated by "pheromones," very few instances of the chemical isolation of putative pheromones have been made. Even in these rare cases, however, the agent or agents that have been isolated have fallen far short of being anything like an insect pheromone, and in a number of cases attempts to replicate the findings have failed (Doty, 2003). In nearly all instances, the putative substances did not meet even a subset of basic criteria inherent in the pheromone concept (e.g., species-specificity, stereotypy, minimal influences from learning), and when effects were seen they were inevitably less salient and reliable than those induced by the original biological secretion. In many instances, learning is involved, and the substitution of "artificial" odorants produced similar results. A classic example of the role of learning is the Bruce effect, where the odor of the stud must be first learned before a strange male odor can block the pregnancy of a recently inseminated female.

That being said, ablation of the VNO of mice, for example, mitigates a number of behavioral or endocrine responses claimed to be due to pheromones, leading some molecular biologists to label the VNO the "pheromone detector." Detection of chemosensory stimuli by the VNO is thought to be mediated by two families of G-protein-coupled receptors (GPCRs) that are distinct from the classical olfactory receptor family originally identified by Buck and Axel (1991). Recently, genes of another family of receptors, also distinct from this olfactory receptor family, have been shown to be expressed on subsets of olfactory receptor cells in mice, fish, and humans (Liberles &

Buck, 2006). These trace amine-associated receptors (TAARs) are not expressed on the same cells as the canonical olfactory receptors, being sparsely expressed in discrete subdomains within the epithelium. The function of this new class of receptors is unknown, but it has been suggested they may serve to detect volatiles, most notably amines, from urine and other sources. If this proves to be the case, they potentially provide an additional substrate for the mediation of chemical signals that some might construe as pheromones.

Putting aside evidence that humans lack a functional VNO and that no chemicals analogous to insect pheromones have been identified in mammals, evidence for the existence of human pheromones – even broadly defined – seems weak. Perhaps the most widely publicized claim for a human phero-mone was made in a *Nature* article published in 1971 (McClintock, 1971). This study suggested that the menstrual cycles of women who are close friends or roommates in a dormitory-living situation tend to synchronize over time. A subsequent *Nature* paper claimed that this effect was attributed to axillary odors (Stern & McClintock, 1998). However, these and other studies on this topic have been roundly criticized on the basis of methodo-logical and statistical considerations, together with the existence of menstrual synchrony itself (e.g., Arden & Dye, 1998; Schank, 1997, 2000; Strassmann, 1997; 1999; Wilson, 1987, 1992).

Strassmann (1997) points out that in most pre-industrialized societies, which likely reflect the norm for much of human evolution, pregnancy and lactation (not menstrual cycling) take up the majority of a female's repro-ductive years, obviating any reason for menstrual synchrony to evolve. In such societies pregnancy occurs in the early teenage years and there is little attempt to control fertility in a parity-dependent manner. In her long-term prospective study of the Dogon of Mali, a society in which menstruating women are segregated at night in special huts, the proportion of women cycling on a given day was about 25 percent; approximately 16 percent were pregnant, 29 percent were in lactational amenorrhea, and 30 percent were postmenopausal. Subfecund women were most common among the cycling women, and conception usually occurred for the most fecund women on one of their first postpartum ovulations, resulting in their dropping out of the pool of regularly menstruating women. Employing statistical procedures that overcame the synchrony calculation problems inherent in the McClintock studies (Wilson, 1987), Strassmann found no evidence for synchrony of the cycling women who habitually ate and worked together or who lived with a particular lineage of related males. Moreover, no evidence for synchrony was observed in any of the remaining cycling women, suggesting to Strassmann (1999) that the "Popular belief in menstrual synchrony stems from a mis-perception about how far apart menstrual onsets should be for two women whose onsets are independent. Given a cycle length of 28 days (not the rule – but an example), the maximum that two women can be out of phase is

14 days. On average, the onsets will be 7 days apart. Fully half the time they should be even closer (Strassmann, 1997; Wilson, 1992). Given that menstruation often lasts 5 days, it is not surprising that friends commonly experience overlapping menses, which is taken as personal confirmation of menstrual synchrony."

Aside from the menstrual synchrony pheromone, the most widely publicized claim for a human pheromone is that of 5α-androst-16-en-3α-one (androstenone). Androstenone is a steroid found in the blood, testes, seminal fluid, and fat of pigs (mainly males) that produces a strong odor. It is the major cause of "boar taint," the bad taste of meat of uncastrated boars. In humans, androstenone is found mainly in axillary secretions, although it is common in the roots of a number of plants and vegetables, including parsnip and celery (Claus & Hoppen, 1979). Androstenone and its related alcohol, androstenol, received considerable study by chemists in the 1960s and 1970s, in light of its commercial implications. At that time, it was shown that the odor of androstenone lowered the threshold for pressure-induced lordosis in sows, making it potentially useful for inducing mating in the sow and in determining her time of estrus. However, this effect may be conditioned, and numerous sensory stimuli can similarly produce this phenomenon (Albone, 1984).

The origin of the belief that androstenone is a human pheromone is obscure. Of humans who can smell it (a significant number cannot), it typically has an unpleasant urine-like or musk-like smell. By most definitions, pheromones are species-specific, so assuming they are the same in humans as in pigs would seem to be an oxymoron. However, even if we drop species-specificity from the pheromone definition, if the behaviors attributed to agents differ markedly between species, it would seem unlikely that they have a homologous relationship. In humans, but not in pigs, androstenone largely depends upon bacterial action of apocrine gland secretions within the axilla for its expression. However, it contributes little to axillary odor, which is largely derived from C_6 to C_{11} straight-chain, branched, and unsaturated acids, with (E)-3-methyl-2-hexenoic acid providing the major odorous component (Spielman et al., 1995; Zeng et al., 1991, 1992). The number of apocrine sweat glands varies across ethnic groups, being nearly non-existent in a number of Asians.

Savic and colleagues (2001) undertook fMRI to study the putative pheromone androstadienone, which is probably synthesized from androstadienol by axillary coryneform bacteria and later transformed into the more odorous compound, androstenone (Mallet et al., 1991; Rennie et al., 1991). They used a somewhat unorthodox definition of a pheromone, namely a chemical that has the ability to activate the human hypothalamus in a sex-specific manner. Androstadienone was found to activate the hypothalamus in women but not in men. Compared to other odors, androstadienone produced larger activations in the anterior part of the inferior lateral prefrontal cortex (PFC), the superior temporal cortex (STP), and olfactory areas (Gulyas *et al.*, 2004). The PFC and STP have been implicated in aspects of attention, visual perception or recognition, and social cognition. These observations were extended further in a study of homosexuality (Berglund *et al.*, 2006). Both heterosexual women and homosexual men responded to smelling androstadienone while heterosexual men did not. Maximal activation was found in the medial preoptic and anterior hypothalamic areas, which are thought to be involved in sexual behavior. Estratetrenol (estrogenic) exposure resulted in hypothalamic activation only in heterosexual men. Tests with putative non-pheromonous odors activated only the classical olfactory pathways.

Whilst these findings are interesting, they beg replication and the use of control odors of similar chemical shape, size, and solubility. In general, large molecules, such as steroids, might be expected to stimulate a greater range of receptors and thereby produce greater CNS activity. Heuristically, it is of considerable interest if certain compounds have unique capabilities of activating brain regions associated with the regulation of hormones. If it can be determined that such effects have functional consequences and play a meaningful role in human social communication or endocrine function, then we might argue that, in fact, agents reasonably defined as pheromones may exist in humans. However, until an abundance of such evidence is presented, it would seem prudent to assume that the existence of pheromones in humans is an open question. The reader is referred elsewhere for more extensive information on the strengths and weaknesses of the pheromone concept (Doty, 2003).

Factors that influence normal function

In light of the plasticity of the olfactory system, it is not surprising that numerous compounds can modify its activity. Although odor training, as well as exposure to some odorants, can positively alter its function (Smith *et al.*, 1993), many factors have the opposite effect. Detailed below are the major subject and environmental factors that influence, under normal circumstances, olfactory function. Pathological effects are described in greater detail in Chapters 3 and 4.

Specific anosmia

(See also Chapter 3.) This is defined usually as the inability to detect one or a few related odorants in the absence of other evidence of smell loss, and probably has a genetic basis. Such anosmias should not be confused with acquired anosmias that bring a patient to the clinic. Specific anosmias about which the subject is usually unaware are present in one form or another in a large segment of the population, and may be viewed as the olfactory equivalent of color blindness. Since most so-called specific anosmias reflect markedly decreased sensitivity to an odorant, rather than anosmia per se, a number of theorists feel the phenomenon is best described as "specific hyposmia." In many cases, the frequency distribution of sensitivity in the population for odorants exhibiting this effect is bimodal.

There are many varieties of specific anosmia. Musk anosmia, which is probably an autosomal recessive trait, afflicts 7 percent of Caucasians but no Blacks (Whissell-Buechy & Amoore, 1973). No genetic locus has so far been identified. Specific anosmia to androsterone (sweaty or urinous) is also thought to be inherited, possibly X-linked, based on raised concordance in identical twins, but again no locus is presently known (Wysocki & Beauchamp, 1984). This condition affects up to 50 percent of otherwise healthy people, but some individuals with an initial specific anosmia can eventually detect the odor after repeated exposure to it (Wysocki *et al.*, 1989). A similar learning or sensitization process applies to furfural (almond-like) and isovaleric acid (sweaty) (Doty *et al.*, 1981; Jacob *et al.*, 2006; Yee & Wysocki, 2001). The specific anosmia to isobutyric acid (cheesy, vomit-like smell) affects about 2.5 percent of apparently healthy individuals, whereas that to isovaleric acid affects about 1.4 percent of Caucasians and 9.1 percent of Blacks (Amoore, 1967). There is one report of a family comprising a mother and three children, all of whom were unable to perceive the smell of n-butylmercaptan (skunk odor; Patterson & Lauder, 1948). There are reportedly many other specific anosmias, although relatively little research is currently being performed on this topic.

Even though specific anosmias generally go unrecognized, they can influence the overall perception of odorants, which depend upon multiple receptors, and, in some cases, eating habits. A classic example is specific anosmia to trimethylamine, a fish-like odor. Individuals who are relatively insensitive to this chemical are more likely to ingest fish whose odors are often repugnant to more sensitive people. Some of the better known specific anosmias are listed in Table 1.1.

Blind smell

"Blind smell" is a term that denotes detection of a subthreshold odor by the brain in the absence of conscious perception. It has to be carefully distinguished from smell blindness or specific anosmia. To demonstrate this phenomenon, fMRI was used to localize brain activation induced by high and low concentrations of estratetrenyl acetate (Sobel *et al.*, 1999b). Although subjects reported verbally that they were unable to detect either concentration, their forced-choice guess was better than chance for the higher concentration, and both concentrations produced significant brain activation on fMRI, mainly in

Table 1.1 Compounds associated with specific anosmia[*]

Compound	Odor quality	Percent anosmic
Androstenone	Sweaty/urinous	47
Isobutyraldehyde	Malty	36
Cineole	Camphorous	33
Pyrroline	Spermous	12
Pentadecalactone	Musky	12
Carvone	Minty	8
Trimethylamine	Fishy	6
Isovaleric acid	Sweaty	3

[*] Adapted from Wysocki and Beauchamp (1991).

the right orbitofrontal cortex. In other words these subjects were able to detect odor at a "subconscious" level without being fully aware they could do so. These observations complement earlier work on subthreshold visual perception and localization, termed "blindsight" (Sanders *et al.*, 1974), where a subject correctly localizes objects that cannot be seen consciously in a blind or even a normal visual field (Weiskrantz, 1990).

Age

Approximately half of the adult population between the ages of 65 and 80 years has demonstrable reduction in smell function, whereas about three-quarters of those over 80 years of age exhibit meaningful decrements (Doty *et al.*, 1984). These numbers may even be conservative depending on the criteria used for olfactory loss (Murphy *et al.*, 2002). There is evidence that not all odorants show the same degree of age-related decline, reflecting such factors as the odorant's threshold and the nature of the function relating odorant concentration to perceived intensity. For example, it was shown that healthy control subjects over the age of 50 years in general had more difficulty in identifying pleasant odors compared with less pleasant ones, an effect that may relate to the intensity of the smells in question (Hawkes *et al.*, 2005). Such effects are complicated, however, given the aforementioned conversion of multiple odorants into odor percepts from which individual odorant components cannot be ascertained. The age-related changes in odor identification ability, as measured by a forced-choice odor identification test, are shown in Figure 1.19. These losses are not culture-specific, and are much more pronounced than the influences of gender, which are shown in the same figure.

Age-related damage to the olfactory epithelium from environmental agents such as viruses, bacteria, toxins, and pollutants is a primary factor that influences human olfactory function. Thus, this epithelium undergoes

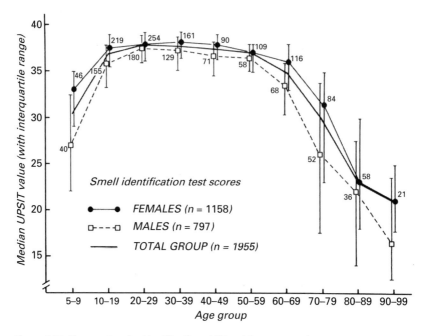

Figure 1.19 Changes in odor identification ability with age. Note that, on average, women perform better on the University of Pennsylvania Smell Identification Test (UPSIT) than men at all ages. (Reproduced with permission from Doty *et al.*, 1984.)

cumulative damage throughout life, resulting in islands of respiratory-like metaplasia that begin to appear soon after birth (Nakashima *et al.*, 1984), decreased epithelial thickness, and decreased numbers of olfactory receptors (Rosli *et al.*, 1999). Such damage appears to be accelerated in environments containing pollutants and industrial chemicals (Hudson *et al.*, 2006). Factors associated with age-related changes in olfactory function include: (1) an epithelium with reduced protein synthesis; (2) fewer neurotrophic factors; (3) altered vascularity; (4) decreased mitotic activity; (5) decreased intramucosal blood flow; (6) increased mucus viscosity; (7) increased secretory gland and lymphatic atrophy; (8) decreased enzymatic capacity to deactivate xenobiotics; and (9) possibly neurodegenerative conditions within CNS structures, as described below and in detail in Chapter 3. As mentioned earlier, the number and cross-sectional area of the foramina of the cribriform plate decrease in many elderly people as a result of bony overgrowth, in effect pinching off the olfactory receptor axons en route from the nasal cavity into the brain (Kalmey *et al.*, 1998; Krmpotic-Nemanic, 1969).

The age-related decrease in olfactory receptor neurons results in declining volume and mitral cell count, as well as reduced bulbar glomeruli number

(Hinds & McNelly, 1981). In a pioneering study, Smith (1942) capitalized on the latter fact to estimate age-related losses of human olfactory receptors. In this study, he counted the glomeruli in 205 olfactory bulbs of 121 cadavers representing a wide range of ages, concluding that loss of olfactory nerves begins soon after birth and continues throughout life at about 1 percent per year. In more recent work, Meisami *et al.* (1998) measured the number of mitral cells and glomeruli in olfactory bulbs from three young adult women, three middle-aged adult women, and three aged women. The number of mitral cells and glomeruli decreased steadily with age at an approximate rate of 10 percent per decade; in the ninth and tenth decades of life, less than 30 percent of these structures were present. Such decreases support the finding of olfactory bulb and tract volume decrement with age (Hinds & McNelly, 1977; Yousem *et al.*, 1998).

As described in Chapter 4, histopathological studies find that older brains inevitably exhibit pathology associated with neurodegenerative disorders such as Alzheimer's disease and Parkinson's disease. Such pathology probably accounts for some age-related olfactory deficits seen in otherwise normally functioning older people. Thus, a number of elderly people have neurofi-brillary tangles, neuropil threads, and Lewy bodies in all layers of their olfactory bulbs, with the possible exception of the olfactory nerve cell axon layer (Kishikawa *et al.*, 1990; Ohm & Braak 1987). In Alzheimer's disease, central limbic structures that receive olfactory bulb projections preferentially exhibit relatively high numbers of neurofibrillary tangles and neuritic plaques (Hooper & Vogel, 1976; Pearson *et al.*, 1985; Reyes *et al.*, 1993). Such structures include the hippocampal formation, periamygdaloid nucleus, prepiri-form cortex, and entorhinal cortex (Braak *et al.*, 1996; Ferreyra-Moyano & Barragan 1989; Jellinger *et al.*, 1991). It appears that the most salient and earliest signs of traditional Alzheimer's neuropathology appear within the transentorhinal cortical region (Braak *et al.*, 1996; Jellinger *et al.*, 1991), a zone containing afferent fibers en route from the sensory association cortex to the entorhinal cortex (Figure 1.20). It is not known to what degree such patho-logical entities contribute to the age-related decline in olfactory function in non-demented elderly people or whether they represent the earliest changes of disease that would be manifest clinically had the subject lived long enough.

Hormonal factors

On average, women outperform men on tests of odor identification, detec-tion, discrimination, and memory. Such effects are seen across a wide range of cultures (Doty *et al.*, 1985; Gilbert & Wysocki 1987). The basis of this finding is not clear, but it is presumed that organizational influences of reproductive hormones are involved, since before puberty girls tend to outperform boys on tests of odor identification and no overall change in performance is observed

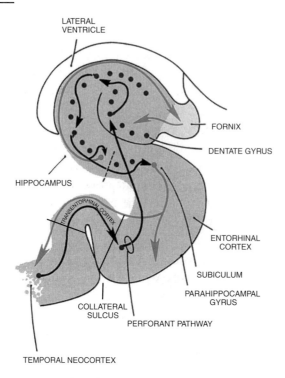

LATERAL
VENTRICLE

FORNIX

DENTATE GYRUS

HIPPOCAMPUS

TRANSENTORHINAL CORTEX

ENTORHINAL
CORTEX

SUBICULUM

PARAHIPPOCAMPAL
GYRUS

COLLATERAL
SULCUS

PERFORANT PATHWAY

TEMPORAL NEOCORTEX

Figure 1.20 (See also Figure 1.20 in the color plate section, p. 82–3.) Coronal section of the hippocampus to show the position of the transentorhinal cortex. This is in the depths of the collateral sulcus between the two straight lines as shown. According to Braak *et al.* (1996) it is the first area to show abnormalities in Alzheimer's disease. (Modified with permission from Gilman and Winans, 2003 © FA Davis.)

across the time of puberty. During the menstrual cycle, women evidence three peaks in detection performance: during the latter half of menses, midcycle near the time of the luteinizing hormone surge, and during the mid-luteal phase (Doty *et al.*, 1981; Figure 1.21). The latter two changes are closely related to circulating levels of both estrone and estradiol.

Although there are anecdotal reports of heightened olfactory sensitivity during pregnancy, particularly during the first trimester (Nordin *et al.*, 2004), empirical data on this topic are inconclusive (for review, see Cameron, 2007). The limited evidence suggests that during pregnancy some odors, such as amyl acetate, may be perceived as stronger, and others, such as androstenone, weaker than before pregnancy (Gilbert & Wysocki, 1987). Interestingly, most female smokers experience an aversion to the taste or smell of tobacco smoke while pregnant, and cease smoking during this time. However, the majority resume smoking within three months after delivery (Pletsch & Kratz, 2004).

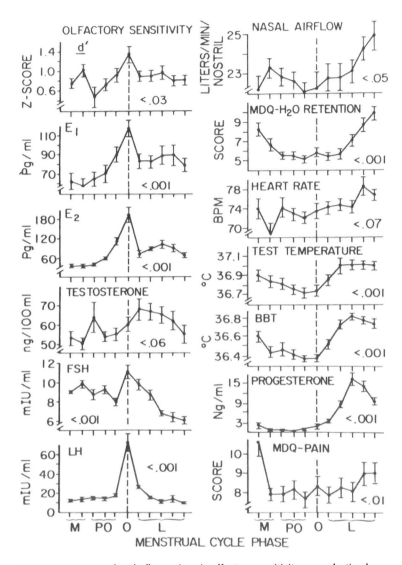

Figure 1.21 Menstrual cycle fluctuations in olfactory sensitivity, reproductive hormones, and several physiological and psychological variables; $n = 17$ menstrual cycles, with sensory data collected every other day. d' denotes signal detection measure reflecting distance between signal + noise and noise distributions. d' based upon 350 trials/test session. E_1, estrone; E_2, estradiol; FSH, follicle stimulating hormone; LH, luteinizing hormone; MDQ, Moos Menstrual Distress Questionnaire; BBT, basal body temperature; M, menstrual phase; PO proliferative (follicular) phase; O, ovulation; L, luteal (secretory) phase. Note strong association between circulating estrogen levels and the olfactory sensitivity measure. (Reproduced from Doty et al., 1981.)

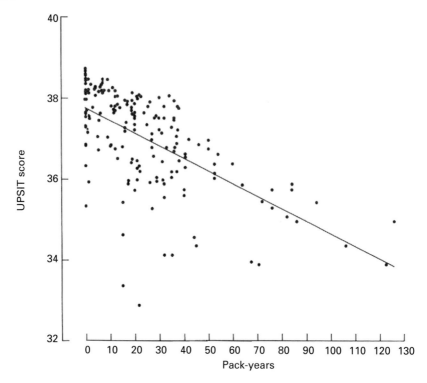

Figure 1.22 Effect of cumulative smoking dose on University of Pennsylvania Smell Identification Test (UPSIT) scores for current smokers. UPSIT scores adjusted for age and sex. The linear regression line indicates the magnitude of the smoking dose effect. Note that subjects with very high smoking doses evidence a four-point difference in UPSIT scores relative to subjects with low smoking doses. (From Frye *et al.*, 1990. With permission. Copyright © 1990, American Medical Association. All rights reserved.)

Cigarette smoking

Animal studies have noted that exposure to volatiles associated with burning tobacco can cause damage to the olfactory neuroepithelium, including squamous metaplasia and atrophy (Vanscheeuwijck *et al.*, 2002). Most studies of humans find that tobacco smoking by itself hardly ever causes anosmia, although hyposmia can occur and odor identification test scores are inversely related to pack-years smoked (Figure 1.22). Previous smokers show gradual improvement of olfaction commensurate with the amount and duration of prior smoking (Figure 1.23; Frye *et al.*, 1990). Thus, a number of hyposmic cigarette smokers can expect to improve if they give up the habit. The degree

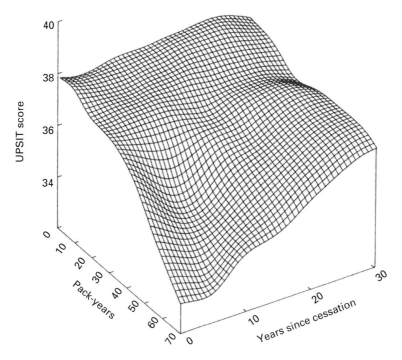

Figure 1.23 Influences of years since cessation and prior smoking history on University of Pennsylvania Smell Identification Test (UPSIT) scores. The individual data were fitted to a distance-weighted least-squares regression to derive the surface plot. Although a few subjects had a smoking dose greater than 70 pack-years, the pack-years scale was limited for clarity of surface presentation. (From Frye *et al.*, 1990. With permission. Copyright © 1990, American Medical Association. All rights reserved.)

of smell identification impairment in current smokers is relatively small (around 1–2 UPSIT points, falling well behind the effect of age in those over 60 years and, to a lesser degree, gender in terms of relative influences (Doty *et al.*, 1984). However these variables may be additive; there will be a large difference (around 3–4 UPSIT points) when comparing, say, a female who has never smoked with a male current smoker of the same age.

Pollution

Recent studies suggest that olfactory function is worse in those living in highly polluted conurbations compared with those in less polluted environments, while those in rural dwellings are affected least of all. For example, Hudson *et al.* (2006) compared olfactory function in residents of Mexico

City, known to have high levels of air contamination, with residents of the Mexican state of Tlaxcala, a region geographically similar to Mexico City but unaccompanied by significant air pollution. The Tlaxcala residents detected the odors of instant coffee and an orange drink at significantly lower concentrations than those in Mexico City. Moreover, they were better in discriminating the odors of two similarly smelling Mexican beverages, horchata and atole. About 10 percent of the Mexico City subjects were judged to have poor olfactory function, in contrast to about 2 percent of the Tlaxcala subjects. The authors concluded that air pollution in Mexico City damages olfactory function of young and middle-aged residents.

Demography

In a massive *National Geographic Magazine* survey, nearly 11 million subscribers were asked about basic demography, their ability to smell, and frequency of their perfume use (Gilbert & Wysocki, 1987). Identification and intensity ratings were given to the following microencapsulated odorants: androstenone (urinous), amyl-acetate (banana-like), galaxolide (musky), eugenol (cloves), mercaptans (sulphurous – often added to natural gas), and rose. With the exception of androstenone and mercaptan, all of these odors were generally rated pleasant by men and women of all nationalities. Androstenone was perceived (if at all) either as stale urine, musk-like, or sweet. People who rated androstenone as unpleasant generally gave this a high intensity rating – especially those from Europe. This observation correlates with other data suggesting that if a subject has a low threshold to androstenone it is rated unpleasant; if the threshold is high then it is rated indifferent or pleasant. Amyl acetate was given a fairly uniform hedonic rating, whereas major differences appeared for the synthetic musk, Galaxolide. Galaxolide received unpleasant ratings by most Asian respondents, and pleasant ratings by Australians, 50 percent of whom indicated they would be prepared to wear it as perfume. Whilst the majority thought that mercaptans were unpleasant, there was one exception – most people from India liked it. Many other regional differences were noted, presumably reflecting cultural and other environmental differences. Four of the six odors evoked a vivid memory, and this was true throughout the world. Galaxolide and mercaptan, to a lesser extent, were the two odorants least likely to evoke graphic memories. The ability to identify the six odors was fairly uniform worldwide. Androstenone gave most difficulty, with only 20 percent responding correctly. Galaxolide was similarly difficult, especially for men. This information concurs with the well-recognized specific anosmia to either androstenone or Galaxolide. Androstenone anosmia was present in 33 percent of males and 24 percent of females from America in contrast with 22 percent of males and 14 percent of females from Africa.

Summary

Apart from playing a critical role in safety, nutrition, and quality of life, olfaction provides a "health index" or probe for relatively inaccessible brain areas. Indeed, olfactory dysfunction is among the first signs of Alzheimer's disease and idiopathic Parkinson's disease. Olfaction has become a model system for neural degeneration and regeneration as it is one of few sensory systems where regeneration occurs. Olfactory ensheathing cells have axonal guidance properties and are being used experimentally to direct spinal nerve cell axons through regions of spinal cord sclerosis.

The olfactory neuroepithelium, located high in the nasal cavity, contains ~6 million receptor cells. Each cell expresses only one of hundreds of receptor types that belong to the largest gene family in the mammalian genome. Olfactory receptors are "generalists," responding to a range of chemical moieties. Even single-molecule odorants, which are the exception rather than the rule, are agonists for multiple receptors, indicating that the "code" for a given odorant sensation reflects a patterned combination of neural activity across different receptor types. The olfactory bulb, the first olfactory relay station in the brain, sharpens and refines the incoming signals from multiple molecules, aiding the ultimate synthesis of information from numerous peripheral inputs into single odor "percepts."

Cortical regions receiving projections from the olfactory bulb include those collectively termed the "primary olfactory cortex"; namely, the anterior olfactory nucleus, the piriform and periamygdaloid cortices, the entorhinal cortex, the olfactory tubercle, and the corticomedial nuclear group of the amygdala. Reciprocal relationships exist among these brain regions, as well as many other brain regions. The PC is no longer viewed as a simple relay station, but, along with the amygdala, responds to odor intensity, valence, and memory.

Many factors influence the ability to smell, including age, gender, cigarette smoking, environmental pollution, and circulating levels of reproductive hormones. Some individuals, for all practical purposes, cannot detect specific odorants, a problem termed "specific anosmia." Preferences for odors are influenced by a number of experiential factors, most notably cultural. Many disorders alter smell function, as described in detail in Chapters 3 and 4.

In the next chapter, we describe practical clinical means for quantifying smell function to help formulate a prognosis and monitor treatment efficacy.

REFERENCES

Ache BW and Restrepo D. Olfactory transduction. In TE Finger, WL Silver, and D Restrepo, eds. *The Neurobiology of Taste and Smell.* New York, NY: Wiley–Liss, 2000, p. 159–77.

Adrian ED. Olfactory reactions in the brain of the hedgehog. *Journal of Physiology*, 1942, **100**, 459–73.

Albone ES. *Mammalian Semiochemistry*. New York, NY: John Wiley & Sons, 1984.

Altman, J. Autoradiographic and histological studies of postnatal neurogenesis. IV. Cell proliferation and migration in the anterior forebrain, with special reference to persisting neurogenesis in the olfactory bulb. *Journal of Comparative Neurology*, 1969, **137**, 433–57.

Amoore JE. Specific anosmia: a clue to the olfactory code. *Nature*, 1967, **214**(5093), 1095–8.

Anderson AK, Christoff K, Stappen I *et al.* Dissociated neural representations of intensity and valence in human olfaction. *Nature and Neuroscience*, 2003, **6**(2), 196–202.

Anholt RR. Molecular physiology of olfaction. *American Journal of Physiology*, 1989, **257**, C1043–54.

Arden MA and Dye L. The assessment of menstrual synchrony: comment on Weller and Weller (1997). *Journal of Comparative Psychology*, 1998, **112**, 323–4.

Aronsohn E. Experimentalle Untersuchungen zur Physiologie des Geruchs. *Archiv Physiol. Leipzig*, 1886, 321–57.

Baylis LL, Rolls ET and Baylis GC. Afferent connections of the caudolateral orbitofrontal cortex taste area of the primate. *Neuroscience*, 1995, **64**(3), 801–12.

Berglund H, Lindstrom P and Savic I. Brain response to putative pheromones in lesbian women. *Proceedings of the National Academy of Science of the United States of America*, 2006, **103**(21), 8269–74.

Bethe A. Vernachlässigte hormone. *Naturwissenschaften*, 1932, **11**, 177–81.

Bhatnagar KP, Smith TD, Winstead W, Bhatnagar KP, Smith TD and Winstead W. The human vomeronasal organ: part IV. Incidence, topography, endoscopy, and ultrastructure of the nasopalatine recess, nasopalatine fossa, and vomeronasal organ. *American Journal of Rhinology*, 2002, **16**, 343–50.

Bond JA. Bioactivation and biotransformation of xenobiotics in rat nasal tissue. In: CS Barrow, ed. *Toxicology of the Nasal Passages*. Washington, DC: Hemisphere Publishing Corporation, 1986, pp. 249–61.

Braak H, Braak E, Yilmazer D, de Vos RAI, Jansen ENH and Bohl J. Pattern of brain destruction in Parkinson's and Alzheimer's diseases. *Journal of Neural Trans*, 1996, **103**, 455–90.

Breer H. Sense of smell: recognition and transduction of olfactory signals. *Biochemical Society Transactions*, 2003, **31**, 113–16.

Breer H and Boekhoff I. Second messenger signalling in olfaction. *Current Opinion in Neurobiology*, 1992, **2**, 439–43.

Brittebo EB, Eriksson VF, Bakke J, and Brandt I. Toxicity of 2,6-dichlorothiobenzamide (Chlorthiamid) and 2,6-dichlorobenzamide in the olfactory nasal mucosa of mice. *Fundamental and Applied Toxicology*, 1991, **17**: 92–102.

Bruch RC. Signal transducing GTP-binding proteins in olfaction. *Comparative Biochemistry and Physiology*, 1990, **95A**, 27–9.

Bryant B and Silver WL. Chemesthesis: the common chemical sense. In: TE Finger, WL Silver and D Restrepo, eds. *The Neurobiology of Taste and Smell* (2nd edition). New York, NY: Wiley–Liss, 2000, p. 73.

Buchanan TW, Tranel D and Adolphs R. A specific role for the human amygdala in olfactory memory. *Learning and Memory*, 2003, **10**(5), 319–25.

Buchel C, Morris J, Dolan RJ and Friston KJ. Brain systems mediating aversive conditioning: an event-related fMRI study. *Neuron*, 1998, **20**(5), 947–57.

Buck L and Axel R. A novel multigene family may encode odorant receptors: a molecular basis for odor recognition. *Cell*, 1991, **65**, 175–87.

Burdach KJ and Doty RL. The effects of mouth movements, swallowing, and spitting on retronasal odor perception. *Physiology and Behavior*, 1987, **41**, 353–6.

Buttery RG, Teranishi R, Ling LC and Turnbaugh JG. Quantitative and sensory studies on tomato paste volatiles. *Journal of Agricultural and Food Chemistry*, 1990, **38**, 336–40.

Cameron EL. Measures of human olfactory perception during pregnancy. *Chemical Senses*, 2007, **32**, 775–82.

Chabaud P, Ravel N, Wilson DA *et al.* Exposure to behaviorally relevant odor reveals differential characteristics in rat central olfactory pathways as studied through oscillatory activities. *Chemical Senses*, 2000, **25**(5), 561–73.

Chuah MI, Schwob JE and Farbman AI. Developmental anatomy of the olfactory system. In: RL Doty, ed. *Handbook of Olfaction and Gustation*. New York, NY: Marcel Dekker, 2003, pp. 115–38.

Claus R and Hoppen HO. The boar-pheromone steroid identified in vegetables. *Experientia*, 1979, **35**, 1674–5.

Cometto-Muniz JE and Cain WS. Olfactory adaptation. In: RL Doty, ed. *Handbook of Olfaction and Gustation* (1st edition). New York, NY: Marcel Dekker, 1995, pp. 257–81.

Coopersmith R, Henderson SR and Leon M. Odor specificity of the enhanced neural response following early odor experience in rats. *Brain Research*, 1986, **392**, 191–7.

Critchley M. The citadel of the senses: the nose as its sentinel. In: M Critchley, ed. *The Citadel of the Senses*. New York, NY: Raven Press, 1986, pp. 1–14.

Dade LA, Zatorre RJ and Jones-Gotman M. Olfactory learning: convergent findings from lesion and brain imaging studies in humans. *Brain*, 2002, **125**, 86–101.

Dahl AR. Possible consequences of cytochrome P-450 dependent monooxygenases in nasal tissues. In: CS Barrow, ed. *Toxicology of the Nasal Passages*. Washington, DC: Hemisphere Publishing Corporation, 1986, pp. 263–73.

Dahl AR. The effect of cytochrome P-450-dependent metabolism and other enzyme activities in olfaction. In: FL Margolis and TV Getchell, eds. *Molecular Neurobiology of the Olfactory System*. New York, NY: Plenum Press, 1988, pp. 51–70.

Davila NG, Blakemore LJ and Trombley PQ. Dopamine modulates synaptic transmission between rat olfactory bulb neurons in culture. *Journal of Neurophysiology*, 2003, **90**, 395–404.

Davis RG. Acquisition and retention of verbal associations to olfactory and abstract visual stimuli of varying similarity. *Journal of Experimental Psychology: Human Learning and Memory*, 1977, **3**, 37–51.

Ding X and Coon MJ. Immunochemical characterisation of multiple forms of cytochrome P-450 in rabbit nasal microsomes and evidence for tissue specific expression of P-450s NMa and NMb. *Cellular Pharmacology*, 1990, **37**, 489–96.

Ding X and Dahl AR. Olfactory mucosa: composition, enzymatic localization, and metabolism. In: RL Doty, ed. *Handbook of Olfaction and Gustation*. New York, NY: Marcel Dekker, 2003, pp. 51–73.

Doty RL. Mammalian pheromones: fact or fantasy? In: RL Doty, ed. *Handbook of Olfaction and Gustation*. New York, NY: Marcel Dekker, 2003, pp. 345–83.

Doty RL and Bromley SM. Olfaction and taste. In: A Crockard, R Hayward and JT Hoff, eds. *Neurosurgery: The Scientific Basis of Clinical Practice.* London: Blackwell Science, 2000, pp. 347–65.

Doty RL and Cometto-Muniz JE. Trigeminal chemosensation. In: RL Doty, ed. *Handbook of Olfaction and Gustation.* New York, NY: Marcel Dekker, 2003, pp. 981–99.

Doty RL and Kerr KL. Episodic odor memory: influences of handedness, sex, and side of nose. *Neuropsychologia*, 2005, **43**, 1749–53.

Doty RL, Brugger WE, Jurs PC, Orndorff MA, Snyder PJ and Lowry LD. Intranasal trigeminal stimulation from odorous volatiles: psychometric responses from anosmic and normal humans. *Physiology and Behavior*, 1978, **20**, 175–85.

Doty RL, Snyder PJ, Huggins GR and Lowry LD. Endocrine, cardiovascular, and psychological correlates of olfactory sensitivity changes during the human menstrual cycle. *Journal of Comparative Physiology and Psychology*, 1981, **95**, 45–60.

Doty RL, Shaman P, Applebaum SL, Giberson R, Siksorski L and Rosenberg L. Smell identification ability: changes with age. *Science*, 1984, **226**, 1441–3.

Doty RL, Applebaum S, Zusho H and Settle RG. Sex differences in odor identification ability: a cross-cultural analysis. *Neuropsychologia*, 1985, **23**, 667–72.

Doty RL, Kreiss DS and Frye RE. Human odor intensity perception: correlation with frog epithelial adenylate cyclase activity and transepithelial voltage response. *Brain Research*, 1990, **527**, 130–4.

Eichenbaum H, Morton TH, Potter H and Corkin S. Selective olfactory deficits in case H.M. *Brain*, 1983, **106**, 459–72.

Engen T and Ross BM. Long-term memory of odors with and without verbal descriptions. *Journal of Experimental Psychology*, 1973, **100**, 221–7.

Eskenazi B, Cain WS, Novelly RA and Mattson R. Odor perception in temporal lobe epilepsy patients with and without temporal lobectomy. *Neuropsychologia*, 1986, **24**(4), 553–62.

Felton DL and Jozefowicz R. *Netter's Atlas of Human Neuroscience.* New York, NY: Elsevier, 2003.

Ferreyra-Moyano H and Barragan E. The olfactory system and Alzheimer's disease. *International Journal of Neuroscience*, 1989, **49**, 157–97.

Flanagan P and Eccles R. Spontaneous changes of unilateral nasal airflow in man. A re-examination of the nasal cycle. *Acta Oto-Laryngologica*, 1997, **117**, 590–5.

Floriano WB, Vaidehi N, Goddard WA III, Singer MS and Shepherd GM. Molecular mechanisms underlying differential odor responses of a mouse olfactory receptor. *Proceedings of the National Academy of Science of the United States of America*, 2000, **97**, 10 712–16.

Frye RE and Doty RL. The influence of ultradian autonomic rhythms, as indexed by the nasal cycle, on unilateral olfactory thresholds. In: RL Doty and D Müller-Schwarze, eds. *Chemical Signals in Vertebrates 6.* New York, NY: Plenum Press, 1992, pp. 595–6.

Frye RE, Schwartz BS and Doty RL. Dose-related effects of cigarette smoking on olfactory function. *JAMA*, 1990, **263**, 1233–6.

Gesteland RC. Speculations on receptor cells as analyzers and filters. *Experientia*, 1986, **42**, 287–91.

Gheusi G, Cremer H, McLean H, Chazal G, Vincent JD and Lledo PM. Importance of newly generated neurons in the adult olfactory bulb for odor discrimination.

Proceedings of the National Academy of Sciences of the United States of America, 2000, **97**, 1823–8.

Gilad Y, Man O and Glusman G. A comparison of the human and chimpanzee olfactory receptor gene repertoires. *Genome Research*, 2005, **15**, 224–30.

Gilbert AN and Rosenwasser AM. Biological rhythmicity of nasal airway patency: a re-examination of the 'nasal cycle'. *Acta Otolaryngologica*, 1987, **104**, 180–6.

Gilbert AN and Wysocki CJ. The Smell Survey results. *National Geographic Magazine*, 1987, **172**, 514–25.

Gillner M, Brittebo EB, Brandt I, Söderkvist P, Appelgren L-E and Gustafsson J-A. Uptake and specific binding of 2,3,7,8-tetrachlorodibenzo-p-dioxin in the olfactory mucosa of mice and rats. *Cancer Research*, 1987, **47**, 4150–9.

Gilman S and Winans S. *Manter and Gatz's Essentials of Clinical Neuroanatomy and Neurophysiology* (10th edition). Philadelphia, PA: FA Davis Publishers.

Glusman G, Yanai I, Rubin I and Lancet D. The complete human olfactory subgenome. *Genome Research*, 2001, **11**, 685–702.

Goel N, Kim H and Lao RP. An olfactory stimulus modifies nighttime sleep in young men and women. *Chronobiology International*, 2005, **22**, 889–904.

Gold GH. Controversial issues in vertebrate olfactory transduction. *Annual Review of Physiology*, 1999, **61**, 857–71.

Goldstein L, Stoltzfus NW and Gardocki JF. Changes in interhemispheric amplitude relationships in the EEG during sleep. *Physiology and Behavior*, 1972, **8**, 811–15.

Gottfried JA. Smell: central nervous processing. *Advances in Oto-Rhino-Laryngology*, 2006, **63**, 44–69.

Gottfried JA and Dolan RJ. The nose smells what the eye sees: crossmodal visual facilitation of human olfactory perception. *Neuron*, 2003, **39**(2), 375–86.

Gottfried JA and Zald DH. On the scent of human olfactory orbitofrontal cortex: meta-analysis and comparison to non-human primates. *Brain Research and Brain Research Reviews*, 2005, **50**(2), 287–304.

Gottfried JA, Deichmann R, Winston JS and Dolan RJ. Functional heterogeneity in human olfactory cortex: an event-related functional magnetic resonance imaging study. *Journal of Neuroscience*, 2002, **22**(24), 10 819–28.

Gottfried JA, Smith AP, Rugg MD and Dolan RJ. Remembrance of odors past: human olfactory cortex in cross-modal recognition memory. *Neuron*, 2004, **42**(4), 687–95.

Gottfried JA, Winston JS and Dolan RJ. Dissociable codes of odor quality and odorant structure in human piriform cortex. *Neuron*, 2006, **49**(3), 467–79.

Gulyas B, Keri S, O'Sullivan BT, Decety J and Roland PE. The putative pheromone androstadienone activates cortical fields in the human brain related to social cognition. *Neurochemistry International*, 2004, **44**(8), 595–600.

Haberly LB and Price JL. Association and commissural fiber systems of the olfactory cortex of the rat. *Journal of Comparative Neurology*, 1978, **178**, 711–40.

Hague C, Uberti MA, Chen Z *et al.* Olfactory receptor surface expression is driven by association with the beta2-adrenergic receptor. *Proceedings of the National Academy of Sciences of the United States of America*, 2004, **101**, 13 672–6.

Haight JJ and Cole P. Reciprocating nasal airflow resistances. *Acta Otolaryngologica*, 1984, **97**(1–2), 93–8.

Halasz N and Shepherd GM. Neurochemistry of the vertebrate olfactory bulb. *Neuroscience*, 1983, **10**, 579–619.

Hawkes CH, Shah M and Fogo A. Smell identification declines from age 36 years and mainly affects pleasant odors. *Neurology*, 2005, Abs. P01.147. Number 6, Supplement 1.

Henley DV, Lipson N, Korach KS and Bloch CA. Prepubertal gynecomastia linked to lavender and tea tree oils. *New England Journal of Medicine*, 2007, **356**(5), 479–85.

Herz RS. Are odors the best cues to memory? A cross-modal comparison of associative memory stimuli. *Annals of the New York Academy of Sciences*, 1998, **855**, 670–4.

Herz RS. A naturalistic analysis of autobiographical memories triggered by olfactory visual and auditory stimuli. *Chemical Senses*, 2004, **29**(3), 217–24.

Hext PM and Lock EA. The accumulation and metabolism of 3-trifluoromethylpyridine by rat olfactory and hepatic tissues. *Toxicology*, 1992, **72**, 61–75.

Hinds JW and McNelly NA. Aging of the rat olfactory bulb: growth and atrophy of constituent layers and changes in size and number of mitral cells. *Journal of Comparative Neurology*, 1977, **72**, 345–67.

Hinds JW and McNelly NA. Aging in the rat olfactory system: correlation of changes in the olfactory epithelium and olfactory bulb. *Journal of Comparative Neurology*, 1981, **203**, 441–53.

Hinds JW, Hinds PL and McNelly NA. An autoradiographic study of the mouse olfactory epithelium: evidence for long-lived receptors. *Anatomical Record*, 1984, **210**, 375–83.

Hirotsune S, Yoshida N, Chen A *et al*. An expressed pseudogene regulates the messenger-RNA stability of its homologous coding gene. *Nature*, 2003, **423**, 91–6.

Höglinger GU, Rizk P, Muriel MP *et al*. Dopamine depletion impairs precursor cell proliferation in Parkinson disease. *Nature Neuroscience*, 2004, **7**, 726–35.

Hooper MW and Vogel FS. The limbic system in Alzheimer's disease. *American Journal of Pathology*, 1976, **95**, 1–13.

Huard JM, Youngentob SL, Goldstein BL, Luskin MB and Schwob JE. Adult olfactory epithelium contains multipotent progenitors that give rise to neurons and non-neural cells. *Journal of Comparative Neurology*, 1998, **400**, 469–86.

Hudry J, Ryvlin P, Royet JP and Mauguiere F. Odorants elicit evoked potentials in the human amygdala. *Cerebral Cortex*, 2001, **11**(7), 619–27.

Hudson R, Arriola A, Martinez-Gomez M and Distel H. Effect of air pollution on olfactory function in residents of Mexico City. *Chemical Senses*, 2006, **31**, 79–85.

Ibrahim A, Li Y, Li D, Raisman G and El Masry WS. Olfactory ensheathing cells: ripples of an incoming tide? *Lancet Neurology*, 2006, **5**(5), 453–7.

Jacob TJ, Wang L, Jaffer S and McPhee S. Changes in the odor quality of androstadienone during exposure-induced sensitization. *Chemical Senses*, 2006, **31**(1), 3–8.

Jellinger K, Braak H, Braak E and Fischer P. Alzheimer lesions in the entorhinal region and isocortex in Parkinson's and Alzheimer's diseases. *Annals of the New York Academy of Sciences*, 1991, **640**, 203–9.

Jones N. The nose and paranasal sinuses: physiology and anatomy. *Advanced Drug Delivery Reviews*, 2001, **51**, 5–19.

Kalmey JK, Thewissen JG and Dluzen DE. Age-related size reduction of foramina in the cribriform plate. *Anatomical Record*, 1998, **251**, 326–9.

Karlson P and Lüscher M. "Pheromones:" a new term for a class of biologically active substances. *Nature*, 1959, **183**, 55–6.

Kaupp UB and Seifert R. Cyclic nucleotide-gated ion channels. *Physiological Reviews*, 2002, **82**(3), 769–824.

Keyhani K, Scherer PW and Mozell MM. Numerical simulation of airflow in the human nasal cavity. *Journal of Biomechanical Engineering*, 1995, **117**(4), 429–41.

Kishikawa M, Iseki M, Nishimura M, Sekine I and Fujii H. A histopathological study on senile changes in the human olfactory bulb. *Acta Pathologica Japonica*, 1990, **40**, 255–60.

Klein R, Pilon D, Prosser S and Shannahoff-Khalsa D. Nasal airflow asymmetries and human performance. *Biological Psychology*, 1986, **23**, 127–37.

Kobal G, Van Toller S and Hummel T. Is there directional smelling? *Experientia*, 1989, **45**, 130–2.

Kobal G, Hummel T and Van Toller S. Differences in human chemosensory evoked potentials to olfactory and somatosensory chemical stimuli presented to left and right nostrils. *Chemical Senses* 1992, **17**, 233–44.

Kratskin IL and Belluzzi O. Anatomy and neurochemistry of the olfactory bulb. In: RL Doty, ed. *Handbook of Olfaction and Gustation*. New York, NY: Marcel Dekker, 2003, pp. 139–64.

Krmpotic-Nemanic J. Presbycusis, presbystasis and presbyosmia as consequences of the analogous biological process. *Acta Otolaryngologica*, 1969, **67**, 217–23.

Laing DG. Natural sniffing gives optimum odor perception for humans. *Perception*, 1983, **12**, 99–117.

Lane RP, Smutzer GS and Doty RL. Sense of smell. In: RA Meyers, ed. *Encyclopeda of Molecular Cell Biology and Molecular Medicine*. Weinheim: Wiley–VCH Verlag GmbH & Co., KGaA, 2005, pp. 637–705.

Larsson M, Lovden M and Nilsson LG. Sex differences in recollective experience for olfactory and verbal information. *Acta Psychologica*, 2003, **112**, 89–103.

Lee HY, Kim HU, Kim SS *et al.* Surgical anatomy of the sphenopalatine artery in lateral nasal wall. *Laryngoscope*, 2002, **112**, 1813–18.

Leopold DA, Hummel T, Schwob JE, Hong SC, Knecht M and Kobal G. Anterior distribution of human olfactory epithelium. *Laryngoscope*, 2000, **110**(3 Pt 1), 417–21.

Leypold BG, Yu CR, Leinders-Zufall T, Kim MM, Zufall F and Axel R. Altered sexual and social behaviors in trp2 mutant mice. *Proceedings of the National Academy of Sciences of the United States of America*, 2002, **99**(9), 6376–81.

Li W, Luxenberg E, Parrish T and Gottfried JA. Learning to smell the roses: experience-dependent neural plasticity in human piriform and orbitofrontal cortices. *Neuron*, 2006, **52**(6), 1097–108.

Liberles SD and Buck LB. A second class of chemosensory receptors in the olfactory epithelium. *Nature*, 2006, **442**(7103), 645–50.

Liman ER, Corey DP and Dulac C. TRP2: a candidate transduction channel for mammalian pheromone sensory signaling. *Proceedings of the National Academy of Sciences of the United States of America*, 1999, **96**, 5791–6.

Lois C, Garcia-Verdugo JM and Varez-Buylla A. Chain migration of neuronal precursors. *Science*, 1996, **271**, 978–81.

Lundstrom JN, Seven S, Olsson MJ, Schaal B and Hummel T. Olfactory event-related potentials reflect individual differences in odor valence perception. *Chemical Senses*, 2006, **31**(8), 705–11.

Mackay-Sim A. Neurogenesis in the adult olfactory neuroepithelium. In: RL Doty, ed. *Handbook of Olfaction and Gustation*. New York, NY: Marcel Dekker, 2003, pp. 93–114.

Mainland J and Sobel N. The sniff is part of the olfactory percept. *Chemical Senses*, 2006, **31**(2), 181–96.

Mallet AI, Holland KT, Rennie PJ, Watkins WJ and Gower DB. Applications of gas chromatography–mass spectrometry in the study of androgen and odorous 16-androstene metabolism by human axillary bacteria. *Journal of Chromatography*, 1991, **562**(1–2), 647–58.

McClintock MK. Menstrual synchrony and suppression. *Nature*, 1971, **229**, 244–5.

Meisami E, Mikhail L, Baim D and Bhatnagar KP. Human olfactory bulb: aging of glomeruli and mitral cells and a search for the accessory olfactory bulb. *Annals of the New York Academy of Sciences*, 1998, **855**, 708–15.

Menco BPM and Morrison EE. Morphology of the mammalian olfactory epithelium: form, fine structure, function, and pathology. In: RL Doty, ed. *Handbook of Olfaction and Gustation*. New York, NY: Marcel Dekker, 2003, pp. 17–49.

Mirza N, Kroger H and Doty RL. Influence of age on the 'nasal cycle'. *Laryngoscope*, 1997, **107**, 62–6.

Mombaerts P. How smell develops. *Nature and Neuroscience*, 2001, **4**(Suppl.), 119–28.

Mombaerts P, Wang F, Dulac C *et al.* Visualizing an olfactory sensory map. *Cell*, 1996, **87**, 675–86.

Moran DT, Rowley JC III, Jafek BW and Lovell MA. The fine structure of the olfactory mucosa in man. *Journal of Neurocytology*, 1982, **11**, 721–46.

Mozell MM, Kent PF and Murphy SJ. The effect of flow rate upon the magnitude of the olfactory response differs for different odors. *Chemical Senses*, 1991, **16**, 631–49.

Murphy C, Shubert CR, Cruickshanks KJ, Klein BE, and Nondahl DM. Prevalence of olfactory impairment in older adults. *JAMA*, 2002, **288**, 2307–12.

Nakashima T, Kimmelman CP and Snow JB Jr. Structure of human fetal and adult olfactory neuroepithelium. *Archives of Otolaryngology*, 1984, **110**, 641–6.

Nordin S, Broman DA, Olofsson JK and Wulff M. A longitudinal descriptive study of self-reported abnormal smell and taste perception in pregnant women. *Chemical Senses*, 2004, **29**, 391–402.

Oberg C, Larsson M and Backman L. Differential sex effects in olfactory functioning: the role of verbal processing. *Journal of the International Neuropsychological Society*, 2002, **8**, 691–8.

Ohm TG and Braak H. Olfactory bulb changes in Alzheimer's disease. *Acta Neuropathologica*, 1987, **73**, 365–9.

Oka Y, Nakamura A, Watanabe H and Touhara K. An odorant derivative as an antagonist for an olfactory receptor. *Chemical Senses*, 2004, **29**, 815–22.

Pager J, Giachetti I, Holley A and LeMagnen J. A selective control of olfactory bulb electrical activity in relation to food deprivation and satiety in rats. *Physiological Behavior*, 1972, **9**, 573–9.

Pain S. Stench warfare. *New Scientist*, 2001, **2298**, 43–5.

Patterson PM and Lauder BA. The incidence and probable inheritance of "smell blindness" to normal butyl mercaptan. *Journal of Heredity*, 1948, **39**, 295–7.

Pearson RCA, Esiri MM, Hiornes RW, Wilcock GK and Powell TPS. Anatomical correlates of the distribution of the pathological changes in the neocortex in Alzheimer's disease. *Proceedings of the National Academy of Sciences of the United States of America*, 1985, **82**, 4531–4.

Pelosi P, Maremmani C and Muratorio A. Purification of an odorant binding protein from human nasal mucosa. *NATO ASI series*, 1990, **H 39**, 125–30.

Pilpel Y and Lancet D. The variable and conserved interfaces of modeled olfactory receptor proteins. *Protein Science*, 1999, **8**, 969–77.

Plailly J, Bensafi M, Pachot-Clouard M *et al.* Involvement of right piriform cortex in olfactory familiarity judgments. *Neuroimage*, 2005, **24**(4), 1032–41.

Pletsch PK and Kratz AT. Why do women stop smoking during pregnancy? Cigarettes taste and smell bad. *Health Care for Women International*, 2004, **25**, 671–9.

Poellinger A, Thomas R, Lio P *et al.* Activation and habituation in olfaction – an fMRI study. *Neuroimage*, 2001, **13**(4), 547–60.

Price JL. The olfactory system. In: G Paxinos and JK Mai, eds. *The Human Nervous System* (2nd edition). New York, NY: Academic Press, Inc., 2004, Chapter 32.

Proust M. *Remembrance of Things Past*. C. K. Scott-Moncrieff and T. Kilmartin, trans. New York, NY: Alfred A. Knoff, 1982.

Rajan R, Clement JP and Bhalla US. Rats smell in stereo. *Science*, 2006, **311**, 666–70.

Rennie PJ, Gower DB and Holland KT. In-vitro and in-vivo studies of human axillary odor and the cutaneous microflora. *British Journal of Dermatology*, 1991, **124**(6), 596–602.

Reyes PF, Deems DA and Suarez MG. Olfactory-related changes in Alzheimer's disease: a quantitative neuropathologic study. *Brain Research Bulletin*, 1993, **32**, 1–5.

Rochefort C, Gheusi G, Vincent JD and Lledo PM. Enriched odor exposure increases the number of newborn neurons in the adult olfactory bulb and improves odor memory. *Journal of Neuroscience*, 2002, **22**, 2679–89.

Rolls ET. The functions of the orbitofrontal cortex. *Brain and Cognition*, 2004, **55**(1), 11–29.

Ronnett GV and Snyder SH. Molecular messengers of olfaction. *Trends in Neuroscience*, 1992, **15**, 508–13.

Rosli Y, Breckenridge LJ and Smith RA. An ultrastructural study of age-related changes in mouse olfactory epithelium. *Journal of Electron Microscopy*, 1999, **48**, 77–84.

Rousselot P, Lois C and Alvarez-Buylla A. Embryonic (PSA) N-CAM reveals chains of migrating neuroblasts between the lateral ventricle and the olfactory bulb of adult mice. *Journal of Comparative Neurology*, 1994, **351**, 51–61.

Royet JP, Hudry J and Zald DH *et al.* Functional neuroanatomy of different olfactory judgments. *Neuroimage*, 2001, **13**(3), 506–19.

Sallaz M and Jourdan F. Apomorphine disrupts odor-induced patterns of glomerular activation in the olfactory bulb. *Neuroreport*, 1992, **3**, 833–6.

Sanders MD, Warrington EK, Marshall J and Wieskrantz L. 'Blindsight': Vision in a field defect. *Lancet*, 1974, **1**(7860), 707–8.

Sassoe-Pognetto M and Ottersen OP. Organization of ionotropic glutamate receptors at dendrodendritic synapses in the rat olfactory bulb. *Journal of Neuroscience*, 2000, **20**, 2192–201.

Savic I, Berglund H, Gulyas B and Roland P. Smelling of odorous sex hormone-like compounds causes sex-differentiated hypothalamic activations in humans. *Neuron*, 2001, **31**, 661–8.

Schank JC. Problems with dimensionless measurement models of synchrony in biological systems. *American Journal of Primatology*, 1997, **41**, 65–85.

Schank JC. Menstrual-cycle variability and measurement: further cause for doubt. *Psychoneuroendocrinology*, 2000, **25**, 837–47.

Schlesinger RB. Comparative deposition of inhaled aerosols in experimental animals and humans: a review. *Journal of Toxicology and Environmental Health*, 1985, **15**, 197–214.

Schneider RA and Wolf S. Relation of olfactory acuity to nasal membrane function. *Journal of Applied Physiology*, 1960, **15**, 914–20.

Serizawa S, Miyamichi K, Nakatani H *et al.* Negative feedback regulation ensures the one receptor–one olfactory neuron rule in mouse. *Science*, 2003, **302**, 2088–94.

Shannahoff-Khalsa DS, Kennedy B, Yates FE and Ziegler MG. Ultradian rhythms of autonomic, cardiovascular, and neuroendocrine systems are related in humans. *American Journal of Physiology*, 1996, **270**, R873–87.

Shepherd GM. In: GM Shepherd, ed. *Neurobiology* (3rd edition). Oxford, UK: Oxford University Press, 2004.

Sklar PB, Anholt RR and Snyder SH. The odorant-sensitive adenylate cyclase of olfactory receptor cells. Differential stimulation by distinct classes of odorants. *Journal of Biological Chemistry*, 1986, **261**, 15 538–43.

Smith CG. Age incident of atrophy of olfactory nerves in man. *Journal of Comparative Neurology*, 1942, **77**, 589–94.

Smith RS, Doty RL, Burlingame GK and McKeown DA. Smell and taste function in the visually impaired. *Perception and Psychophysics*, 1993, **54**, 649–55.

Smith TD, Bhatnagar KP, Shimp KL *et al.* Histological definition of the vomeronasal organ in humans and chimpanzees, with a comparison to other primates. *Anatomical Record*, 2002, **267**, 166–76.

Sobel N, Prabhakaran V, Desmond JE *et al.* Sniffing and smelling: separate subsystems in the human olfactory cortex. *Nature*, 1998, **392**, 282–6.

Sobel N, Khan RM, Saltman A, Sullivan EV and Gabrieli JD. The world smells different to each nostril. *Nature*, 1999a, **402**, 35.

Sobel N, Prabhakaran V, Hartley CA *et al.* Blind smell: brain activation induced by an undetected air-borne chemical. *Brain*, 1999b, **122**, 209–17.

Spielman AI, Zeng XN, Leyden JJ and Preti G. Proteinaceous precursors of human axillary odor: isolation of two novel odor-binding proteins. *Experientia*, 1995, **51**, 40–7.

Stern K and McClintock MK. Regulation of ovulation by human pheromones. *Nature*, 1998, **392**, 177–9.

Strassmann BI. The biology of menstruation in *Homo sapiens*: total lifetime menses, fecundity, and nonsynchrony in a natural-fertility population. *Current Anthropology*, 1997, **38**, 123–9.

Strassmann BI. Menstrual synchrony pheromones: cause for doubt. *Human Reproduction*, 1999, **14**, 579–80.

Stott WT, Ramsey JC and McKenna MJ. Absorption of chemical vapors by the upper respiratory tract of rats. In: CS Barrow, ed. *Toxicology of the Nasal Passages*. Washington, DC: Hemisphere Publishing Corporation, 1986, pp. 191–210.

Tirindelli R, Mucignat-Caretta C and Ryba NJ. Molecular aspects of pheromonal communication via the vomeronasal organ of mammals. *Trends in Neurosciences*, 1998, **21**, 482–6.

Vanscheeuwijck PM, Teredesai A and Terpstra PM *et al.* Evaluation of the potential effects of ingredients added to cigarettes. Part 4: subchronic inhalation toxicity. *Food and Chemical Toxicology*, 2002, **40**, 113–31.

von Skramlik E. Uber die Lokalisation der Empfindungen bei den niederen Sinnen. *Zeitschrift fur Sinnesphysiologie*, 1925, **56**, 69–140.

Weiskrantz L. The Ferrier Lecture, Outlooks for blindsight: explicit methodologies for implicit processes. *Proceedings of the Royal Society London B Biological Science*, 1990, **239**(1296), 247–78.

Werntz DA, Bickford RG, Bloom FE and Shannahoff-Khalsa DS. Alternating cerebral hemispheric activity and the lateralization of autonomic nervous function. *Human Neurobiology*, 1983, **2**, 39–43.

Whissell-Buechy D and Amoore JE. Odor-blindness to musk: simple recessive inheritance. *Nature*, 1973, **242**(5395), 271–3.

Whitten W. Comment on: Pheromones and regulation of ovulation. *Nature*, 1999, **401**(6750), 232–3.

Wilson DA. Comparison of odor receptive field plasticity in the rat olfactory bulb and anterior piriform cortex. *Journal of Neurophysiology*, 2000, **84**, 3036–42.

Wilson DA and Stevenson RJ. The fundamental role of memory in olfactory perception. *Trends in Neurosciences*, 2003, **26**, 243–7.

Wilson DA and Sullivan RM. The D2 antagonist spiperone mimics the effects of olfactory deprivation on mitral/tufted cell odor response patterns. *Journal of Neuroscience*, 1995, **15**, 5574–81.

Wilson HC. Female axillary secretions influence women's menstrual cycles: a critique. *Hormones and Behavior*, 1987, **21**, 536–46.

Wilson HC. A critical review of menstrual synchrony research. *Psychoneuroendocrinology*, 1992, **17**, 565–91.

Winston JS, Gottfried JA, Kilner JM and Dolan RJ. Integrated neural representations of odor intensity and affective valence in human amygdala. *Journal of Neuroscience*, 2005, **25**(39), 8903–7.

Wysocki CJ and Beauchamp GK. Ability to smell androstenone is genetically determined. *Proceedings of the Nationall Academy of Science of the United States of America*, 1984, **81**(15), 4899–902.

Wysocki CJ and Beauchamp GK. Individual differences in olfaction. In: CJ Wysocki and MR Kare, eds. *Genetics of Perception and Communications*. New York, NY: Marcel Dekker, 1991, pp. 353–73.

Wysocki CJ, Dorries KM and Beauchamp GK. Ability to perceive androstenone can be acquired by ostensibly anosmic people. *Proceedings of the National Academy of Science of the United States of America*, 1989, **86**(20), 7976–8.

Yano Y, Saito R, Yoshida N *et al.* A new role for expressed pseudogenes as ncRNA: regulation of mRNA stability of its homologous coding gene. *Journal of Molecular Medicine*, 2004, **82**, 414–22.

Yee KK and Wysocki CJ. Odorant exposure increases olfactory sensitivity: olfactory epithelium is implicated. *Physiology and Behavior*, 2001, **72**, 705–11.

Yousem DM, Geckle RJ, Bilker WB and Doty RL. Olfactory bulb and tract and temporal lobe volumes. Normative data across decades. *Annals of the New York Academy of Science*, 1998, **855**, 546–55.

Zaborszky L, Carlsen J, Brashear HR and Heimer L. Cholinergic and GABAergaic afferents to the olfactory bulb in the rat with special emphasis on the projection neurons in the nucleus of the horizontal limb of the diagonal band. *Journal of Comparative Neurology*, 1986, **243**, 488–509.

Zald DH and Pardo JV. Emotion, olfaction, and the human amygdala: amygdala activation during aversive olfactory stimulation. *Proceedings of the Natioanal Academy of Science of the United States of America*, 1997, **94**(8), 4119–24.

Zatorre RJ, Jones-Gotman M, Evans AC and Meyer E. Functional localization and lateralization of human olfactory cortex. *Nature*, 1992, **360**(6402), 339–40.

Zelano C, Bensafi M and Porter J *et al.* Attentional modulation in human primary olfactory cortex. *Nature and Neuroscience*, 2005, **8**, 114–20.

Zeng XN, Leyden JJ, Lawley HJ, Sawano K, Nohara I and Preti G. Analysis of characteristic odors from human male axillae. *Journal of Chemical Ecology*, 1991, **17**, 1469–91.

Zeng XN, Leyden JJ, Brand JG, Speilman AI, McGinley KJ and Preti G. An investigation of human apocrine gland secretion for axillary odor precursors. *Journal of Chemical Ecology*, 1992, **18**, 1039–1055.

Zhao K, Scherer PW, Hajiloo SA and Dalton P. Effect of anatomy on human nasal air flow and odorant transport patterns: implications for olfaction. *Chemical Senses*, 2004, **29**, 365–79.

Zhao K, Dalton P, Yang GC and Scherer PW. Numerical modeling of turbulent and laminar airflow and odorant transport during sniffing in the human and rat nose. *Chemical Senses*, 2006, **31**, 107–18.

Zola E. *Les Oeuvres Completes. Correspondence. 1858–1871. Notes et Commentaires de Maurice Leblond.* Paris: Renouard, 1928.

Clinical evaluation

Introduction

We begin this chapter by providing guidelines for the assessment of patients complaining of olfactory disturbances. Such information includes advice on how to structure the history and examination to identify better the underlying cause, how to quantify the dysfunction, and how to assess nasal function in general (e.g., nasal airway patency). Included is information about structural and functional imaging. The strengths and weaknesses of various procedures are examined, with a focus on validity and practicality. The chapter is concluded with a short discussion about how the sense of smell itself can aid medical diagnosis. Although, in the clinical setting, there is declining use of odors in diagnosing disease, there is growing interest in the electronic nose (E-nose) which, as discussed in this chapter, may become a key tool in the diagnostic armamentarium of the future clinician.

Medical history and examination

The etiology of most taste or smell disorders may be deduced from the history. Specifically, questions about the nature, onset, duration, and pattern of symptoms, as well as a historical account of antecedent events, such as head trauma, upper respiratory infections, toxic exposures, radiation or chemotherapy, and nasal or oral surgery, can usually establish etiology. The physician should attempt to identify exacerbating or relieving foods or products, prior treatment and its efficacy, and co-morbid medical conditions (e.g., liver disease, kidney disease, hypothyroidism, diabetes, vitamin deficiencies). Remission of symptoms during exercise, showering, or during periods of treatment with systemic steroids, implicates a conductive problem, since these procedures alter nasal congestion and turbinate engorgement. A history of epistaxis, nasal discharge (clear, purulent, or bloody), nasal obstruction, and somatic symptoms, including headache or irritation, should be sought.

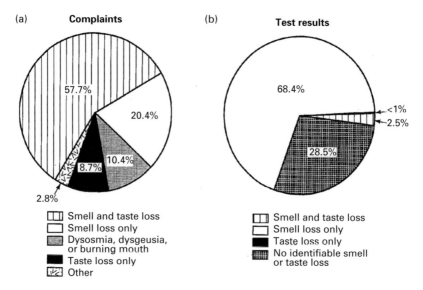

(a) **Complaints**   (b) **Test results**

☐☐ Smell and taste loss
☐ Smell loss only
▦ Dysosmia, dysgeusia,
  or burning mouth
■ Taste loss only
▨ Other

☐☐ Smell and taste loss
☐ Smell loss only
■ Taste loss only
▦ No identifiable smell
  or taste loss

Figure 2.1 Distribution of primary chemosensory complaints (a) and test results (b) from a study of 750 consecutive patients evaluated at the University of Pennsylvania Smell and Taste Center. (Reproduced with permission from Deems *et al.*, 1991 Copyright © 1991, American Medical Association. All rights reserved.)

Delayed puberty associated with anosmia, variably related to midline craniofacial abnormalities, deafness, mirror movements, and renal anomalies, suggests the possibility of Kallmann syndrome or one of its variants. Those who have never been able to smell typically lack normal olfactory bulbs or tracts. This can be demonstrated by specialized magnetic resonance imaging (MRI) (see Chapter 3, Figure 3.1). Although distorted smell sensations (dysosmias) or illusionary smells (phantosmias) can reflect pathology at the level of the olfactory epithelium, they may signify a lesion of the temporal lobe – in particular a tumor or seizure focus.

It should be emphasized that patients presenting with "taste loss" most commonly have olfactory, not gustatory, dysfunction, and a key goal of the history and medical examination should be to establish whether this is, in fact, the case (Figure 2.1). Insight can usually be obtained by asking the patient whether he or she can still detect the sweetness of sugar, the sourness of grapefruit, or the saltiness of potato chips. Many true taste deficits, including dysgeusias (distorted taste sensations), reflect side-effects of medication, some of which appear only after long-term usage. As described in detail in Chapter 3, such widely used agents as statins, antifungal agents, antiviral agents, and angiotensin-converting enzyme (ACE) inhibitors have been associated with chemosensory disturbances, particularly gustatory. Problems with articulation, salivation, chewing, swallowing, oral pain or burning, dryness of the mouth, periodontal disease, foul breath, dental work, or bruxism may aid in distinguishing between a true taste problem and an olfactory one, although the rare coincidence of a taste and smell problem should not be ruled out. Questions about hearing, tinnitus, and balance are important since the vestibulocochlear nerve (cranial nerve (CN) VIII) is close to the facial nerve and can be damaged at the same time (e.g., from cerebellopontine angle tumors). Gastric problems such as gastro-esophageal reflux may be relevant as they can compromise the sense of taste. Constitutional symptoms, such as fever, malaise, headache, and body pains, often accompany cancers or systemic inflammatory conditions (e.g., lupus). Unexplained anosmia presenting, as it usually does, during the winter months, suggests a viral origin, even if other elements of an upper respiratory infection are not present or recognized.

Before commencing physical examination it should be noted whether the patient has a cold, allergic rhinitis, or migraine attack, all of which are associated with nasal congestion and preclude reliable assessment of smell function. Physical examination should start with basic inspection of the nose for external evidence of poor nasal air entry. It may be abnormally narrow, or blunted from previous trauma. This is especially common in boxers. Saddle-nose deformity is typical of congenital syphilis but may occur in any granulomatous disorder such as sarcoidosis, leprosy, tuberculosis, or Wegener's granulomatosis. We should be alert to patients who mouth-breathe, as they may have local nasal disease that could affect their ability to smell.

Simple anterior rhinoscopy with a pair of nasal forceps will help determine whether gross nasal problems are present. Referral to an ear nose and throat specialist for detailed nasal endoscopy is highly recommended in unexplained cases and when signs of nasal inflammation, polyposis, severe septal deviation with adhesions, mucosal atrophy or erosion, or exudates are noted. Pallor of the mucosa usually reflects allergies and edema within the lamina propria. Purulent rhinorrhea stemming primarily from the middle meatus suggests maxillary, anterior ethmoid, or frontal sinusitis, whereas rhinorrhea localized to the superior meatus suggests posterior ethmoid or sphenoid sinusitis.

Ideally, all cranial nerves should be examined in someone with a smell problem. Apart from CN I, the more essential cranial nerves for valuation are the optic and trigeminal nerves. An abnormal visual field, pupillary defect, optic disk swelling, or atrophy in conjunction with anosmia may signify a frontal lobe tumor or related structural pathology. The Foster Kennedy syndrome is occasionally overlooked. In its complete form it is characterized by an ipsilateral central scotoma, optic atrophy, anosmia, and contralateral papilledema. Classically, it is caused by a large frontal neoplasm, but other lesions include a meningioma of the olfactory groove or medial third of the sphenoid wing. The sensory component of the trigeminal nerve is of particular relevance. Common sensation should be assessed over the face with cotton wool and a pin. Corneal reflex testing evaluates the first division of the trigeminal nerve and it is of relevance to sensation in the upper regions of the nose, but the procedure carries risk of corneal damage and is best avoided. Nasal tickle is a less well known but useful stimulant of maxillary (trigeminal) nerve sensation. It is examined by moving gently a wisp of cotton wool inside one nostril. Most normal people respond by flinching rapidly; loss or asymmetry would suggest a disorder of trigeminal fine nerve fibers.

The following blood tests are of potential relevance to olfactory disorders, particularly of the central (neurogenic) type: blood count (for anemia, drug effects); sedimentation rate (vasculitic disease, malignancy); B_{12} and folate level (nutritional state); glucose (diabetes and pituitary disease); calcium and phosphate (parathyroid function, Paget's disease); thyroid function (myxoedema); electrolytes (renal disease, Addison's or Cushing's disease); liver function tests (cirrhosis); autoimmune tests such as anti-neutrophil cytoplasmic antibodies (ANCA) for Wegener's granulomatosis; anti-Ro and anti-La for Sjögren's disease; IgE (allergic rhinitis). Further investigation depends on complexity and whether there is a question of malingering, as may be the case in compensation claims.

Olfactory testing

The astute clinician of yesteryear tested CN I by presenting an odorant (e.g., tobacco or perfume) to a patient and asking whether it can be smelled and, if so, what it smells like. Although better than performing no testing at all, this approach is akin to shining a flashlight into a patient's eye and asking whether it is seen and, if so, what is its color. More sophisticated approaches, such as measuring olfactory thresholds, were reserved for the laboratory. Fortunately, practical and reliable psychophysical tests of olfactory function are now generally available, as described later in this chapter.

It is critical to establish the nature and validity of a patient's complaint by quantitative testing. A common error made by clinicians is to accept at face value a patient's report of chemosensory disturbance and to neglect formal measurement of the presence or magnitude of the problem. Most patients are poor at assessing the acuity of their sense of smell unless this faculty is essential for their work or hobbies, e.g., chef, perfumer, or wine taster. The elderly or those with dementia are poor self-evaluators (Doty et al., 1987; Nordin et al., 1995), and a number of patients presenting with olfactory dysfunction have no meaningful smell function at all (London et al., 2008). It is rare for those with unilateral anosmia to be aware of any defect; a situation that can be detected by proper clinical assessment. Moreover, as noted above, many patients, as well as their physicians, confuse loss of flavor sensations derived from decreased retronasal stimulation of the olfactory system, with loss of taste. Some patients, particularly those involved in litigation, malinger or overstate the nature of their dysfunction. Quantitative testing addresses the nature and degree of the chemosensory problem, detects malingering, and tracks changes in function over time. The latter is important for determining the efficacy of any future medical or surgical intervention.

Some physicians, as well as lawyers seeking to denigrate or enhance the results of examinations, divide sensory procedures into "subjective" and "objective." The former usually refers to tests where a conscious subject response is required and the latter where some presumed involuntary reaction is assessed, such as altered electrical or autonomic nervous system activity. The so-called "objective" procedures are presumed to be harder to manipulate by the determined malingerer. Unfortunately, this dichotomy is misleading and laden with a value judgment, since objective always trumps subjective. As pointed out by the Nobel Laureate Georg von Békésy in the case of hearing science, so-called subjective tests are often more sensitive and reliable than so-called objective tests (von Békésy, 1968), contrary to the underlying suggestion of superiority of the latter class of tests. In view of these difficulties, the terms subjective and objective are not used in this volume and tests are categorized according to the operational classes into which they fall.

Olfactory tests may be classified into three broad categories: psychophysical, electrophysiological, and psychophysiological. *Psychophysical tests*, described in more detail below, are those where stimuli are varied in some manner (e.g., in concentration or quality) and the patient is required to indicate whether the stimulus is perceived (e.g., as in a detection threshold test) or changes in some way relative to other stimuli, such as intensity. Included in this category are measures of odor detection, discrimination, memory, and identification. *Electrophysiological tests* evaluate either summated electrical activity at the surface of the olfactory receptor epithelium (i.e., the electro-olfactogram or EOG) or integrated electrical activity at the surface of the scalp (e.g., odor event-related potentials or OERPs). These tests typically require complex stimulus presentation and recording equipment. *Psychophysiological tests*, a number of which also employ electrical recording methods, measure autonomic nervous system responses to odorants, such as changes in blood pressure, heart rate, respiratory rate, or galvanic skin responses. Given their poor reliability, and in some cases dependence upon non-olfactory sensory afferents (e.g., trigeminal activation), psychophysiological tests are not described in this chapter. Most psychophysical tests measure overlapping physiological determinants of perceptual function, despite being operationally distinct or having different names (e.g., tests of detection, identification, memory, and so on). Such overlap, as well as differences in reliability and validity, can complicate the comparison of findings across test measures.

It should be emphasized that it is rarely possible to localize the anatomical site of a deficit based upon olfactory tests of any type. Although the EOG can detect, in some instances, specific peripheral pathology, such pathology will also influence tests of more central brain function, making it difficult to ascertain whether a deficit is present in peripheral or central structures, or both. Importantly, as described in more detail later in this chapter, the results of the EOG must be interpreted with caution, as some patients with marked hyposmia or anosmia will exhibit EOGs even when no odor is perceived (Hummel *et al.*, 2006). Animal studies clearly demonstrate that the EOG lasts for several hours after death and it is not abolished following pharmacological blockage of olfactory receptor action potentials (Scott & Scott-Johnson, 2002). Moreover, EOGs can differ markedly in magnitude, depending upon the integrity of the epithelial region that is sampled. Functional imaging and OERPs are rarely capable of localizing a smell problem to the nose, epithelium, olfactory tract, or more central structures.

Odorant presentation procedures

Before any type of olfactory assessment can be made, an odorant must be presented reliably to the patient. Attempts to achieve this go back hundreds of years and include: (1) the draw tube olfactometer (Zwaardemaker, 1889, 1925); (2) glass sniff bottles (Cheeseman & Townsend, 1956; Doty *et al.*, 1986); (3) odorized glass rods, wooden sticks, felt-tipped pens, alcohol pads, or strips of blotter paper (Davidson & Murphy, 1997; Hummel *et al.*, 1997; Semb, 1968; Takagi, 1989; Toyota *et al.*, 1978); (4) plastic squeeze bottles (Amoore & Ollman, 1983; Cain *et al.*, 1983; Doty, 2001; Guadagni *et al.*, 1963); (5) bottles from which blasts of saturated air are presented (Elsberg & Levy, 1935); (6) microencapsulated "scratch and sniff" odorized strips (Doty *et al.*, 1984); and (7) air-dilution olfactometers (Cheeseman & Kirby, 1959; Doty *et al.*, 1988; Kobal & Plattig, 1978; Lorig *et al.*, 1999; Punter, 1983; Walker *et al.*, 1990; Wenzel, 1948; Figure 2.2).

In addition to presenting stimuli for sniffing, odorants can be delivered into the mouth (so-called retronasal odor perception; Heilmann *et al.*, 2002), as well as intravenously (Nakashima *et al.*, 2006). The intra-oral approach, in which odorants are placed in small containers slipped to the rear of the tongue, may discern subtle differences in the perception of flavor sensations dependent upon so-called retronasal stimulation of the olfactory receptors. However, it is extremely difficult to quantify and establish the influences of odorants presented in this way, given the complexities of absorption and the difficulty mimicking the air currents generated during normal chewing and swallowing (Burdach & Doty, 1987). Intravenous odorant presentation, a procedure employed primarily in Japan, attempts to determine whether the olfactory receptors are working when nasal

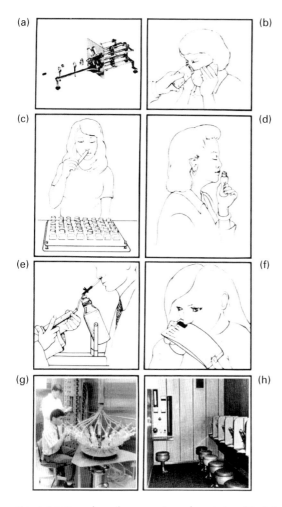

Figure 2.2 Procedures for presenting odorants to subjects for assessment. (a) Laboratory version of the draw-tube olfactometer of Zwaardemaker. In its simplest version, an outer tube, made of rubber or another odorous material, slides along a calibrated inner tube, which is connected to a sniffing tube. When the odorized tube is slid toward the patient, less of its internal surface is exposed to the inspired airstream, resulting in a weaker olfactory sensation. In the pictured version, several stimuli can be presented simultaneously at varying concentrations. (b) Sniff bottle. (c) Perfumer's strip. (d) Squeeze bottle. (e) Blast injection device. The experimenter injects a given volume of air into the odorant-containing bottle and releases the pressure by squeezing a clamp on the tube leading to the nostril, producing a stimulus pulse. (f) Microencapsulated "scratch-and-sniff" test. (g) An air-dilution olfactometer connected to sniff ports located on a rotating table. (h) An odor evaluation room where subjects sit in front of sniff ports to sample odorants. (From Doty and Laing, 2003. With permission.)

congestion or blockage eliminates or mitigates airflow to the receptor region. The assumption underlying this technique is that the stimulus makes its way to the olfactory receptors via the bloodstream and that if odor is perceived, the receptors are still functional. Most commonly, thiamine propyldisulfide (also termed Alinamin or Prosultiamine) is injected into the median cubital vein, and recordings are made of the duration and latency of the onset of a garlic-like sensation experienced by the patient (see Takagi (1989) for review). Although this procedure may have some merit, its physiological basis is controversial (i.e., whether the stimulus reaches the receptors via diffusion from nasal capillaries, from lung air, or both; see Maruniak *et al.*, 1983). Thus, measurable quantities of the odorant appear in the nasal cavity within 20 seconds of an injection (Nakashima *et al.*, 2006). Given its invasive nature and difficulties in interpretation, this procedure is not widely used.

Psychophysical tests

Traditional psychophysics, developed in the nineteenth century, sought to establish mathematical functions that relate events in the physical world to their psychological counterparts; that is, how measurable changes in stimuli relate to measurable changes in the magnitude of psychological sensations. This approach led to the understanding, for example, that logarithmic or power functions describe the relationship between changes in physical energy, such as luminance, and the perception of these changes, such as brightness (e.g., the Weber–Fechner Law; Weber, 1834). Today, any procedure that provides a quantitative measure of sensory function and requires a verbal or conscious overt response on the part of the examinee is generally considered a psychophysical procedure. Since scores from tests of odor identification, detection, and discrimination are generally correlated with one another, simple identification tests are usually adequate for an overall assessment of olfactory function (Doty *et al.*, 1994).

Although most olfactory problems are bilateral, bilateral testing reflects the better-functioning side of the nose. Thus, in some instances unilateral testing is warranted. Total anosmia may be present on one side of the nose and will be overlooked completely by a bilateral test. To assess olfaction accurately and unilaterally, the nostril contralateral to the tested side should be occluded without distorting the cross-sectional area or shape of the nasal valve (the narrowed area of the nasal cavity about 2 cm posterior to the opening of the naris). This prevents crossing of inhaled or exhaled air within the naso-pharynx. An easy way of doing this is to seal the contralateral nostril using a piece of Microfoam^{TM} tape (3M Corporation, Minneapolis, MN) cut to fit the borders of the nostril. The patient is instructed to sniff the stimulus normally and to exhale through the mouth.

Odor identification tests

The most widely used procedures for assessing smell function involve stimulus quality identification. Three types of identification tests are common: naming tests, yes/no identification tests, and multiple-choice identification tests. The responses required for these three classes are: (1) to provide a name for the quality of the stimulus; (2) to signify whether or not a given odorant smells like an object named by the examiner (e.g., "Does this smell like a rose?"); and (3) to identify a stimulus from a list of names or pictures.

Odor-naming tests in which no response choices are presented have been the mainstay for olfactory testing by physicians, but their value is diminished because most normal individuals have difficulty naming or identifying even familiar odors without cues. Moreover, such tests lack normative referents and are easy to malinger. A more useful test is to ask a patient to indicate whether or not each of a set of stimuli smells like a particular odor named by the experimenter (yes/no identification test). Two trials per stimulus are usually given, with the correct alternative provided on one trial and an incorrect one on the other trial (e.g., rose odor is presented and the subject is asked on one trial whether the odor smells like rose and on another trial whether the odor smells like apple). Although such a test requires the patient to keep the percept in memory long enough to compare it with the target word (which, of course, must also be recalled from memory), some proponents argue that this type of test is minimally influenced by cognitive and memory demands. Since chance performance on this type of test is 50 percent, a considerable number of trials are usually needed to obtain reliable findings.

The most popular tests for assessing olfactory function in the clinic are multiple-choice odor identification tests. The most widely used odor identification test, the 40-odorant University of Pennsylvania Smell Identification Test (UPSIT), is available in 11 languages and has been administered to many thousands of patients worldwide (Doty et al., 1984; Doty, 1995). This test examines the ability of subjects to identify, from sets of four descriptors, each of 40 "scratch and sniff" odorants (Figure 2.3a). The number of correct items that are answered serves as the test measure. This value is compared to norms and a percentile rank is determined, depending on the age and gender of the subject, based upon a group of nearly 4000 normal subjects (Figure 2.4 and Doty, 1995). The UPSIT is amenable to self-administration, can be sent through the post for self-completion at home, has excellent test–retest reliability (r values >0.90), and provides a means of detecting malingering on the basis of improbable responses. Shorter versions of the UPSIT, including 3- and 12-item versions (Doty et al., 1996), are available for brief screening (Figure 2.3b). If dysfunction is found on the shorter screening tests, more extensive evaluation is recommended.

In keeping with other odor identification tests and most other psychophysical measures, the UPSIT may assess indirectly some elements of

(a)

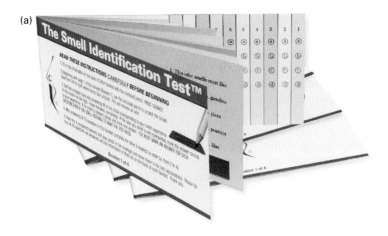

(b)

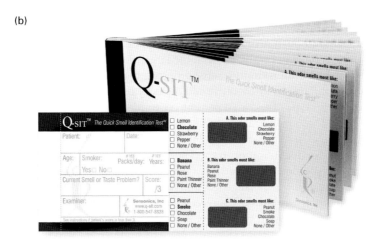

Figure 2.3 (a) Booklet 1 of the four-booklet University of Pennsylvania Smell Identification Test (UPSIT). Each page of each 10-page booklet contains a microencapsulated odorant that is released by scratching it with a pencil tip, along with a multiple-choice question about which of four possibilities is correct. Forced-choice answers are recorded on the last page of the booklet and assessed with a simple scoring key.
(b) The Quick Smell Identification Test (Q-SIT). The right side of each page of this three-item test is torn off and presented to a patient. The patient scratches the microencapsulated label with a fingernail or coin and indicates which of four options is most like the odor, if the odor smells unlike any given possibility, or has no smell. A score of 2 or more wrong on this test is highly suggestive of a smell problem.
(Copyright © 2004, Sensonics, Inc., Haddon Heights, New Jersey, USA.)

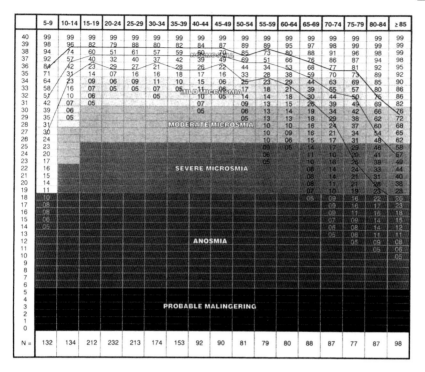

Figure 2.4 Female normative data for the UPSIT (males have separate norms). UPSIT scores are indicated on the ordinate, and age of the subject on the abscissa. Numbers at bottom indicate sample sizes within each five-year age group. A patient's test score is categorized into absolute categories of probable malingering, anosmia, severe microsmia, moderate microsmia, mild microsmia, and normosmia. Percentile ranks indicated for each age group. (From Doty, 1995. Copyright © 1995, Sensonics, Inc., Haddon Heights, New Jersey, USA.)

cognitive function unrelated to olfaction, e.g., the more intelligent person may not recognize the correct odor but might identify those which are wrong, and deduce the correct answer by elimination. This rare, but potential, problem can be overcome to some extent by administering a 40-item visual test, analogous to the UPSIT, that uses pictures, rather than odorants, as test stimuli (the Picture Identification Test; PIT) (Vollmecke & Doty, 1985). If a patient scores normally on the PIT, then we may assume that poor performance on the UPSIT is not due to lack of understanding of the concepts of the test procedure. Some argue that non-olfactory elements of the UPSIT may aid in its usefulness for assessing Alzheimer's disease where, for example, smell memory, concentration, and reasoning may be affected.

A recurrent criticism of the UPSIT concerns the presence of odorants or response options unfamiliar to patients outside of the USA, such as root beer, skunk, fruit punch, and pumpkin pie. This is the case only with the American version of the test, not with the various European and Asian versions. For research purposes and particularly for countries outside the USA, it is nonetheless advisable to obtain local norms. This controls for cultural effects, education, social class, and numerous environmental factors that may not be evident to the investigator.

Among other commercially available psychophysical tests are shorter versions of the UPSIT (e.g., the three-item Quick Smell Identification Test (Q-SIT) (Jackman et al., 2005) and the 12-item Brief Smell Identification Test (B-SIT) (Doty et al., 1996), the Smell Diskettes Olfaction Test (Simmen et al., 1999), the T&T Olfactometer (Toyota et al., 1978), and the Sniffin' Sticks Test (SST) (Figure 2.5). The latter employs felt tip pen dispensers to present different odorants (Kobal et al., 1996). The identification (screening) version has 16 sticks (12 odors and blanks). Although the reliability of the identification component of this test is less than that of the 40-odor UPSIT, it is comparable with the 12-odor B-SIT (Hummel et al., 1997). The SST is available in a longer version ("Extended" Test) which combines identification with elements of threshold and discrimination, resulting in a reliable heuristic "TDI" index. Normative data are available for this index based on several thousand healthy subjects (Hummel et al., 2007; Pause et al., 1997). The standard 12-odor SST is rapid and can be self-administered (Mueller et al., 2006), but the extended version, which requires threshold measurement, is time-consuming and has to be administered by a trained technician. Where the two tests (UPSIT and screening SST) have been compared directly (Silveira-Moriyama et al., 2006; Wolfensberger et al., 2000) correlations have been found to be moderate (e.g., r's ~ 0.75). Although these procedures are amenable to unsupervised completion, it is our view that unless healthy control subjects are being studied, it is prudent to supervise the testing, especially in patients with upper limb problems or attention difficulties. A full list of olfactory test procedures that includes non-commercial varieties can be found in Doty (2007).

Odor discrimination tests establish the degree to which a patient can differentiate between different odorants, but do not require naming or formal identification of the odors. On one such test, a patient indicates on a given trial whether two stimuli are the same or different. The number of same-odorant and different-odorant trials that are correctly differentiated serves as the dependent measure (Eichenbaum et al., 1983; Potter & Butters, 1980). More sophisticated analyses of such data, based upon signal detection theory (see below), can also be made but are beyond the scope of this chapter. Variants on this general theme include picking the "odd" stimulus from a set from which only the "odd" stimulus differs (e.g., the so-called triangle test; Frijters, 1980) and the classical match-to-sample test with or without differing delay intervals between the target and inspection odorants (Choudhury et al., 2003).

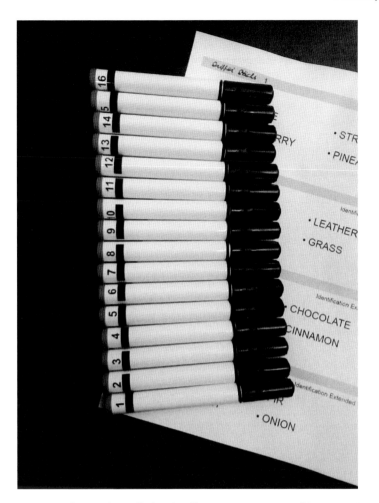

Figure 2.5 The 12-odor Sniffin' Sticks Olfactory Screening Test. This test consists of 16 felt-tip pens of which 12 are filled with odors and four are blanks. The patient is asked to smell the tip and name the odor from multiple choice cards containing four items for each pen. For more detailed testing an "Extended" test is available which has 48 sticks. This produces a threshold, discrimination, and identification score (TDI index). (Photograph courtesy of Dr. L. Silveira-Moriyama.)

Another approach to odor discrimination is that of multidimensional scaling (MDS). MDS provides a spatial representation of the perceived similarities of odorants. In one application of MDS, ratings are made for all possible pairs of stimuli (or selected subsets of pairs) on a scale anchored with descriptors like "completely different vs. exactly the same." The correlations among the ratings are subjected to an algorithm that places the stimuli in two or more dimensional space relative to their perceived similarities (e.g., Schiffman *et al.*, 1981). The degree to which groupings of odorants established for a patient differ in space from those obtained from normal subjects reflects the perceptual alterations of the patient. Because MDS requires considerable time to perform and statistical procedures for comparing one person's MDS spaces to another's (or to a norm) are poorly worked out, MDS is not used routinely. Interestingly, when subjects are asked to rate the similarity of stimuli that are only indicated to them by name (i.e., the odorants, per se, are never presented), stimulus spaces derived by MDS are analogous to those obtained by the actual use of the odorants (Carrasco & Ridout, 1993). This implies that well-defined conceptual representations of odors are present in humans, and stresses the importance of semantic processes in odor recognition.

Odor threshold tests

Next to odor identification tests, odor threshold tests are the most common means of assessing olfactory function clinically. The *absolute* or *detection threshold* is the lowest odorant concentration where such a presence is reliably detected, whereas the *recognition threshold* is the lowest concentration where odor quality is reliably discerned. The *difference threshold* (also termed the "differential threshold") seeks to establish the smallest amount by which a stimulus must be changed to make it perceptibly stronger or weaker (i.e., the "just noticeable difference" or JND). The increment in odorant concentration (ΔI) required to produce a JND increases as the comparison concentration (I) increases, with the ratio approximating a constant; i.e., $\Delta I/I = K$ (Weber's law) (Weber, 1834).

For a number of reasons, detection thresholds are more commonly measured in the clinic than either recognition or differential thresholds. Their values are usually lower than recognition thresholds, since a qualitative odor sensation (e.g., "rose-like") is rarely perceived at very low odorant concentrations, where only the faint presence of something is noted. They are also more reliable and straightforward to obtain than recognition or differential thresholds, with the latter not always conforming to Weber's law across the entire stimulus continuum.

Several threshold tests are commercially available, including the T&T olfactometer (Toyota *et al.*, 1978), the extended version of the Sniffin' Sticks test (Hummel *et al.*, 1997), and the Smell Threshold Test (STT) (Doty, 2000) (see Figure 2.6). In these and most other modern threshold tests, the subject is instructed to indicate, on a given trial, which of two or more stimuli (e.g., a low-concentration odorant and one or more blanks) smells strongest, rather than to report whether an odor is perceived. Such forced-choice procedures are less susceptible than non-forced choice procedures to confounding by

(a)

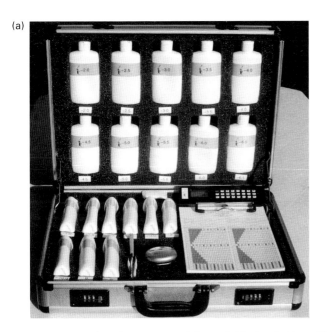

Figure 2.6a Examples of two commercially available threshold test kits. (a) The Smell Threshold Test (STT; Sensonics Inc, Haddon Hts., NJ, USA). The rose-like CN I stimulant, phenyl ethyl alcohol, is provided in 17 half-log concentration steps ranging from −10 log vol/vol to −2 log vol/vol. The stimulus is delivered with squeeze bottles and a single staircase method is used to present the stimuli – see Figure 2.7.

response biases (i.e., the conservatism or liberalism in reporting the presence of an odor under uncertain conditions), and are generally more reliable and produce lower threshold values (Doty & Laing, 2003). Furthermore, like the UPSIT, they can provide a statistical means for assessing malingering.

Psychophysical procedures most commonly used in the clinic to measure detection thresholds are the ascending method of limits (AML) and single-staircase (SS) procedures. In the AML procedure, odorants are presented sequentially from low to high concentrations (ascending series; Cain *et al.*, 1983). The point of transition between detection and no detection is estimated. In the SS method (a variant of the method of limits technique; see Cornsweet, 1962), an initial, usually ascending, stimulus series is used to reach the peri-threshold region. Additional trials are then presented, with the concentration of the stimulus being increased following trials in which a subject fails to detect the stimulus and decreased after trials where correct detection occurs (Doty *et al.*, 1986). Numerous variations on this theme have been employed to decrease the number of trials required to establish a

(b)

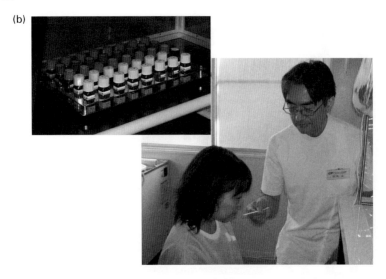

Figure 2.6b The T&T Olfactometer (Daiichi Yakuhin Sangyo Co. Ltd, Tokyo, Japan). This is a non-forced-choice test of odor recognition and detection thresholds for five different odorants. The odorants are presented to the subject on perfumer's blotter strips, which are dipped into the test solution for each trial and then discarded. (Figure courtesy of Dr. Tadashi Ishimaru, Japan.)

reliable detection measure. For example, in some SS paradigms larger concentration steps are made initially until the first reversal occurs to facilitate reaching the peri-threshold region. Examples of data from subjects using an SS procedure are shown in Figure 2.7, where the first element of the staircase ascends (i.e., goes from weak to strong stimuli) in log steps and five correct trials at a given concentration are required before a lower concentration is presented (Doty, 2000). After the initial staircase reversal, movements of the staircase are made in half-log steps and only two sets of trials are presented under the "two down, one up rule." Under this rule, a miss on either the first or the second of two sets of pairs that are presented results in the next trial being at a higher concentration, whereas perform-ance on both sets of pairs must be correct for the next trial to occur at a lower odorant concentration. The geometric mean of the last four of seven staircase reversals serves as the threshold estimate.

A recent variant of the SS procedure, termed the maximum-likelihood adaptative staircase procedure, has been employed clinically (Linschoten et al., 2001). In this paradigm, an estimate is made continuously on the basis of responses to prior trials about where the threshold is most likely to be and the next odorant concentration is presented at the estimated value. This

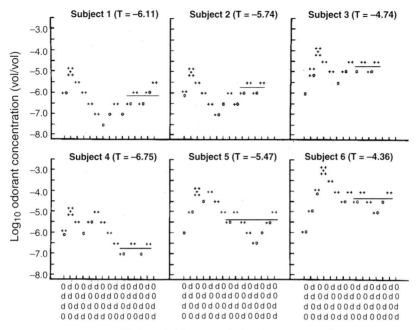

Figure 2.7 Graph illustrating single-staircase detection threshold determinations. Each plus (+) indicates a correct detection when on odorant versus a blank is presented. Each zero (0) indicates an incorrect response. Threshold value (T; vol/vol phenyl ethyl alcohol concentration in USP grade light mineral oil) is calculated as the mean of the last four of seven staircase reversals. The o's and d's on the abscissa indicate the counterbalancing order of the presentation sequences for each trial and are read downward (o – odorant presented first, then diluent; d – diluent presented first than odorant). At the first reversal point (where five correct sets of pairs at the same concentration are required before the staircase can move to a lower concentration), the fifth-order sequence is determined by the first o or d of the subsequent column of four order sequences. Before reaching the first reversal, the staircase is moved in full log steps; after this reversal, all movements are made in half-log steps and only two trials, each consisting of a blank and odorant, are presented at each concentration. If the first trial is missed, the second one is not given and the next highest concentration is presented. (From Doty and Laing, 2003. With permission.)

results in a quicker convergence on to the threshold value than the SS pro-cedure, but requires a computer to calculate the threshold. Whilst somewhat more economical in terms of time, this technique arrives at threshold values very similar to those of the traditional SS procedure.

It is important to realize that threshold values are relative and both their magnitude and stability depend upon factors such as the method of stimulus dilution, volume of presented stimulus, species of molecule, type of psychophysical task, interstimulus duration, stimulus step size and number of trials presented (Pierce *et al.*, 1996). Some authors report that threshold values exhibit marked variability (Brown *et al.*, 1968; Stevens *et al.*, 1988; Yoshida, 1984). In most cases, however, such variability arises from stimulus presentation techniques with too few trials, (e.g., the single series ascending method of limits technique), failure to instruct the subject to distinguish between detection and recognition of the stimulus, and the lack of forced-choice testing.

Signal detection tests

Although threshold tests are clinically useful, some scientists argue convincingly that there is no such entity as a threshold (Tanner & Swets, 1954). Adherents to signal detection theory (SDT) reject the threshold concept, whether absolute or differential. Instead, SDT focuses on (1) noise and signal plus noise as the milieu of the detection situation and (2) the influences of subject expectancies and rewards on the detection decision. SDT provides both a measure of sensory sensitivity and the subject's response criterion or bias, the latter being an index of the subject's liberalism or conservatism for reporting the presence or absence of a sensation under uncertain circumstances. For example, two patients may experience the same subtle degree of sensation from a very weak stimulus. However, one may report that no sensation was perceived (perhaps because of lack of self-confidence), whereas the other may report the presence of the sensation. In both cases, the stimulus was perceived to the same degree, but the two subjects had different criteria for reporting its presence. In a traditional non-forced-choice detection threshold paradigm, the investigator would conclude that these two subjects differed in sensitivity to the stimulus, when, in fact, they only differed in regards to their response criterion (Figure 2.8).

Signal detection measurement is very useful when subtle variations in an individual's sensitivity are sought, or when a distinction between sensitivity and response bias is of interest, as in evaluating small changes in olfactory sensitivity across phases of the menstrual cycle (Doty *et al.*, 1981). Because signal detection tests typically require a large number of trials, and normative data are lacking for clinical application, they are rarely used in the clinical setting. The interested reader is referred for more detailed descriptions of this approach to olfactory measurement (Doty & Laing, 2003).

Odor memory tests

Odor memory tests require a subject to smell a target stimulus (or set of target stimuli) and then identify, after a delay, the target stimulus from foils. For example, on a given trial in one standardized odor memory test, the

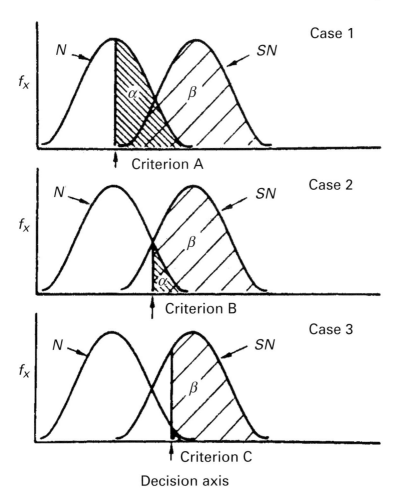

Figure 2.8 Examples of how the response criterion can vary when sensory sensitivity (d′) remains constant, i.e., the distance between the noise (N) and signal plus noise (SN) distributions. In Case 1, a liberal criterion was chosen by the subject in which a relatively large number of false positive responses occurred (i.e., α, reports of the presence of an odor when a blank which represents noise (N) is presented). In Cases 2 and 3, more conservative criteria were chosen, decreasing both the number of false positives (α) and hits (β). Traditional threshold measures confound the influences of sensory or perceptual sensitivity and the setting of the response criterion. (From Doty and Laing, 2003. With permission.)

patient is required to smell a microencapsulated odorant and keep the odor in memory for either 10, 30, or 60 seconds, after which the target odor is selected from a set of four choices (Doty, 2003). During the delay periods of this 12-trial test, the patient is required to count aloud backward in threes from 260, a task designed to minimize the rehearsal of verbal labels that the examinee may attempt to apply to the target stimulus. The proportion of trials where correct performance occurs at each delay interval, as well as the total number of correct trials, serve as the dependent measures.

Odor memory tests are sensitive to the effects of gender and age in a manner similar to that seen with threshold and odor identification tests (Choudhury *et al.*, 2003), and may be more sensitive than such tests to the influences of some drugs and hormones (Patel *et al.*, 2004). However, delay interval effects are rarely seen, complicating the degree to which we may assume that odor memory, per se, is the trait being specifically assessed. Given that normal people show little decline in remembering odors across rather extensive delay intervals (Engen & Ross, 1973; Engen *et al.*, 1973), clear evidence of a delay-related decrement of performance is needed to confirm that odor memory, per se, is abnormal. Odor memory tests such as that described by Choudhury *et al.* (2003) can be viewed as match-to-sample odor discrimination tests, with varying time periods between the target and inspection odors.

Odor rating and magnitude estimation tests

A number of olfactory tests seek to establish how well a subject can perceive changes in the magnitude of such psychological attributes as odorant quality, intensity, and pleasantness. The most common quantified attribute is odorant intensity, which varies as a function of stimulus concentration. Although perceived pleasantness or unpleasantness of an odor also can change with concentration, it is more variable and idiosyncratic (Doty, 1975; Figure 2.9). Only rarely is odor quality influenced significantly by odorant concentration within the suprathreshold concentration range. Conceptually, ratings of odorant intensity could reflect the extent of neural damage present in the afferent pathway, given that the intensity of a stimulus is typically related to the number of neurons that are recruited and the frequency at which they fire (Drake *et al.*, 1969). Nonetheless, tests employing suprathreshold rating scales are less sensitive to olfactory dysfunction than odor identification and threshold tests, and are rarely used clinically. In some cases, such scales have completely missed major effects observed by other methods (e.g., the influences of age on olfactory function) (see Rovee *et al.*, 1975).

One problem that may occur with traditional rating scales is that patients tend to bunch responses in the extreme ends of the scale, limiting their fidelity. When present, attempts to eliminate categories and to provide continua with disparate descriptors (e.g., "weak," "strong") at their extreme ends (e.g., visual analog scales) only partially correct this problem. Some rating scales now place descriptors at logarithmic points along the scale continuum in an effort to overcome ceiling effects and produce more linear

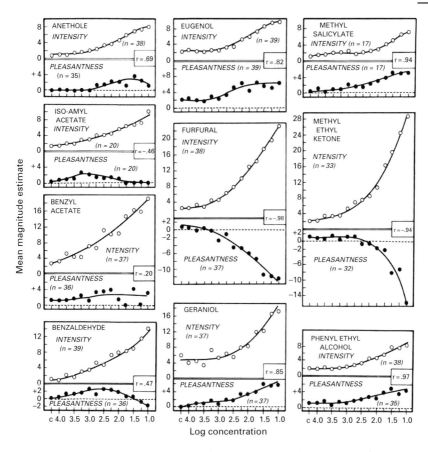

Figure 2.9 Relationship of pleasantness and intensity magnitude estimates to log volume concentration in propylene glycol diluent for 10 compounds. $r =$ Pearson's correlation coefficient between pleasantness and intensity estimates across data points differing significantly in intensity from control (c). Lines fitted to data points by visual inspection. (From Doty, 1975.)

responses (e.g., Green *et al.*, 1996; Neely *et al.*, 1992; Figure 2.10). In general, investigators need to examine the distribution of responses on a rating scale. If it is normally distributed, then we can usually assume there is no meaningful clustering or other problem.

Another means for overcoming non-linearities in scaling is cross-modal matching, the most popular of which is termed "magnitude estimation" (Marks, 1988). Unlike rating scales, ratio relationships among the intensities of the different stimuli are defined, and responses are not confined to a few categories or a short response line. In the most common magnitude estimation procedure, numbers are assigned in proportion to the perceived

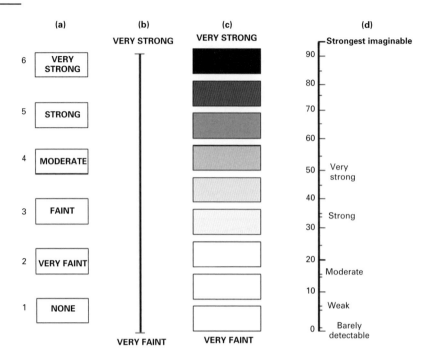

Figure 2.10 Examples of four types of rating scales. From left to right: (a) A standard category scale in which the subject provides answers in discrete categories; (b) a visual analog or graphic scale with anchors (descriptors) at each end; (c) a category scale with logarithmic visual density referents to denote non-linear increasing magnitudes of sensation, with verbal anchors at each end; (d) a labeled magnitude scale with labels or anchors positioned in logarithmic fashion. In these examples the scales are oriented in a vertical position; in many cases, such scales are presented in a horizontal (left–right) configuration. (Copyright © 2002, Richard L. Doty.)

intensity of a set of odors differing in concentration (Stevens & Marks, 1980). For example, if the number 10 is assigned to the perceived intensity of one concentration of an odorant, a concentration that smells ten times as intense would be assigned the number 100. If another concentration is perceived to be half as strong as the initial one, it would be assigned the value 5, and so on. In some cases, a standard for which a number has been pre-assigned (often the middle stimulus of the series) is initially provided to the subject in an effort to make his or her responses more reliable. In other cases, the individual can choose any desired number system, as long as the numbers are made proportional to the magnitude of the attribute (the "free modulus method"). The important point is that the absolute values of the numbers are not important, only the ratios between them.

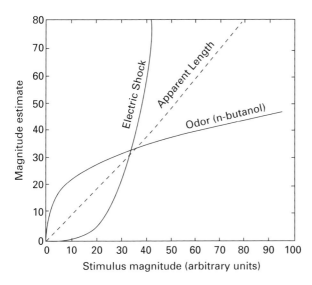

Figure 2.11 Relationship between perceived magnitude of three types of stimuli, as measured by magnitude estimation and stimulus magnitude. Note that the perceived intensity of the example odorant increases in a negatively accelerated fashion, indicating a power function exponent less than 1 (in this case, 0.33). (From Doty and Laing, 2003. With permission.)

The primary measure of sensory function determined by magnitude estimation is the degree of build-up of sensation relative to increases in odorant concentration. Magnitude estimation data are typically plotted on log–log coordinates (log magnitude estimates on the ordinate and log odorant concentrations on the abscissa) and the best line of fit determined using linear regression. The resulting function, $\log P = n \log \Phi + \log k$, where P = perceived intensity, k = the Y intercept, Φ = stimulus concentration, and n = the slope, can be represented in its exponential form as a power function, $P = k\Phi^n$. The exponent, n, is the slope of the function on the log–log plot and serves as the index of sensory function. The larger the value of n, the greater the increase in perceived intensity as concentration is increased. This value varies in magnitude from odorant to odorant, but is generally less than 1, reflecting a negatively accelerated function on linear–linear coordinates (Figure 2.11).

Like other types of scaling, magnitude estimation is not immune to bias from procedural or subject factors (Marks, 1974). For example, a moderately intense odor is reported to be more intense when presented with weak comparison stimuli than with strong comparison stimuli (Eyman et al., 1975; Helson, 1964). The estimation task is relatively complex, in that accurate responses to a stimulus require a good memory for the prior stimulus. If too much time lapses between the presentations of the stimuli, the memory of the prior stimulus fades. On the other hand, if the trials are spaced too closely together, adaptation can distort the relationship. Not all subjects consistently provide ratio estimates of stimuli, and a number do not understand the concept of producing ratios (Baird *et al.*, 1970; Moskowitz, 1977). Comparative assessments of nine-point rating scales, line scales, magnitude estimation scales, and a hybrid of category and line scales suggest that, for untrained or mathematically unsophisticated subjects, category scales and line scales are often superior when such factors as variability, reliability, and ease of use are considered (Lawless & Malone, 1986a, b).

In conclusion, there is a wide variety of psychophysical olfactory tests available for quantifying olfactory dysfunction. However, many are applicable only in the research setting. From a clinical perspective, the choice of test depends on the nature of the disease, the time available for testing, the degree to which high sensitivity and specificity of testing is needed, and the ability of the subject to cooperate. For rapid screening in a neurological or ENT clinic, relatively brief identification tests containing 3–16 items can be useful, although such screening needs to be followed up with more complete testing if abnormal results are found. For research purposes, longer tests are desirable. Although psychophysical testing is reliable early in cognitive disorders such as Alzheimer's disease, such evaluation is questionable where moderate or advanced dementia precludes an understanding of the test requirements. In such cases, non-olfactory tests such as the PIT (Vollmecke & Doty, 1985) should be employed to assess whether patients are capable of being adequately evaluated by a given test procedure or, in experimental paradigms, as covariates to minimize or control for the influences of cognitive state on test performance.

Electrophysiological tests

The electro-olfactogram

As mentioned earlier in this chapter, when an odorant activates the receptor cells, a negative potential, followed by a rebound potential, is generated and this can be measured using electrodes placed on or near the surface of the epithelium. The magnitude of this generator potential, termed the "electro-olfactogram" (EOG), varies with stimulus concentration (Figure 2.12) and shows little evidence of adaptation, supporting the notion that adaptation is largely a central phenomenon (Zwaardemaker, 1927).

Since the EOG can be measured for some time after death or following pharmacological blocking of axonal transmission of the olfactory receptors, results from EOG recordings must be interpreted with caution (Scott & Scott-Johnson, 2002). Given that there can be considerable heterogeneity of damage

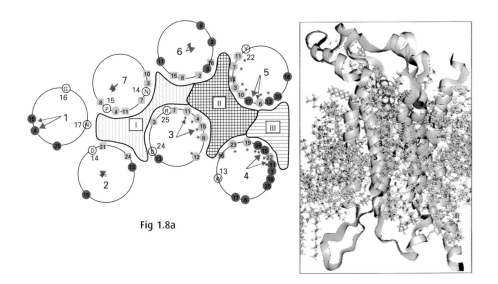

Fig 1.8a

Fig 1.8b

(a)

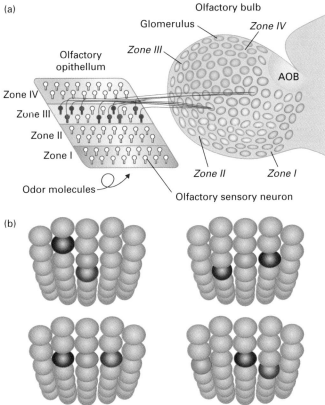

Olfactory bulb

Glomerulus

Zone IV

Zone III

AOB

Olfactory
opithellum

Zone IV

Zone III

Zone II

Zone I

Odor molecules

Olfactory sensory neuron

Zone III

Zone II

Zone I

(b)

Fig 1.9

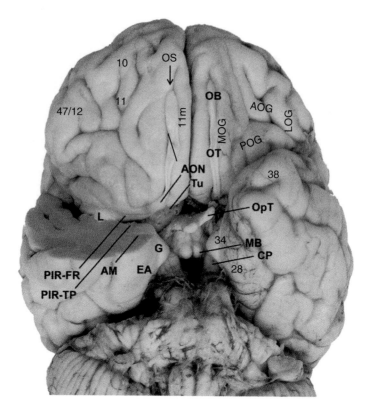

Fig 1.11

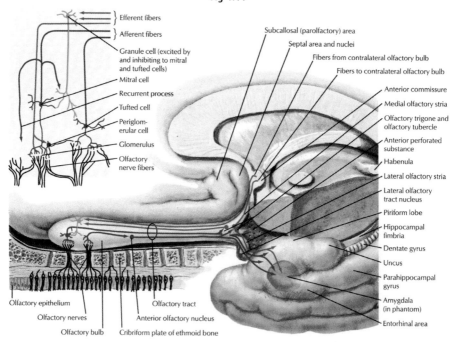

Efferent fibers

Afferent fibers

Granule cell (excited by and inhibiting to mitral and tufted cells)

Mitral cell

Recurrent process

Tufted cell

Periglomerular cell

Glomerulus

Olfactory nerve fibers

Olfactory epithelium

Olfactory nerves

Olfactory bulb

Olfactory tract

Anterior olfactory nucleus

Cribriform plate of ethmoid bone

Subcallosal (parolfactory) area

Septal area and nuclei

Fibers from contralateral olfactory bulb

Fibers to contralateral olfactory bulb

Anterior commissure

Medial olfactory stria

Olfactory trigone and olfactory tubercle

Anterior perforated substance

Habenula

Lateral olfactory stria

Lateral olfactory tract nucleus

Piriform lobe

Hippocampal fimbria

Dentate gyrus

Uncus

Parahippocampal gyrus

Amygdala (in phantom)

Entorhinal area

Fig 1.15

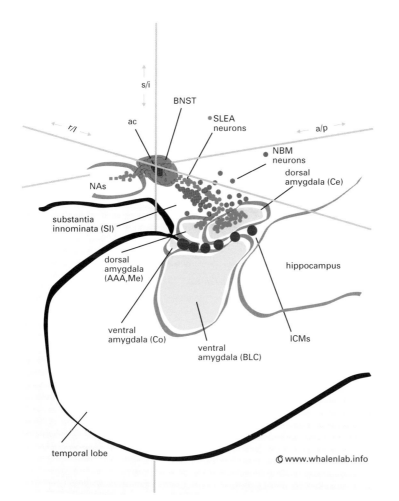

Fig 1.16

© www.whalenlab.info

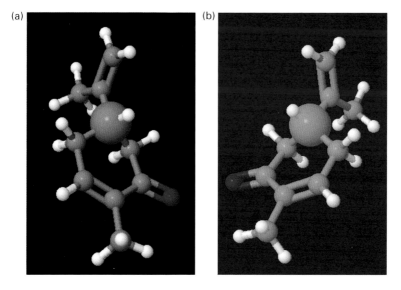

(a) (b)

Fig 1.18

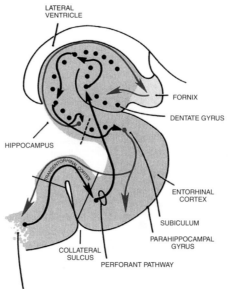

Fig 1.20

LATERAL
VENTRICLE

FORNIX

DENTATE GYRUS

HIPPOCAMPUS

TRANSENTORHINAL CORTEX

ENTORHINAL
CORTEX

SUBICULUM

PARAHIPPOCAMPAL
GYRUS

COLLATERAL
SULCUS

PERFORANT PATHWAY

TEMPORAL NEOCORTEX

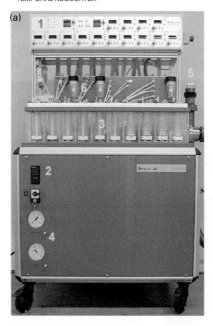

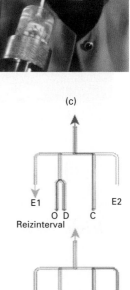

(a)

(b)

(c)

E1   E2

O D   C
Reizinterval

E1   E2

O D   C
Reiz

Key:
1. Temperature controller
2. Warming chamber for odor
   and humidification
3. Pressure and vacuum control
4. Switching device
5. Main exhaust

Fig 2.13

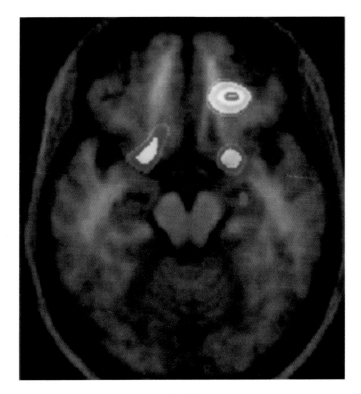

Fig 2.20

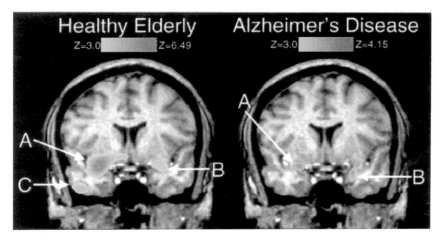

Fig 2.21

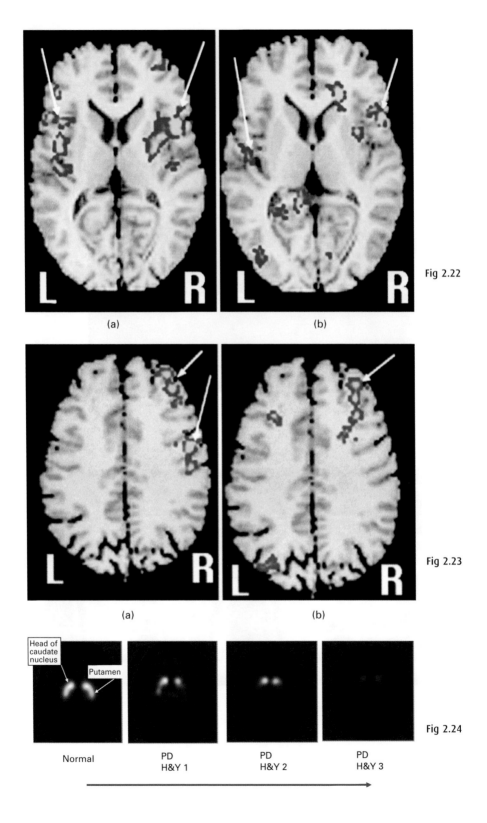

Fig 2.22

(a)   (b)

Fig 2.23

(a)   (b)

Fig 2.24

Head of caudate nucleus

Putamen

Normal   PD   PD   PD
                H&Y 1   H&Y 2   H&Y 3

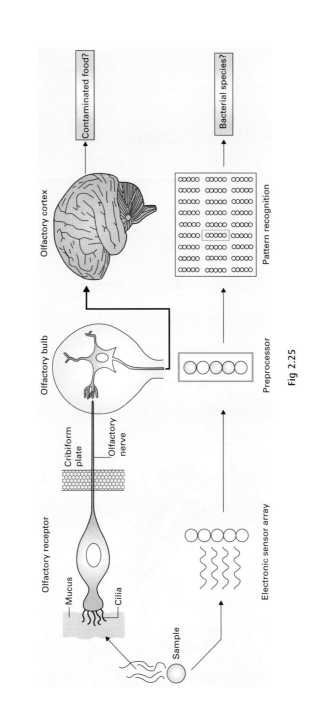

Olfactory receptor

Mucus

Cilia

Olfactory bulb

Cribiform plate

Olfactory nerve

Olfactory cortex

Contaminated food?

Sample

Electronic sensor array

Preprocessor

Pattern recognition

Bacterial species?

Fig 2.25

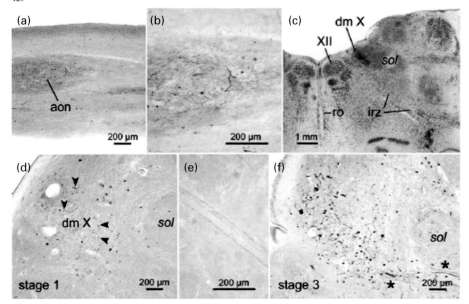

Fig 4.3

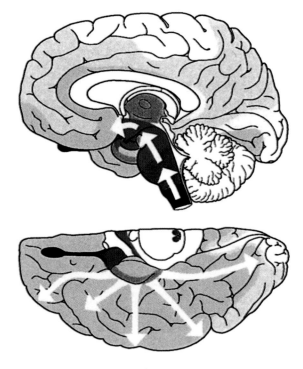

Fig 4.4

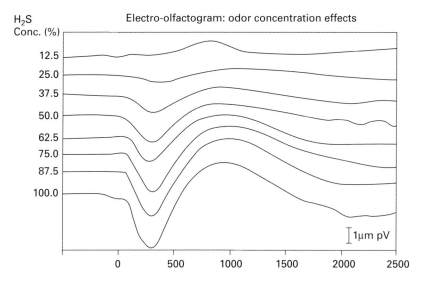

Figure 2.12 Examples of the electro-olfactogram (EOG), a summated potential measured from the surface of the olfactory epithelium. The size of the EOG is proportional to the concentration of the stimulus, in this case H_2S. (Photo courtesy of Dr. Bruce Turetsky, University of Pennsylvania.)

within the olfactory epithelium, an abnormal EOG response can reflect sampling issues rather than the lack of functioning olfactory tissue. EOGs have received only scant application in the clinic, in part because a significant number of patients cannot tolerate electrodes positioned in their unanesthetized noses. Electrodes can be placed only on limited regions of the epithelium, and maintaining reliable EOG responses over even brief periods of time can be tedious. Recently, investigators at Cardiff University, UK, have shown that *surface electrodes* located at the top of the nose can reliably measure potentials that correspond to the EOG (Wang *et al.*, 2004). Although such potentials correlate positively with the EOG, their amplitudes are markedly attenuated relative to EOG measurements from intranasal electrodes.

Olfactory event-related and evoked potentials

Event-related potentials (ERPs) are changes induced in electrical fields generated by large populations of neurons during or after a sensory or internal psychological event (Gevins & Remond, 1987). *Evoked potentials* (EPs) reflect those aggregate stimulus-induced neural events that occur during the earliest stages of sensory processing. In contrast to ERPs, they are little influenced by non-sensory mental events (e.g., attention, ideation). Olfactory event-related olfactory potentials (OERPs), which arise from cortical structures and are considered "late near-field event-related potentials," can be measured reliably

(a)

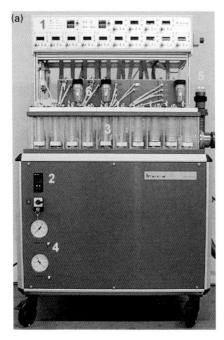

(b)

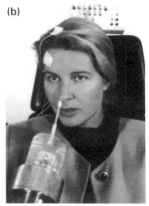

(c)

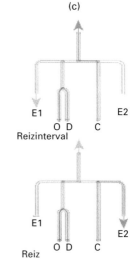

Key:

1. Temperature controller
2. Warming chamber for odor and humidification
3. Pressure and vacuum control
4. Switching device
5. Main exhaust

Figure 2.13 (See also Figure 2.13 in the color plate section, p. 82–3.) (a) a commercially available six-odor olfactometer (Burghart OM6b). (b) Recording setup showing a thin piece of Teflon tubing inserted about 1 cm into the nose. (c) Technique of creating an odorant bolus without disturbing the main airflow. The main odorless airstream, (C, in blue) is continually blown into the nose in resting conditions (Reizinterval). The odor-containing air (O, in red) is sucked away by vacuum E1. To achieve an olfactory stimulus the odorless airstream C is vented away by vacuum E2 while E1 is closed simultaneously. This allows the odor-containing gas to reach the nose imperceptibly, without disturbing the main inflow and therefore avoiding trigeminal stimulation (Reiz). (Reproduced with permission from H. Burghart Medizintechnik, Hamburg, Germany.)

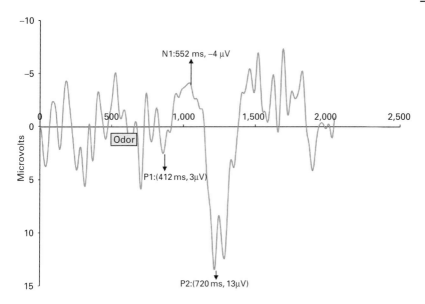

Figure 2.14 Normal olfactory event-related potential evoked by a 200 ms pulse of H2S (2 ppm) shown as gray bar. Trace is derived from A1 – Pz. Filters are set at 1–50 Hz. (Copyright © 2007, Christopher H. Hawkes.)

from the surface of the scalp and have been used clinically (for review, see Kobal, 2003).

To overcome the difficulty of detecting a very weak signal ($<50\ \mu V$) embedded in a melody of seemingly random background signals, multiple stimulus trials must be averaged to cancel out the background activity. To enhance the synchronous onset of a large population of olfactory receptor cells and optimize the stimulus signal, elaborate olfactometers have been developed that introduce pulses of odorants into the nose with rapid rise times (<100 ms; Figure 2.13) and if properly calibrated, no trigeminal co-stimulation. Using such devices, multiple presentations of well-defined stimulus pulses can be made, although only at 30-s intervals or longer, since briefer presentations can induce confounding from adaptation. Mass–flow controllers determine the airflow rates and a computer initiates the stimulus pulse. Some odors, even in low concentration, may induce trigeminal ERPs that confound the OERP, thus care must be taken to select odors and odor concentrations with minimal trigeminal involvement (Geisler & Murphy, 2000).

An example of an OERP is shown in Figure 2.14. The first positive peak, P1, occurs at latencies >250 ms, which is considerably longer than the latencies observed for auditory and visual evoked potentials. Chemical stimulation is delayed by 100–200 ms at the receptor site, reflecting absorption and other physiochemical phenomena within the mucosa. When this time is subtracted from the overall latencies, N1 and P2 latencies become comparable to the N100 and P200/P300 latencies seen in other sensory systems. Although the perceived intensity of the stimulus increases as the duration of the stimulus increases, at least across 100 ms to 700 ms durations, the form of the OERP stays the same, i.e., amplitudes and latencies to the peaks do not change (Kobal, 1981). This reflects, in part, the fact that the ERP largely indicates stimulus onset. Nevertheless, latency decreases and the amplitude increases when stronger stimuli are presented (Covington *et al.*, 1999; Pause *et al.*, 1997). The earlier components of the OERP (e.g., N1) are related to perceptions less dependent upon central modulation (e.g., intensity and quality), whereas the later components (e.g., P2) are more reflective of processes associated with the meaning of the stimulus (Donchin & Coles, 1988).

The amplitude of the OERP is positively correlated with the number of activated neurons and, hence, with such factors as stimulus airflow and the perceived intensity of the stimulus (Tateyama *et al.*, 1998). OERP latencies, but not amplitudes, correlate moderately with olfactory threshold measures. For example, correlations ranging from −0.45 to −0.58 between n-butanol thresholds and peak latencies induced by vanillin for P1, N1, P2, and P3 components measured at the Cz scalp position have been reported (Tateyama *et al.*, 1998). The late positive OERP amplitudes and latencies also correlate weakly with scores on neuropsychological tests of visual-motor attention (Trail Making Test) and verbal memory (Geisler *et al.*, 1999). To date, attempts to relate odorant qualities to differences in the shape of olfactory ERPs have not been successful (e.g., Kobal & Hummel, 1988). Although some odor-related differences in topography of the pattern of potentials across the surface of the scalp have been observed, such alterations are not well defined and likely reflect, in addition to odor quality, such properties as odor intensity, pleasantness, saliency, and emotional significance (Kobal, 2003).

It is uncertain whether OERPs add significantly to basic psychophysical clinical assessment. Even the best commercially available olfactometers are unstable and need daily attention and recalibration, although there is no doubt that with effort an olfactory potential can be derived. The OERP is of theoretical value in assessment of malingerers, assuming a real cheat can be persuaded to cooperate. However, even those with genuine anosmia or hyposmia may become upset with the procedure and this can affect recording quality and interpretation.

Like psychophysical measures, changes in OERP amplitudes or latencies are sensitive to airway obstruction or neural damage anywhere from the olfactory epithelium to the cortex. This reduces the value of OERP, although recordings of the EOG can be made at the same time in some patients from either intranasal electrodes or surface electrodes placed at the base of the nose

(Wang *et al.*, 2004). Abnormal late OERP components, and normal early OERP components, might theoretically signify a central problem, although clinical examples of such differentiation are not available.

Nasal airway patency and airflow measurement

Subtle differences in the internal anatomy of the human nose can influence smell function, presumably by directing more airflow toward the olfactory epithelium (Frye, 1995; Hornung, 2006). In a classical study, Leopold (1988) obtained computed tomography (CT) scans from 34 patients with conductive or idiopathic hyposmia. The volume of nine three-dimensional sections of the nasal cavity above the middle turbinate was defined and entered into a stepwise regression analysis to see which volumes were most strongly related to odor identification ability. A larger volume in the nasal region 10–15 mm below the cribriform plate and a smaller volume 1–5 mm below and anterior to the cribriform plate were associated with higher odor identification test scores. A larger volume in the region 10–15 mm below and posterior to the cribriform plate potentiated both effects.

Unfortunately, the translation of such observations to specific clinical cases is difficult, and it is not clear if such measures correlate with more practical clinical measures of nasal anatomy and function, such as acoustic rhinometry and rhinomanometry, respectively (see below). Many patients do report "nasal stuffiness" related to smell loss that is associated with measures of nasal congestion secondary, for example, to abnormal engorgement of the nasal turbinates (see Chapter 1). It should be pointed out, however, that a patient's perception of nasal blockage need not be congruous with actual airway blockage, given that nerve fibers which mediate sensations of airflow can be damaged (Eccles *et al.*, 1990). Also, subtle inflammation within the nasal mucosa can influence olfactory function adversely even in the presence of a normally patent and functioning airway (Kern, 2000).

Acoustic rhinometry

Acoustic rhinometry assesses elements of nasal anatomy (Figure 2.15). In this procedure, sound waves in the form of a series of clicks are projected into each nasal chamber and their reflections, picked up by a microphone, are analyzed to assess dimensional elements of the nasal cavity. This procedure is analogous to sonar, which is used to identify the distance of objects under water. Volumetric assessment using this procedure takes only a few minutes, and requires minimal cooperation on the part of the patient. An example of an acoustic rhinometry waveform is shown in Figure 2.16. As shown, the cross-sectional area of the cavity is smallest in the region of the nasal valve, and largest in the more posterior regions of the cavity.

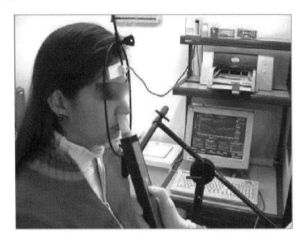

Figure 2.15 Picture of a computerized acoustic rhinometer system. The long vertical tube is attached to one nostril. The sound waves sent into the nose via this tube are reflected back into the same tube and analyzed by computer. (Figure reproduced with permission from the Scientific Electronic Library Online (Scielo) Brazil.)

Acoustic rhinometry is widely used, in part because of its simplicity. Its usefulness in regard to assessing olfaction has not been explored fully. Nasal volumes do not appear to correlate meaningfully with olfactory thresholds in normal subjects (Nordin *et al.*, 1998) or in patients responding to an acute nasal allergen (Lane *et al.*, 1996), although general associations have been reported when severe congestion is present (Akerlund *et al.*, 1995). When obstructions are located in the anterior nose, the accuracy of this procedure in quantifying more posterior cross-sectional areas and volumes is diminished.

Rhinomanometry

Rhinomanometry assesses flow and pressure changes during breathing. In *anterior rhinomanometry*, one nostril is occluded with an adhesive patch that is connected to a small tube to measure pressure changes during inhalation and exhalation. Airflow through the opposite nasal chamber is simultaneously measured using a pneumotachometer (Figure 2.17). Resistance is calculated from a flow/pressure plot (Figure 2.18). In *posterior rhinomanometry*, the pressure-sensing tubing is placed via the mouth near the nasopharynx. A facemask connected to a pneumotachometer is then employed to measure airflow through both nostrils and the total nasal resistance is calculated from the flow/pressure plot. Anterior rhinomanometry is more widely used than the posterior type since some individuals do not tolerate the tube near the nasopharynx, some training is involved, and the pressure tube

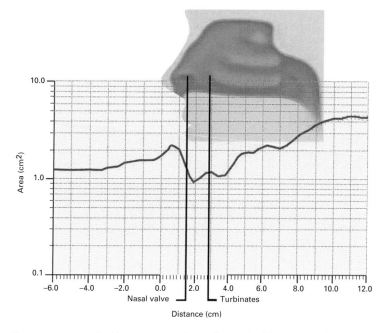

Figure 2.16 Acoustic rhinometry waveforms from a healthy patient. The first dip in the curve represents the position of the nasal valve approximately 2.4 cm from front of the naris and the second peak is the anterior part of the inferior turbinate. (Figure reproduced with permission from the Scientific Electronic Library Online (Scielo) Brazil.)

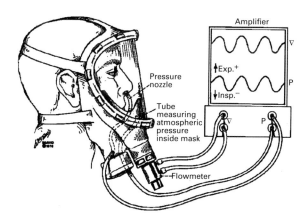

Figure 2.17 Anterior rhinomanometry with mask flow measurement. Transnasal pressure is measured by a pressure catheter occluding one nostril. Airflow is measured by a pneumotachograph attached to a mask placed over the face. (From McCaffrey, 1991.)

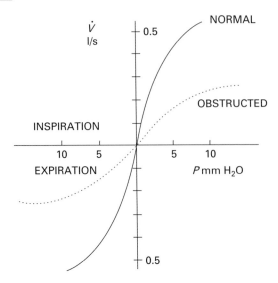

Figure 2.18 Pressure flow curve using rhinomanometry. Since nasal airflow is turbulent, the relationship between pressure and flow as shown by the "S"-shaped line in this figure is curvilinear. Since there is not a unique value for $R = P/V$, resistance must be determined at a specific pressure or flow point. The nasal resistance is shown at a pressure of 2 cm H_2O (200 Pa). (From McCaffrey, 1991.)

can easily become clogged with saliva. Also, unlike anterior rhinomanometry, resistance in each nasal chamber is not assessed.

Whilst rhinomanometry provides an indication of nasal resistance within the lower regions of the nasal cavity, it is not clear whether this measure is meaningfully associated with olfactory function in most patients. To our knowledge, significant correlations between olfactory and nasal resistance measures have not been demonstrated. Nonetheless, septoplasty with partial inferior turbinectomy has been reported to enhance both olfactory function and nasal patency (Damm *et al.*, 2003).

Structural imaging

Computerized axial tomography
Computerized axial tomography (CAT; also known as computed tomography or CT), reconstructs images from X-rays passed through the body from multiple angles. In effect, CT triangulates every point in a plane from many different directions, allowing for computer reconstruction of an image. CT is excellent at evaluating sinonasal tract inflammatory disorders, since it is sensitive to soft tissue inflammatory responses and bony changes. Such

imaging is indicated if nasal obstruction is suspected owing to anatomical deformity, polyps, or tumors, or if an intranasal mass is present for which extension into the cranium is possible. The CT of someone complaining of smell loss should assess all of the nasal cavity, paranasal sinuses, hard palate, anterior skull base, orbits, and nasopharynx in both axial and coronal planes. Coronal scans are essential to visualize appropriately the anterior naso-ethmoid (osteomeatal) region, but demonstration of the olfactory bulb and tract requires magnetic resonance imaging (MRI).

Magnetic resonance imaging

Like CT, MRI produces cross-sectional images in many planes and is visually equivalent to a slice of anatomy. In T1-weighted images of the brain, fiber tracts appear as high intensity (white), congregations of neurons as inter-mediate density (gray), and cerebrospinal fluid as low intensity (black). In T2- and T2*-weighted images, cerebrospinal fluid is high intensity (white), fiber tracts low (black), and congregations of neurons intermediate (gray).

The resolution of MRI is generally superior to CT, and it is usually more effective at detecting inflammation. It cannot be used in patients with pacemakers, intracranial metallic clips, or other potentially mobile metal objects in their bodies. However, it is the method of choice when central nervous system (CNS) lesions are suspected, and has the distinct advantage of not subjecting the patient to ionizing radiation. It is also the method of choice for visualizing directly the olfactory bulbs and tracts, skull base (particularly for invasion by tumor), and brain inflammatory lesions asso-ciated with smell impairment such as multiple sclerosis or encephalitis. Injection of gadolinium-DTPA, a paramagnetic contrast agent, is particularly useful at the skull base to detect dural or leptomeningeal involvement, as well as differentiating enhancing sino-nasal mucosa from secretions and distinguishing solidly enhancing tumors from rim-enhancing inflammatory processes.

Most patients presenting with olfactory loss do not require structural imaging. In general, brain tumors are rarely the basis of smell loss unaccompanied by other clinical signs. Smell distortions, hallucinations, or other features suggestive of complex partial seizures are perhaps more frequent and require MRI to detect neoplasia or vascular lesions. Those with a history of anosmia secondary to head injury need careful evaluation. Gradient echo (T2 or T2*) MRI sequences are sensitive to hemosiderin deposits, the tell-tale sign of petechial hemorrhages that might otherwise be overlooked by con-ventional sequences. Such lesions are common in the temporal and frontal polar zones in head trauma victims, and defects in either region may result in central olfactory dysfunction – a point of medicolegal significance as described in Chapter 3. With an adequate number of slices through the anterior cranial fossa, MRI provides reasonably clear images of the olfactory bulb and

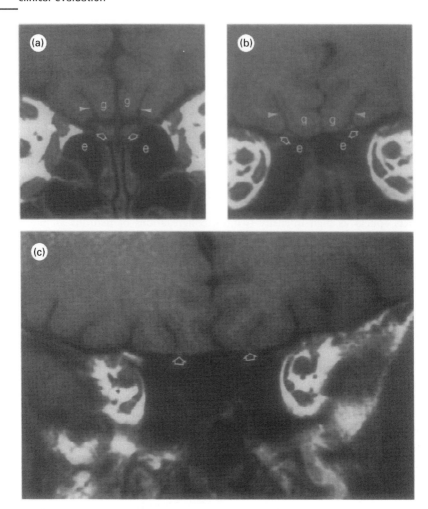

Figure 2.19 MRI of normal olfactory bulbs and tracts. (a) The olfactory bulbs (open arrows), olfactory sulci (arrowheads), and gyri recti (g) are well seen on coronal T1-weighted surface coil images (e, ethmoid sinuses). (b) At a more posterior cut, the open arrows now show the olfactory tracts sitting in the olfactory sulci (arrowheads). (c) Even more posteriorly, normal small tracts (arrows) are seen in the sulci. (Reproduced with permission from Yousem *et al.*, 2001.)

tracts sufficient to detect agenesis or Kallmann syndrome (Figure 2.19 and Chapter 3, Figure 3.1). With sequential imaging, regression of the bulbs and tracts induced by damage from head trauma or viral infection can be demonstrated.

Functional imaging

Unlike traditional lesioning or recording procedures usually performed only in animals, functional imaging requires no anesthesia, does not damage brain cells, and is relatively non-invasive (Sobel *et al.*, 2003). A considerable amount of new information about the olfactory system has accrued using such procedures. For example, we now know that sectors of the cerebellum, parietal lobe, occipital lobe, and the inferior and superior temporal gyri are involved to some degree in higher-order odor processing. However, functional imaging has been used very little in clinical assessment of olfactory disturbances, largely because of practicality, cost, and the fact that most olfactory disturbances are easily detected and quantified through less expensive means. Although functional imaging has tremendous research potential, its clinical potential in regards to olfaction has yet to be realized.

Positron emission tomography

Positron emission tomography (PET) indirectly measures brain function. Specific tracers are chosen to illustrate particular brain functions of interest. For example, ^{18}F-2-deoxyglucose (^{18}FDG) is used to investigate cerebral glucose metabolism, whereas $H_2^{15}O$ is used to examine cerebral blood flow. In this procedure, specific biological compounds tagged with a positron-emitting radioisotope (e.g., ^{15}O, ^{18}F, or ^{11}C) are injected into the bloodstream while the patient is relatively quiescent. As the unstable tracer decays, it emits positrons that are annihilated by negatively charged electrons within the tissue. This results in the emission of two photons per tracer molecule in exactly opposite directions from the point of annihilation. An array of radiation detectors located around the head, coupled via coincidence circuits, localizes the brain regions emitting the photons, with representation proportional to the amount of blood flow. Since the half-life of most tracers is relatively short (e.g., in the case of ^{15}O, ~2 minutes), the patient's brain can be scanned repeatedly in a single session with relatively minimal radiation exposure.

While PET displays brain regions activated by stimulants or function of specific neurotransmitter systems, injection of radioactive tracers is nonetheless invasive and such scanning requires complex and expensive equipment, including a cyclotron to produce the isotopes (Sobel *et al.*, 2003). With longer-life isotopes such as ^{18}F the cyclotron does not need to be onsite as in the case of ^{15}O. Relative to the neural events, which occur in milliseconds, PET requires the integration of signals over tens of seconds. Furthermore, images with no greater than ~3 mm^3 of spatial resolution are obtained under the best of circumstances. PET is time-consuming, particularly since MRI

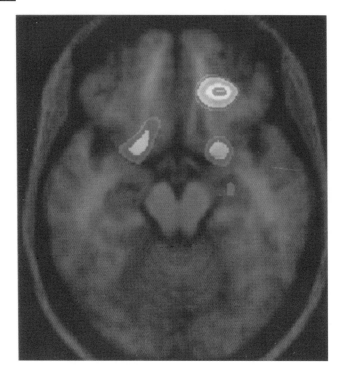

Figure 2.20 (See also Figure 2.20 in the color plate section, p. 82–3.) PET scan showing odorant-induced activation as indicated by areas of increased blood flow. The activation is seen bilaterally (blue) in the piriform cortex and unilaterally in the right orbitofrontal cortex (OFC; red, yellow, and blue). This led to the proposal that the right OFC is dominant for high-level olfactory processing, a concept that is now thought to be only partially correct. (Reprinted with permission from Zatorre *et al.*, 1992.)

scans are often required to provide a template for localization of activated brain structures, although it is possible to perform simultaneous PET–CT imaging. PET has some advantages over functional magnetic resonance imaging (fMRI), described in the next section, including the ability to visualize structures at the skull base. It has the unique advantage of providing *in vivo* measurement of specific brain function, such as dopamine storage capacity within the presynaptic dopaminergic terminals or dopamine receptor availability.

An example of a PET scan in which the orbitofrontal cortex and piriform cortices are activated is shown in Figure 2.20. Figure 2.21 shows PET scan abnormalities in response to phenyl ethyl alcohol in Alzheimer's disease compared with healthy controls (Karaken *et al.*, 2001).

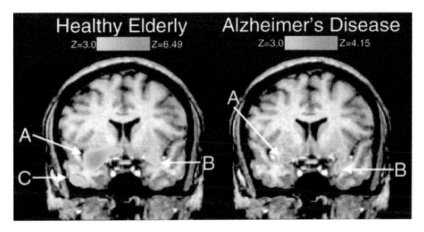

Figure 2.21 (See also Figure 2.21 in the color plate section, p. 82–3.) PET imaging of blood flow in Alzheimer's disease. *Left image*: Controls. A, Right frontotemporal junction (piriform area); B, Left piriform area; C, Right anterior ventral temporal lobe (Brodmann area 20). Number of controls: 7; mean UPSIT = 32.4; mean threshold to phenyl ethyl alcohol, –5.5 log vol/vol in light mineral oil. *Right image*: Alzheimer's disease. A, 7 mm anterior to frontotemporal junction; B, left amygdala-uncus. Number of patients: 6. Mean UPSIT = 18.7 (severe microsmia); mean threshold to phenyl ethyl alcohol = –5.1 log vol/vol in light mineral oil (normal). (From Kareken *et al.*, 2001. Copyright © 2001 by the American Psychological Association. Reproduced with permission.)

Functional magnetic resonance imaging

Functional MRI is the most widely employed functional imaging procedure. Brain oxygen level-dependent (BOLD) fMRI, the most popular of the fMRI procedures, capitalizes on the fact that local changes in neural activity produce neighboring changes in the amount of oxygen carried in hemoglobin (i.e., in the ratio of oxyhemoglobin to deoxyhemoglobin) – changes that disturb the magnetic field. Thus, T2 relaxation times differ relative to the amount of deoxyhemoglobin in the blood, generating signals that indirectly reflect the amount of neural activity within the more activated brain regions. Other fMRI methodologies increase the signal:noise ratio in the target regions by use of contrast agents.

Unlike PET, fMRI is non-invasive, requiring no injection of radioactive materials into the circulatory system. fMRI can be performed in most hospital or medical center settings where MRI machines are available, in contrast to PET imaging, whose isotopes must be generated by cyclotrons available only in large research centers. Since MRI provides accurate identification of brain structures, there is no need for additional scanning to map activity to identifiable brain regions, as is the case with PET. Relative to PET, fMRI has the further advantage of high spatial and temporal resolution. Where bone and

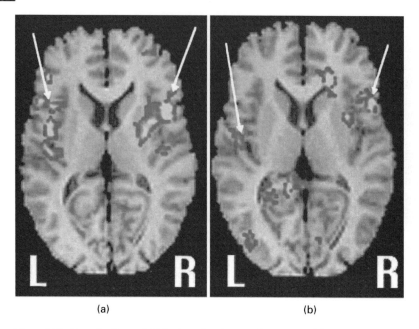

(a)   (b)

Figure 2.22 (See also Figure 2.22 in the color plate section, p. 82–3.) fMRI activation within the peri-insular regions of the brain (arrows) induced by the odorants eugenol and phenyl ethyl alcohol, alternating with hydrogen sulfide. Pictures represent group-averaged data. Note that both peri-insular regions of women (a) show a large number of activated voxels in the group-averaged map which are larger than the number of activated voxels of the men (b). (From Yousem *et al.*, 1999. Copyright © 1999. Reproduced with permission from Elsevier.)

brain are adjacent, as they are at the skull base, there is a tendency for so-called susceptibility artifacts, which can limit image clarity. This problem applies particularly to the olfactory bulbs and tracts, but with a special head coil placed over the nasion reasonable images may be obtained (see Figure 2.19). Figure 2.22 presents an fMRI scan showing functional activation of the perisylvian regions by odorants in eight right-handed women (a) and eight right-handed men (b)(respective mean ages = 25.3 and 30.4 years). A similar fMRI scan showing right frontal lobe activation in the same subjects is shown in Figure 2.23.

Early investigators experienced considerable difficulties in obtaining reliable images of the major olfactory components, notably the piriform cortex (PC) (e.g., Yousem *et al.*, 1997; Zald & Pardo, 1997). This arose because the most widely employed analysis paradigm, where odorants are presented in relatively lengthy blocks (block designs), assumed that the signal was maintained during the entire period of odorant stimulation. Subsequent work

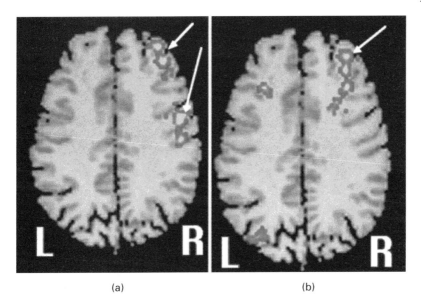

(a)   (b)

Figure 2.23 (See also Figure 2.23 in the color plate section, p. 82–3.) fMRI activation of the frontal lobes (arrows) the odorants eugenol and phenyl ethyl alcohol, alternating with hydrogen sulfide. Note that both women (a) and men (b) evidence greater activation in the right than in the left lobes. Overall, women showed more than a fourfold greater number of activated voxels on the right. (From Yousem *et al.,* 1999. Copyright © 1999. Reproduced with permission from Elsevier.)

showed this was not the case, and that the odorant signal rapidly habituated (Sobel *et al.,* 2000). Thus, robust activation is seen only when data are either analyzed for only a brief initial segment of the odorant "ON" period or when the underlying habituation is modeled using an exponentially decaying reference waveform (Tabert *et al.,* 2007)

Single photon emission computed tomography

Single photon emission computed tomography (SPECT) is an imaging procedure similar to PET; it is a technically simpler imaging method and uses radioactive tracers that do not require an onsite cyclotron. Hence, SPECT images are less expensive. SPECT utilizes radionuclides that emit a single photon with lower energy (about 140 keV) than those employed in PET. A large sheet of perforated lead, known as a "collimator," allows the radiation to be controlled so that only those photons parallel to the holes can pass through to the crystal to be recorded as an event. The spatial resolution of SPECT is three or four times less than PET, the tracers need to have much longer half-lives, and in many instances long image acquisition periods are required depending on the

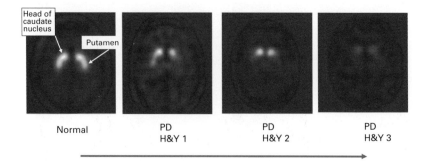

Figure 2.24 (See also Figure 2.24 in the color plate section, p. 82–3.) DATScan using a dopamine transporter ligand (FP-CIT). This displays the level of presynaptic dopamine transporter, which is highest in the caudate and putamen. The left figure is from a healthy control subject and shows the "full-stop" sign from the head of the caudate nucleus and the "comma" sign from the putamen. The scans to the right show progressive reduction of tracer uptake, which usually commences in the putamen. PD, Parkinson's disease; H&Y, Hoehn and Yahr disability stage.

type of tracer and the resolution required. SPECT has been shown to be of value in assessing cortical responses to odor (Di Nardo *et al.*, 2000). It also detects striatal dopaminergic deficiency using a labeled presynaptic dopamine transporter ligand. Dopamine transporter imaging SPECT using [^{18}F] FP-CIT (Figure 2.24) or [^{99m}Tc]TRODAT-1 has now become a major cost-effective investigation for many extrapyramidal disorders.

Other

Ciliary motility tests
The nose, paranasal sinuses, and tracheobronchial tree are lined with ciliated columnar epithelial cells. The cilia of these cells are essential for the movement of the mucous blanket, which serves a critical host defense mechanism, trapping and removing particulate matter, bacteria, and other exogenous agents from the region. The top layer of this blanket, termed the "gel layer," is derived from mucous glands and goblet cells, whereas the bottom layer, the "sol layer," is made up of a water transudate that emanates from the underlying fenestrated capillaries. The function of the cilia, which move rapidly forward and slowly backward at a beat rate of ~10 Hz, can be slowed by rhinosinusitis, dehydration, and a wide range of drugs and irritants, including constituents of tobacco smoke, sulfur dioxide, nitrogen dioxide, various local anesthetics, neurotransmitter neuropeptide Y, beta$_2$-adrenergic agents, and the preservative benzalkonium chloride (Doty *et al.*, 2004).

A practical, albeit somewhat variable, clinical means to assess the effectiveness of mucociliary transport within the nose is to measure saccharin transport time. A small amount of saccharin is placed on the inferior turbinate, approximately 0.5 cm past its most anterior portion, and the time required for the patient to taste the sweetness or bitterness of the saccharin is measured. Healthy subjects typically have a transport time less than 15 minutes, while patients with chronic nasal and sinus disease have delayed transport time, often longer than 20 minutes. Ciliary beat frequency can also be measured *in vivo* using other procedures, including photoelectric methods and laser light scattering. In rhinoscintigraphy a weak gamma-emitting isotope, Technetium-99m, is deposited on the floor of the nasal meatus and its transport followed by a gamma camera. Such techniques, however, require specialized equipment and are generally not practical in the clinic.

Although ciliary motility tests can provide information about the overall health of the nose, their value in assessing problems with olfactory function is unclear. One exception is those disorders associated with ciliary dysfunction, such as cystic fibrosis, which are accompanied by smell loss, presumably because of poor clearance of bacteria and other agents detrimental to the olfactory epithelium (Weiffenbach & McCarthy, 1984).

Body odor in medical diagnosis and development of the electronic nose

In this section we discuss the detection of body odors by clinicians in their diagnosis of medical disorders and the development of specialized electronic sensors, known as the electronic nose ("E-nose"), for recognizing infection-, cancer-, and other disease-related volatiles.

Instinctively, many clinicians evaluate body odor in making a diagnosis, and readily will detect the odor of ketones in the breath of a diabetes sufferer or someone malnourished. Unpleasant breath (halitosis), often caused by the odor of sulfides, is usually a feature of poor oral hygiene. Halitosis may also be secondary to bacterial or fungal colonization elsewhere, such as *Helicobacter pylori* infection of the stomach. The odor of alcohol or cigarettes is often detectable as soon as the patient begins to relate their history. This aspect of clinical examination is highlighted by Bomback (2006), who reports being able to tell whether a patient is going to need intravenous or oral antibiotics by the stench that follows removal of dressings. The odor from a tracheotomy site may indicate the need for antibiotics and those requiring colonoscopy usually have a strong fecal odor if they have taken the correct dose of GoLytely (a strong purgative). A rare, often fatal, syndrome is that of calciphylaxis, where systemic calcification of cutaneous blood vessels leads to widespread necrotic skin ulcers. This usually affects those on dialysis for

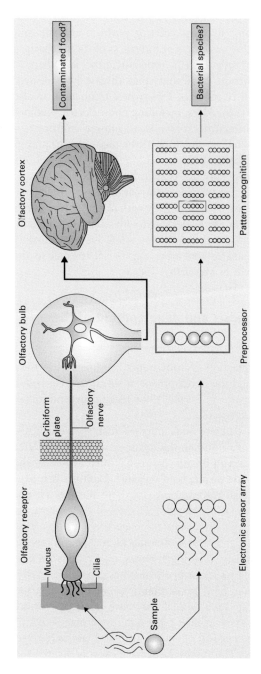

Figure 2.25 (See also Figure 2.25 in the color plate section, p. 82–3.) Comparison of the elements of the human olfactory system with those of the E-nose. Volatile odor recognition may be achieved using pattern recognition techniques. (Reproduced with permission from Macmillan Publishers Ltd: Turner and Magan, 2004 Copyright © 2004.)

chronic renal failure. The severe malodor arising from the multiple necrotic skin lesions – the stench of dead and infected tissue – is composed of cadaverine and putrescine, foul-smelling molecules produced by protein hydrolysis during putrefaction of animal tissue.

Other less well-known conditions that reportedly can be diagnosed on the basis of odors include gout, yellow fever, pellagra, scrofula, cirrhosis of the liver, uremia, typhoid, diphtheria, scurvy, rubella, and some respiratory and gastrointestinal disorders (Hayden, 1980). As summarized by Mace *et al.* (1976) and Cuestas *et al.* (2005), there are several rare metabolic disorders associated with specific odors which constitute a sizeable portion of acute life-threatening illnesses in infancy. These include phenylketonuria (horse-like), maple syrup urine disease (burnt sugar), isovaleric and butyric acidaemia (cheesy or sweaty feet), glycinuria (cat's urine), trimethylaminuria (fish-like), methionine malabsorption (malty or yeast-like), and the odor of rancid butter syndrome. In such cases, an astute physician could make a presumptive diagnosis and initiate life-saving therapy while awaiting confirmatory laboratory results (Mace *et al.*, 1976).

Preliminary evidence suggests that dogs can detect melanoma, prostate, or bladder cancer by an unusual odor on the skin or urine, respectively (Welsh, 2004; Williams & Pembroke, 1989). Comparable studies have not been performed with humans, so it is unknown whether they can be trained to perform similar tasks.

A breakthrough in the field of sensor technology came in 1982 with the first model of an electronic nose that emulated the various stages of the human olfactory system (Figure 2.25) (Persaud & Dodd, 1982). Since then, there have been multiple modifications, but most have three components; namely, a microarray sensor (such as a conducting polymer, metal-oxide, piezo-electric, optical), a pre-processor, and a pattern recognition unit using neural networks (Figure 2.25). Although still in their infancy, E-noses are now marketed that can detect disease-related vapors arising from microorganisms in human excretions and secretions. While such vapors can be identified by gas chromatography or mass spectrometry, E-noses are less expensive, less time-consuming, more portable and, in some instances, more sensitive to the detection of specific agents.

E-noses are presently capable of distinguishing *H. pylori*, *Escherichia coli*, and *Enterococcus* species that co-exist in a mixture, by estimating the amounts of terpenes (citrus, pine), trimethylamines (fishy), and ketones (acetone) that are released (Pavlou *et al.*, 2000). The E-nose may be of value in diagnosing tuberculosis in sputum specimens (Fend *et al.*, 2006), ventilator-associated pneumonia (Hockstein *et al.*, 2005), and bacterial sinusitis (Thaler & Hanson, 2006). This technology may allow the distinction of serum from cerebrospinal fluid where there is cerebrospinal rhinorrhoea (Aronzon *et al.*, 2005) and, in future, it may allow the diagnosis of various forms of metabolic myopathy by urine analysis (K Persaud, personal communication, 2006). Compared with laboratory cultures, the E-nose provides a rapid and inexpensive diagnosis and it is likely that this technology will have considerable value, particularly in developing countries where inexpensive, large-scale and rapid screening is needed for disorders such as pulmonary tuberculosis.

Summary

Numerous means allow the clinician to detect, assess, and diagnose olfactory disorders with accuracy, but often the cause of dysfunction can be established by taking a careful history. Confusion of smell loss with taste makes it important to perform at least a basic quantitative measure of smell function. Straightforward olfactory tests are available to measure the degree of impairment, and special imaging protocols are on hand for assessing whether the olfactory bulbs are intact. CT imaging can identify most cases of sino-nasal inflammatory disease, whereas MRI imaging is uniquely sensitive to CNS tumors and inflammatory processes associated with central olfactory disturbance. Functional imaging, which is still a research procedure, has shown that multiple brain regions are involved in the perception of odors. Specialized tests are available to evaluate general aspects of nasal function, such as ciliary motility, although their use at present is largely laboratory-based. The hitherto lost art of diagnosing a disease by its odor has received added impetus with the advent of the E-nose.

REFERENCES

Akerlund A, Bende M and Murphy C. Olfactory threshold and nasal mucosal changes in experimentally induced common cold. *Acta Otolaryngologica*, 1995, **115**, 88–92.

Amoore JE and Ollman BG. Practical test kits for quantitatively evaluating the sense of smell. *Rhinology*, 1983, **21**, 49–54.

Aronzon A, Hanson CW and Thaler ER. Differentiation between cerebrospinal fluid and serum with electronic nose. *Otolaryngology – Head and Neck Surgery*, 2005, **133**(1), 16–19.

Baird JC, Lewis C and Romer D. Relative frequencies of numerical responses in ratio estimation. *Perception and Psychophysics*, 1970, **8**, 358–62.

Bomback A. The physical exam and the sense of smell. *New England Journal of Medicine*, 2006, **354**(4), 327–9.

Brown KS, MacLean CM and Robinette RR. The distribution of the sensitivity to chemical odors in man. *Human Biology*, 1968, **40**, 456–72.

Burdach KJ and Doty RL. The effects of mouth movements, swallowing, and spitting on retronasal odor perception. *Physiology and Behavior*, 1987, **41**, 353–6.

Cain WS, Gent J, Catalanotto FA. and Goodspeed RB. Clinical evaluation of olfaction. *American Journal of Otolaryngology*, 1983, **4**, 252–6.

Carrasco M and Ridout JB. Olfactory perception and olfactory imagery: a multidimensional analysis. *Journal of Experimental Psychology: Human Perception and Performance*, 1993, **19**, 287–301.

Cheeseman GH and Kirkby HM. An air dilution olfactometer suitable for group threshold measurements. *Quarterly Journal of Experimental Physiology*, 1959, **11**, 115–23.

Cheeseman GH and Townsend MJ. Further experiments on the olfactory thresholds of pure chemical substances using the "sniff-bottle method". *Quarterly Journal of Experimental Psychology*, 1956, **8**, 8–14.

Choudhury ES, Moberg P and Doty RL. Influences of age and sex on a microencapsulated odor memory test. *Chemical Senses*, 2003, **28**, 799–805.

Cornsweet TN. The staircase-method in psychophysics. *American Journal of Psychology*, 1962, **75**, 485–91.

Covington JW, Geisler MW, Polich J and Murphy C. Normal aging and odor intensity effects on the olfactory event-related potential. I*nternational Journal of Psychophysiology*, 1999, **32**, 205–14.

Cuestas E, Busso R, Barcudi S and Tapia N. A case of a child with bad odor. *Medicina*, 2005, **65**(4), 341–4.

Damm M, Eckel HE, Jungehulsing M and Hummel T. Olfactory changes at threshold and suprathreshold levels following septoplasty with partial inferior turbinectomy. *Annals of Otology, Rhinology & Laryngology*, 2003, **112**, 91–7.

Davidson TM and Murphy C. Rapid clinical evaluation of anosmia. The alcohol sniff test. *Archives of Otolaryngology, Head and Neck Surgery*, 1997, **123**: 591–4.

Deems DA, Doty RL, Settle RG *et al.* Smell and taste disorders, a study of 750 patients from the University of Pennsylvania Smell and Taste Center. *Archives of Otolaryngology, Head and Neck Surgery*, 1991, **117**, 519–28.

Di Nardo W, Di Girolamo W, Galli A, Meduri G, Paludetti G and De Rossi G. Olfactory function evaluated by SPECT. *American Journal of Rhinology*, 2000, **14**, 57–61.

Donchin E and Coles MGH. Is the P300 a manifestation of context updating? *Behavioral and Brain Sciences*, 1988, **11**, 357–428.

Doty RL. An examination of relationships between the pleasantness, intensity, and concentration of 10 odorous stimuli. *Perception and Psychophysics*, 1975, **17**, 492–6.

Doty RL. *The Smell Identification Test™ Administration Manual* (3rd edition). Haddon Hts., NJ: Sensonics, Inc., 1995.

Doty RL. *The Odor Threshold Test™ Administration Manual*. Haddon Hts., NJ: Sensonics, Inc., 2000.

Doty RL. Olfaction. *Annual Review of Psychology*, 2001, **52**, 423–52.

Doty RL. *The Odor Memory Test™ Administration Manual*. Haddon Hts., NJ: Sensonics, Inc., 2003.

Doty RL. Office procedures for quantitative assessment of olfactory function. *American Journal of Rhinology*, 2007, **21**, 460–73.

Doty RL and Laing DG. Psychophysical measurement of olfactory function, including odorant mixture assessment. In: RL Doty, ed. *Handbook of Olfaction and Gustation*. New York, NY: Marcel Dekker, 2003, pp. 203–28.

Doty RL, Snyder PJ, Huggins GR and Lowry LD. Endocrine, cardiovascular, and psychological correlates of olfactory sensitivity changes during the human menstrual cycle. *Journal of Comparative Physiology and Psychology*, 1981, **95**, 45–60.

Doty RL, Shaman P and Dann M. Development of the University of Pennsylvania Smell Identification Test: a standardized microencapsulated test of olfactory function. *Physiology and Behavior*, 1984, **32**, 489–502.

Doty RL, Gregor TP and Settle RG. Influence of intertrial interval and sniff-bottle volume on phenyl ethyl alcohol odor detection thresholds. *Chemical Senses*, 1986, **11**, 259–64.

Doty RL, Reyes PF and Gregor T. Presence of both odor identification and detection deficits in Alzheimer's disease. *Brain Research Bulletin*, 1987, **18**, 597–600.

Doty RL, Deems DA, Frye RE, Pelberg R and Shapiro A. Olfactory sensitivity, nasal resistance, and autonomic function in patients with multiple chemical sensitivities. *Archives of Otolaryngology, Head and Neck Surgery*, 1988, **114**, 1422–7.

Doty RL, Smith R, McKeown DA and Raj J. Tests of human olfactory function: principal components analysis suggests that most measure a common source of variance. *Perception and Psychophysics*, 1994, **56**, 701–7.

Doty RL, Marcus A and Lee WW. Development of the 12-item cross-cultural smell identification test (CC-SIT). *Laryngoscope*, 1996, **106**, 353–6.

Doty RL, Cometto-Muniz JE, Jalowayski AA, Dalton P, Kendal-Reed M and Hodgson M. Assessment of upper respiratory tract and ocular irritative effects of volatile chemicals in humans. *Critical Reviews in Toxicology*, 2004, **34**, 85–142.

Drake B, Johansson B, von Sydow D and Doving KB. Quantitative psychophysical and electrophysiological data on some odorous compounds. *Scandinavian Journal of Psychology*, 1969, **10**, 89–96.

Eccles R, Jawad MS and Morris S. The effects of oral administration of (-)-menthol on nasal resistance to airflow and nasal sensation of airflow in subjects suffering from nasal congestion associated with the common cold. *Journal of Pharmacy and Pharmacology*, 1990, **42**, 652–4.

Eichenbaum H, Morton TH, Potter H and Corkin S. Selective olfactory deficits in case H.M. *Brain*, 1983, **106**, 459–72.

Elsberg CA and Levy I. The sense of smell: I. A new and simple method of quantitative olfactometry. *Bulletin of the Neurological Institute of New York*, 1935, **4**, 5–19.

Engen T and Ross BM. Long-term memory of odors with and without verbal descriptions. *Journal of Experimental Psychology*, 1973, **100**, 221–7.

Engen T, Kuisma JE and Eimas PD. Short-term memory of odors. *Journal of Experimental Psychology*, 1973, **99**, 222–5.

Eyman RK, Kim PJ and Call T. Judgment error in category vs. magnitude scales. *Perception and Motor Skills*, 1975, **40**, 415–23.

Fend R, Kolk AH, Bessant C, Buijtels P, Klatser PR and Woodman AC. Prospects for clinical application of electronic-nose technology to early detection of Mycobacterium tuberculosis in culture and sputum. *Journal of Clinical Microbiology*, 2006, **44**(6), 2039–45.

Frijters JE. Three-stimulus procedures in olfactory psychophysics: an experimental comparison of Thurstone-Ura and three-alternative forced-choice models of signal detection theory. *Perception and Psychophysics*, 1980, **28**, 390–7.

Frye RE. Nasal airway dynamics and olfactory function. In: RL Doty, ed. *Handbook of Olfaction and Gustation.* New York, NY: Marcel Dekker, 1995, pp. 471–91.

Geisler MW and Murphy C. Event-related brain potentials to attended and ignored olfactory and trigeminal stimuli. *International Journal of Psychophysiology,* 2000, **37**, 309–15.

Geisler MW, Morgan CD, Covington JW and Murphy C. Neuropsychological performance and cognitive olfactory event-related brain potentials in young and elderly adults. *Journal of Clinical and Experimental Neuropsychology,* 1999, **21**, 108–26.

Gevins AS and Remond A. *Methods of Analysis of Brain Electrical and Magnetic Signals.* New York, NY: Elsevier, 1987.

Green BG, Dalton P, Cowart B, Shaffer G, Rankin K and Higgins J. Evaluating the "Labeled Magnitude Scale" for measuring sensations of taste and smell. *Chemical Senses,* 1996, **21**, 323–34.

Guadagni DG, Buttery RG and Okano S. Odor thresholds of some organic compounds associated with food flavors. *Journal of Food Science and Agriculture,* 1963, **14**, 761–5.

Hayden GR. Olfactory diagnosis in medicine. *Postgraduate Medicine,* 1980, **67**, 110–16.

Heilmann S, Strehle G, Rosenheim K, Damm M and Hummel T. Clinical assessment of retronasal olfactory function. *Archives of Otolaryngology – Head and Neck Surgery,* 2002, **128**, 414–18.

Helson H. *Adaptation-Level Theory: An Experimental and Systematic Approach to Behavior.* New York, NY: Harper & Row, 1964.

Hockstein NG, Thaler ER, Lin Y, Lee DD and Hanson CW. Correlation of pneumonia score with electronic nose signature: a prospective study. *Annals of Otology, Rhinology and Laryngology,* 2005, **114**(7), 504–8.

Hornung DE. Nasal anatomy and the sense of smell. *Advances in Oto-RhinoLaryngology,* 2006, **63**, 1–22.

Hummel T, Sekinger B, Wolf SR, Pauli E and Kobal G. "Sniffin' sticks:" olfactory performance assessed by the combined testing of odor identification, odor discrimination and olfactory threshold. *Chemical Senses,* 1997, **22**, 39–52.

Hummel T, Mojet J and Kobal G. Electro-olfactograms are present when odorous stimuli have not been perceived. *Neuroscience Letters,* 2006, **397**(3), 224–8.

Hummel T, Kobal G, Gudziol H and Mackay-Sim A. Normative data for the "Sniffin' Sticks" including tests of odor identification, odor discrimination, and olfactory thresholds: an upgrade based on a group of more than 3000 subjects. *European Archives of Otorhinolaryngology,* 2007, **264**(3), 237–43.

Jackman AH and Doty RL. Utility of a 3-item smell identification test in detecting olfactory dysfunction. *Laryngoscope,* 2005, **115**, 2209–12.

Kareken DA, Doty RL, Moberg P J *et al.* Olfactory-evoked regional cerebral blood flow in Alzheimer's disease *Neuropsychology,* 2001, **15**(1), 18–29.

Kern RC. Chronic sinusitis and anosmia: pathologic changes in the olfactory mucosa. *Laryngoscope,* 2000, **110**, 1071–7.

Kobal G. *Elektrophysiologische Untersuchungen des menschlichen Geruchssinns.* Stuttgart, Germany: Thieme, 1981.

Kobal G. Electrophysiological measurement of olfactory function. In: RL Doty, ed. *Handbook of Olfaction and Gustation.* New York, NY: Marcel Dekker, 2003, pp. 229–49.

Kobal G and Hummel C. Cerebral chemosensory evoked potentials elicited by chemical stimulation of the human olfactory and respiratory nasal mucosa. *Electroencephalography and Clinical Neurophysiology*, 1988, **71**, 241–50.

Kobal G and Plattig KH. Methodische Anmerkungen zur Gewinnung olfaktorischer EEG-Antworten des wachen Menschen (objektive Olfaktometrie). *Zeitschrift fur Elektroenzephalographie Elektromyographie und Verwandte Gebiete*, 1978, **9**, 135–45.

Kobal G, Hummel T, Sekinger B, Barz S, Roscher S and Wolf S. "Sniffin' sticks": screening of olfactory performance. *Rhinology*, 1996, **34**, 222–6.

Lane AP, Zweiman B, Lanza DC *et al*. Acoustic rhinometry in the study of the acute nasal allergic response. *Annals of Otology, Rhinology and Laryngology*, 1996, **105**, 811–18.

Lawless HT and Malone GT. The discrimination efficiency of common scaling methods. *Journal of Sensory Studies*, 1986a, **1**, 85–98.

Lawless HT and Malone GT. A comparison of rating scales: sensitivity, replicates and relative measurement. *Journal of Sensory Studies*, 1986b, **1**, 155–74.

Leopold DA. The relationship between nasal anatomy and human olfaction. *Laryngoscope*, 1988, **98**, 1232–8.

Linschoten MR, Harvey LO Jr, Eller PM and Jafek BW. Fast and accurate measurement of taste and smell thresholds using a maximum-likelihood adaptive staircase procedure. *Perception and Psychophysics*, 2001, **63**, 1330–47.

London B, Nabet B, Fisher AR, White B, Sammel MD and Doty RL. Predictors of prognosis in patients with olfactory disturbances. *Annals of Neurology*, 2008, **63**, 159–66.

Lorig TS, Elmes DG, Zald DH and Pardo JV. A computer-controlled olfactometer for fMRI and electrophysiological studies of olfaction. *Behavior Research Methods, Instruments, and Computers*, 1999, **31**, 370–5.

Mace JW, Goodman SI, Centerwall WR and Chinnock RF. The child with an unusual odor. *Clinical Pediatrics*, 1976, **15**, 57–62.

Marks LE. *Sensory Processes*. New York, NY: Academic Press, 1974.

Marks LE. Magnitude estimation and sensory matching. *Perception and Psychophysics*, 1988, **43**, 511–25.

Maruniak JA, Mason JR and Kostelc JG. Conditioned aversions to an intravascular odorant. *Physiology and Behavior*, 1983, **30**(4): 617–20.

McCaffrey TV. Rhinomanometry and vasoactive drugs affecting nasal patency. In: TV Getchell, RL Doty, LM Bartoshuk and JB. Snow Jr, eds. *Smell and Taste in Health and Disease*. New York, NY: Raven Press, 1991, pp. 493–502.

Moskowitz HR. Magnitude estimation: notes on what, how, when, and why to use it. *Journal of Food Quality*, 1977, **3**, 195–227.

Mueller CA, Grassinger E, Naka A, Temmel AF, Hummel T and Kobal G. A self-administered odor identification test procedure using the "Sniffin' Sticks". *Chemical Senses*, 2006, **31**, 595–8.

Nakashima T, Kidera K, Miyazaki J, Kuratomi Y and Inokuchi A. Smell intensity monitoring using metal oxide semiconductor odor sensors during intravenous olfactoin test. *Chemical Senses*, 2006, **31**, 43–7.

Neely G, Ljunggren G, Sylven C and Borg G. Comparison between the Visual Analogue Scale (VAS) and the Category Ratio Scale (CR-10) for the evaluation of leg exertion. *International Journal of Sports Medicine*, 1992, **13**, 133–6.

Nordin S, Monsch AU and Murphy C. Unawareness of smell loss in normal aging and Alzheimer's disease: discrepancy between self-reported and diagnosed smell sensitivity. *Journal of Gerontology*, 1995, **50**, 187–92.

Nordin S, Lotsch J, Kobal G and Murphy C. Effects of nasal-airway volume and body temperature on intranasal chemosensitivity. *Physiology and Behavior*, 1998, **63**, 463–6.

Patel SJ, Bollhoefer AD and Doty RL. Influences of ethanol ingestion on olfactory function in humans. *Psychopharmacology*, 2004, **171**, 429–34.

Pause BM, Sojka B and Ferstl R. Central processing of odor concentration is a temporal phenomenon as revealed by chemosensory event-related potentials (CSERP). *Chemical Senses*, 1997, **22**, 9–26.

Pavlou AK, Magan N, Sharp D, Brown J, Barr H and Turner AP. An intelligent rapid odour recognition model in discrimination of *Helicobacter pylori* and other gastrooesophageal isolates in vitro. *Biosensors and Bioelectronics*, 2000, **15**(7–8), 333–42.

Persaud K and Dodd G. Analysis of discrimination mechanisms in the mammalian olfactory system using a model nose. *Nature*, 1982, **299**(5881), 352–5.

Pierce JD Jr, Doty RL and Amoore JE. Analysis of position of trial sequence and type of diluent on the detection threshold for phenyl ethyl alcohol using a single staircase method. *Perceptual and Motor Skills*, 1996, **82**, 451–8.

Potter H and Butters N. An assessment of olfactory deficits in patients with damage to prefrontal cortex. *Neuropsychologia*, 1980, **18**, 621–8.

Punter PH. Measurement of human olfactory thresholds for several groups of structurally related compounds. *Chemical Senses*, 1983, **7**, 215–35.

Rovee CK, Cohen RY and Shlapack W. Life-span stability in olfactory sensitivity. *Developmental Psychology*, 1975, **11**, 311–18.

Schiffman SS, Reynolds ML and Young FW. *Introduction to Multidimensional Scaling: Theory, Methods, and Applications*. Orlando, FL: Academic Press, 1981.

Scott JW and Scott-Johnson PE. The electroolfactogram: a review of its history and uses. *Microscopy Research and Technique*, 2002, **58**(3), 152–60.

Semb G. The detectability of the odor of butanol. *Perception and Psychophysics*, 1968, **4**, 335–40.

Silveira-Moriyama L, Williams DR, Evans AH, Katzenschlager R, Watt H and Lees AJ. A UK comparison of Sniffin' Sticks (SS) and University of Pennsylvania (UPSIT) Smell Identification Tests in Parkinson's disease. *Movement Disorders*, 2006, **21** (Supplement 15), P814.

Simmen D, Briner HR and Hess K. Screening of olfaction with smell diskettes. *Laryngorhinootologie*, 1999, **78**(3), 125–30.

Sobel N, Pabhakaran V, Zhao Z *et al.* Time course of odorant-induced activation in the human primary olfactory cortex. *Journal of Neurophysiology*, 2000, **83**, 537–51.

Sobel N, Johnson BN, Mainland J and Yousem DM. Functional neuroimaging of human olfaction. In: RL Doty, ed. *Handbook of Olfaction and Gustation*. New York, NY: Marcel Dekker, 2003, pp. 251–73.

Stevens JC and Marks LE. Cross-modality matching functions generated by magnitude estimation. *Perception and Psychophysics*, 1980, **27**, 379–89.

Stevens JC, Cain WS and Burke RJ. Variability of olfactory thresholds. *Chemical Senses*, 1988, **13**, 643–53.

Stevens SS. The psychophysics of sensory function. *American Scientist*, 1960, **48**, 226–53.

Tabert MH, Steffener J, Albers MMW *et al*. Validation and optimization of statistical approaches for modeling odorant-induced fMRI signal changes in olfactory-related brain areas. *NeuroImage*, 2007, **34**, 1375–90.

Takagi SF. *Human Olfaction*. Tokyo: University of Tokyo Press, 1989.

Tanner WP Jr and Swets JA. A decision-making theory of visual detection. *Psychological Reviews*, 1954, **61**, 401–9.

Tateyama T, Hummel T, Roscher S, Post H and Kobal G. Relation of olfactory event-related potentials to changes in stimulus concentration. *Electroencephalography and Clinical Neurophysiology*, 1998, **108**, 449–55.

Thaler ER and Hanson CW. Use of an electronic nose to diagnose bacterial sinusitis. *American Journal of Rhinology*, 2006, **20**(2), 170–2.

Toyota B, Kitamura T and Takagi SF. *Olfactory Disorders – Olfactometry and Therapy*. Tokyo: Igaku-Shoin, 1978.

Turner AP and Magan N. Electronic noses and disease diagnostics. *Nature Reviews. Microbiology*, 2004, **2**(2), 161–6.

Vollmecke T and Doty RL. Development of the Picture Identification Test (PIT): a research companion to the University of Pennsylvania Smell Identification Test. *Chemical Senses*, 1985, **10**, 413–14.

von Békésy G. Problems relating psychological and electrophysiological observations in sensory perception. *Perspectives in Biology and Medicine*, 1968, **11**, 179–94.

Walker JC, Kurtz DB, Shore FM, Ogden MW and Reynolds JH. Apparatus for the automated measurement of the responses of humans to odorants. *Chemical Senses*, 1990, **15**, 165–77.

Wang L, Hari, C, Chen L and Jacob T. A new non-invasive method for recording the electro-olfactogram using external electrodes. *Clinical Neurophysiology*, 2004, **115**(7), 1631–40.

Weber EH. *De Pulsu, Resorptione, Auditu et Tactu: Annotationes Anatomicae et Physiologiae*. Leipzig, Germany: Koehler, 1834.

Weiffenbach JM and McCarthy VP. Olfactory deficits in cystic fibrosis: distribution and severity. *Chemical Senses*, 1984, **9**, 193–9.

Welsh JS. Olfactory detection of human bladder cancer by dogs: another cancer detected by "pet scan". *British Medical Journal*, 2004, **329**(7477), 1286–7.

Wenzel BM. Techniques in olfactometry. A critical review of the last one hundred years. *Psychological Bulletin*, 1948, **45**, 231–47.

Williams H and Pembroke A. Sniffer dogs in the melanoma clinic? *Lancet*, 1989, **1**(8640): 734.

Wolfensberger M, Schnieper I and Welge-Lussen A. Sniffin' Sticks: a new olfactory test battery. *Acta Otolaryngologica*, 2000, **120**(2), 303–6.

Yoshida M. Correlation analysis of detection threshold data for "standard test" odors. *Bulletin of the Faculty of Sciences and Engineering of Cho University*, 1984, **27**, 343–53.

Yousem DM, Williams SC, Howard RO *et al*. Functional MR imaging during odor stimulation: preliminary data. *Radiology*, 1997, **204**, 833–8.

Yousem DM, Maldjian JA, Siddiqi F *et al*. Gender effects on odor-stimulated functional magnetic resonance imaging. *Brain Research*, 1999, **818**(2), 480–7.

Yousem DM, Oguz KK, Li C. Imaging of the olfactory system. *Seminars in Ultrasound CT MR*, 2001, **22**(6), 456–72.

Zald DH and Pardo JV. Emotion, olfaction and the human amygdale: amygdale activation during aversive olfactory stimulation. *Proceedings of the National Academy of Science of the United States of America*, 1997, **94**, 4119–24.

Zatorre RJ, Jones-Gotman M, Evans AC and Meyer E. Functional localization and lateralization of human olfactory cortex. *Nature*, 1992, **360**(6402), 339–40.

Zwaardemaker H. On measurement of the sense of smell in clinical examination. *Lancet*, 1889, 1300–2.

Zwaardemaker H. *L'Odorat*. Paris: Doin, 1925 (monograph).

Zwaardemaker H. The sense of smell. *Acta Otolaryngologica*, **1927**, **11**, 3–15.

3

General disorders of olfaction

This chapter deals with olfactory disorders of relevance to the clinician and describes, from the olfactory perspective, the major non-degenerative diseases such as head injury, tumor, infection and inflammation, endocrine disease, epilepsy, and multiple sclerosis. Neurodegenerative diseases, such as Alzheimer's and Parkinson's diseases, and their associated syndromes, are discussed in Chapter 4.

Patients whose only defect is loss of smell regularly complain that they have lost their sense of taste. This is the source of recurrent confusion in the minds of patients and indeed their medical advisers. The answer lies in retronasal olfaction. When we ingest food, there is taste appreciation from taste buds over the tongue and pharynx but, simultaneously, odorants released from food escapes into the retropharyngeal space and enter the nasal cavity where they are detected. Thus any food entering the mouth will evoke a sensation of both taste and smell, unless it is a pure odorless tastant evoking solely sweet, sour, salt, bitter, or umami taste qualities. Sensations such as chocolate, meat sauce, strawberry, cola, lime, walnut, and lemon are mediated principally by smell, not taste.

Types of olfactory disturbance

Like other sensory disorders, disturbances of the olfactory system can present in many ways. *Anosmia* can be total, where there is inability to perceive all odors, or partial, where some but not all odors are detected. Decreased sensitivity to odors, termed *hyposmia* or *microsmia*, may present either unilaterally or bilaterally. *Dysosmia* is distorted smell perception, sometimes termed *parosmia* or, when of a fetid character, *cacosmia*. *Phantosmias* are olfactory hallucinations, and *olfactory agnosia* is failure to identify odors in the presence of generally normal ability to detect and discriminate differences among them. *Accelerated* or *prolonged adaptation* may cause temporary anosmia, for example in long-term chronic exposure to vanillin or industrial

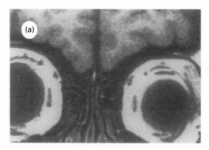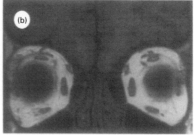

Figure 3.1 Congenital anosmia. T1-weighted coronal magnetic resonance imaging (MRI) at the level of the olfactory bulbs in two patients who had never experienced the sense of smell. The bulbs and tracts are absent. (Reproduced from Yousem *et al.*, 2001. With permission from Elsevier.)

gases such as hydrogen sulfide. Thus, many Icelanders report being anosmic to sulfur, which is present in the domestic water supply, but when they leave the country for a few days, normal perception returns. *Hyperosmia* is defined as enhanced smell sensitivity to one or more odorants but, in many instances, this reflects hyperreactivity, rather than a true change in sensitivity.

Congenital anosmia is characterized by lack of smell function from the time of birth. In a Japanese family, Yamamoto *et al.* (1966) found tremor and/or anosmia or hyposmia in 14 people and proposed that the two traits were independent dominants. In the Faroe Islands, Lygonis (1969) found a large kindred in which 9 males and 19 females in four generations had anosmia but no other abnormality. Male-to-male transmission was observed several times. Singh *et al.* (1970) observed anosmia in six males in three generations. One male who transmitted the trait had only partial anosmia. Mainland (1945) and Joyner (1963) recorded dominant inheritance, and several instances of male-to-male transmission were observed. One of the patients of Hockaday (1966) with anosmia-hypogonadism (Kallman syndrome) had a father and a brother with anosmia alone. Ghadami *et al.* (2004) performed genome-wide linkage analysis in two large unrelated Iranian families of whom seven individuals had isolated congenital anosmia. In both families, the trait appeared to be inherited as an autosomal dominant trait with incomplete penetrance. All affected individuals shared a common haplotype in the 18p11.23-q12.2 region but no mutations were detected. In one magnetic resonance imaging (MRI) study of 25 patients presenting to the University of Pennsylvania Smell and Taste Center with congenital anosmia there was absence or hypoplasia of the olfactory bulbs or tracts, but no cortical changes. (Yousem *et al.*, 1996b, 2001; Figure 3.1).

Specific anosmia

(See also Chapter 1.) This is defined usually as the inability to detect one or a few related odorants in the absence of other evidence of smell loss, and probably has a genetic basis. Such anosmias should not be confused with acquired generalized anosmias which bring a patient to the clinic. Like color blindness there are potential risks associated with this apparently benign condition. An extreme example is specific anosmia to cyanide (almond-like), which reportedly affects about 1 percent of otherwise healthy people (Sayek, 1970). Around 1 percent of the general population is reportedly anosmic to pyridine (acrid, shellfish odor), a known neurotoxin which is present in many herbicides (Hirsch, 1992). Speculatively, it is possible that someone with pyridine anosmia might develop a neurodegenerative disorder by long-term exposure to this agent. In one study all of 12 Alzheimer's disease (AD) patients were either anosmic or had raised threshold to pyridine and there was a correlation between threshold and progression of dementia (Nordin *et al.*, 1997). Unfortunately, this study did not examine the specificity of pyridine hyposmia. Other studies report that patients with idiopathic Parkinson's disease (PD) have a greater reduction in the ability to detect certain odors in the University of Pennsylvania Smell Identification Test (UPSIT) such as pizza, mint, licorice, and wintergreen (Hawkes & Shephard, 1993; Silveira-Moriyama *et al.*, 2005), although such stimuli are composed of multiple chemicals (see Chapter 4 for further discussion of this topic).

Agnosia

Olfactory agnosia may be defined as a disorder affecting cognitively intact individuals who lose the ability to identify an aroma in the presence of an intact detection threshold and normal ability to distinguish differences between various odors. In such cases the peripheral portion (epithelium, bulb, and tract) of the olfactory system are assumed to be intact. Extremely few cases of olfactory agnosia have been described, which is surprising in view of the well-recognized forms of agnosia in the visual and auditory spheres. To be certain a patient has agnosia there must be a thorough assessment of olfactory thresholds. Agnosia was observed in a 53-year-old male patient with predominantly right inferior temporal lobe atrophy (presumably degenerative) in association with prosopagnosia, i.e., agnosia for familiar faces (Mendez & Ghajarnia, 2001) and in another patient with complex partial seizures localized to the right medial temporal lobe (Lehrner *et al.*, 1997). Although one group reported that 50 percent of the male patients with schizophrenia had olfactory agnosia (Kopala et al., 1989; Kopala & Clark, 1990), that is, identification deficits independent of threshold problems, patients with schizophrenia usually have threshold deficits as well (Moberg *et al.*, 1999). The prediction that patients with semantic dementia (SD) would have difficulty in naming smells in the presence of normal discrimination was confirmed recently in a study of eight patients with SD (Luzzi *et al.*, 2007).

Hyperosmia

This disorder of perception is characterized by varying degrees of increased sensitivity to one or more aromas, in the presence of lowered threshold to the odor in question. Some consider that hyperosmia more often represents hyperreactivity, i.e., simply an emotional response associated with normal threshold, rather than a distinct condition. Many researchers have not made this distinction and have simply relied on patient feedback. The concept now has a more scientific footing as a result of gene knockout experiments. Mice with gene-targeted deletion of the Kv 1.3 channel had a 1000- to 10 000-fold lower threshold for detection of odors, and increased ability to discriminate between odorants in comparison with their wild-type littermates, earning the title of "supersmeller" mice (Fadool *et al.*, 2004). Thresholds to a number of odorants exhibit a bimodal distribution in the general population. For example, Amoore and Steinle (1991) reported that about 2 percent of healthy individuals are hyperosmic to pyridine as measured by odor-detection threshold tests, and Lundstrom and colleagues (2003) documented a bimodal distribution of sensitivity to androstadienone with a small group which was very sensitive to this compound. Apparent hyperosmia has been observed in Addison's disease (adrenocortical insufficiency) and following abrupt drug withdrawal from benzodiazepines (Pelissolo & Bisserbe, 1994) or antidepressants (Mourad *et al.*, 1998). In some patients with a pituitary tumor studied by Sherman *et al.* (1979), there was reportedly a 100 000-fold increase of detection threshold sensitivity to pyridine in some patients. During or before migraine attacks, sufferers may describe temporary heightened and unpleasant smell perception (osmophobia) in a manner comparable to photophobia and phonophobia (Kelman, 2004a, b). As described later, those with migraine are reported to have inter-ictal hyperosmia to vanillin and acetone (Snyder & Drummond, 1997). During the early months of pregnancy some women report hypersensitivity to odors, although reliable psychophysical documentation is lacking (Cameron, 2007). Oversensitivity to smells in the early months of pregnancy has been claimed to be the basis of hyperemesis gravidarum, and estrogen excess is suggested as a potential uniting factor for some types of hyperosmia (Heinrichs, 2002). Patients who become hyperosmic or hyperreactive are often depressed initially, but if not they soon become so. Certainly, some neurotic individuals complain of undue sensitivity to odors when there is no proof of actual change in odor perception threshold. Although numerous studies have reported cyclic fluctuations in olfactory sensitivity across the phases of the menstrual cycle (Doty *et al.*, 1981), such changes are not large and at no point is there significant hypersensitivity.

Hyperosmia or overreactivity may form part of a more generalized syndrome of multiple chemical hypersensitivity where there are numerous symptoms connected with repeated exposure to environmental chemicals. Quantitative evaluation of these individuals showed no difference in olfactory detection thresholds (Doty *et al.*, 1988; Hummel *et al.*, 1996), but in some there was a high level of depression, increased nasal resistance, and altered respiratory rate following olfactory stimulation. This suggested there was a complex mixture of physical, psychiatric, and autonomic problems.

Hallucinations, dysosmias, and phantosmias

An *olfactory hallucination* (OH), also termed *phantosmia* or *unstimulated dysosmia*, is the perception of an odor in the absence of a smell in the environment; the subject claims to smell something that no one else can. Traditional teaching holds that most hallucinations, including olfactory ones, are indicative of organic disease. These phenomena are quite common and, in the case of smell, usually reflect degeneration or attempts at regeneration within the olfactory membrane or cribriform plate. Such patients complain of a continuous or intermittent unpleasant smell in the absence of any external stimulus. Olfactory hallucinations were considered initially to originate from disorder anywhere from the nose to the medial temporal lobe, but it is now recognized that lesions of the orbitofrontal cortex, an olfactory association area, may produce olfactory illusions, hallucinations, other autonomic signs, or gestural automatisms as part of a seizure complex (Chabolla, 2002).

Apart from uncinate seizures and local nasal disease, OH and delusions may signify psychiatric illness. Although a variety of smells may be reported, usually the OH is foul or unpleasant. A patient may believe mistakenly that a fetid smell emanates from his or her own body ("intrinsic hallucination") attributing the smell to the skin or breath. In others, the odor is believed to stem from an external source ("extrinsic hallucination"). In a review of depressed patients, Pryse-Phillips (1971, 1975) found olfactory symptoms were an early and predominating complaint in half of his patients with typical endogenous depression and termed this the "olfactory reference syndrome." They usually suffered from intrinsic hallucinations, whereas the OH of schizophrenia was usually extrinsic, sometimes believed to be induced by someone in order to upset the patient. Patients reacted variably to the hallucinations, from doing nothing to petitioning police and neighbors about the malodor; others indulged in continual washing and social withdrawal. Pryse-Phillips also maintained that OH of episodic nature was more likely to be organically based than continuous hallucinations, which related to psychiatric illness.

Olfactory hallucinations were recorded in one case of cluster headache (Silberstein *et al.*, 2000). The patient complained of a bad citrus fruit odor, which preceded the headache by 3–4 minutes. Migraine aura may be associated with OH, nearly always unpleasant, such as decaying animals, burning cookies, cigars, peanut butter, and cigarette smoke (Fuller & Guiloff 1987). Olfactory hallucinations have been noted in PD, sometimes predating the onset of motor symptoms (Sandyk, 1981), and it has been suggested that development of hallucinations (including olfactory) in those with established PD may indicate a comorbid psychotic illness or Parkinsonism (Goetz *et al.*, 1998). Chronic cocaine abuse has been associated with olfactory and other hallucinations (Siegel, 1978). Finally, OH and delusions are seen rarely in cases of dementia in the absence of significant depression as well as in alcohol withdrawal syndromes (Gauntlett-Gilbert and Kuipers, 2003).

Localization of olfactory disorder

Some olfactory disturbances reflect peripheral influences (e.g., blockage of airflow to the receptors, damage to the receptors themselves), others central factors (e.g., tumors that compromise the olfactory bulbs or higher-order structures), and still other systemic factors (e.g., metabolic changes that generally influence olfactory system functioning). One cannot always localize a given disturbance to a peripheral, central, or systemic cause. For example, anosmia, which is less common than hyposmia or microsmia, can result from damage to the olfactory epithelium (as in toxic exposures, chronic rhinosinusitis, or upper respiratory infections), damage to the axons of the receptor cells or sectors of the olfactory bulb (as in head trauma-related shearing of the olfactory filaments), or injury to regions of the olfactory cortex (as in multiple sclerosis or Alzheimer's disease). Similarly, dysosmia can be attributed to peripheral, central, systemic, or some combination of these factors. Usually, dysosmia is accompanied by some diminution of olfactory function, regardless of its locus. As mentioned in Chapter 2, threshold measurements do not necessarily reflect peripheral disorders of the olfactory tract, nor do problems with smell identification automatically indicate a more centrally mediated problem. With these caveats, and purely as a general rule, impairment of smell that is continuous is more likely to be neurogenic in origin, whereas fluctuating hyposmia with intermittent recovery in between often indicates inflammation-related within the nose or sinuses. Also as a general rule, complete lack of smell early in the course of disease is more likely to be caused by a peripheral than central lesion because of the considerable redundancy in central olfactory areas.

Disorders affecting olfaction

As indicated in Table 3.1 and Figure 3.2, a large number of relatively common diseases may compromise the sense of smell, in many cases permanently.

Table 3.1 List of main categories of disease causing smell disturbance with typical examples; "neurodegenerative" causes are given separately in Chapter 4

Disease	Examples
Local nasal	Polyps; allergic rhinitis; sinus disease
Infection	Common cold; influenza; herpes encephalitis; AIDS; prion disease; fungi, e.g., aspergillosis, mucormycosis
Head injury	Usually severe posterior or lateral impact
Epilepsy	Olfactory aura; complex partial seizure (CPS)
Migraine	Before, during, or after attack
Multiple sclerosis (MS)	During relapse or in more advanced disease; rarely may be a presenting feature
Tumors and inflammatory disease	Nasopharyngeal carcinoma; Wegener's granulomatosis; olfactory groove meningioma or neuroblastoma; facial Paget disease; Sjögren syndrome
Endocrine	Diabetes; Addison's disease; Cushing and Klinefelter syndromes; pseudohypoparathyroidism; Kallman syndrome; septo-optic dysplasia
Neurodegenerative	See Chapter 4, Table 4.1

These range from the simple cold to extremely debilitating central nervous system (CNS) diseases. Non-neurodegenerative disorders known to cause olfactory dysfunction are described below, beginning with those that are most frequent (i.e., local nasal disease, upper respiratory infections, and head trauma).

Local nasal disease

This is one of the most common causes of olfactory disturbance. Nasal disease can prevent air from reaching the olfactory neuroepithelium (conductive problem), as well as produce nasal inflammation, which inhibits function. Any obstructive or inflammatory process can be responsible for decreased smell ability, including seasonal rhinitis (hay fever), allergic rhinitis, polyposis (particularly in the nasal vault), and inflammatory disease of the ethmoid or maxillary sinuses, osteomeatal deformity owing to trauma, and malignant disease of the nose, paranasal sinuses, or nasopharynx. If there is chronic nasal sinus infection, the mucus clearance rate may be reduced because of disordered ciliary motility. This, along with inflammation, contributes to smell loss and, if left unchecked, can ultimately result in permanent damage to the olfactory receptors.

Recent studies indicate that the nasal airway remains patent in up to 70 percent of those with olfactory disturbance due to local nasal disease. In such instances, the loss is attributed to micro-inflammatory changes within

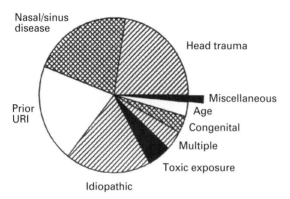

Figure 3.2 Proportion of patients in various diagnostic categories of olfactory impairment among 200 patients at University of Cincinnati Taste and Smell Center. Four categories (nasal/sinus disease, head trauma, upper respiratory infection (URI), and idiopathic) account for 83 percent of all patients. (Reproduced from Duncan HJ and Smith DV, 1995. With permission.)

the olfactory mucosa (Kern, 2000). Oddly enough, mild or moderate congestion of the turbinates in the absence of disease does not necessarily cause impairment of smell function and may actually enhance it, perhaps by shunting more air up into the olfactory cleft (Doty & Frye, 1989; Zhao *et al.*, 2006). In general, the variation of nasal resistance across the two sides of the nose (i.e., the so-called nasal cycle) does not result in noticeable hyposmia on the less patent side, except in cases where the nasal septum is extremely deformed or when adhesions occur between the turbinate and the septum. Nevertheless, subtle influences on odor quality based upon differential absorption patterns may occur when testing is confined to a single nasal chamber (Sobel *et al.*, 1999). Nasal dryness, which can develop after repeated surgery, atrophic rhinitis, or Sjögren syndrome, has been associated with hyposmia or anosmia since – like taste – normal perception depends upon a moist receptor area.

When there is a peripheral cause for the smell problem, variability in olfactory sensitivity over the course of days is often reported. Such fluctuations reflect varying degrees of odorant molecule access to the receptors, either by frank alterations in airflow or by more subtle inflammation within the olfactory membrane. These variations may help to differentiate anosmia caused by nasal inflammatory processes from that due to damage of the olfactory receptors or more central structures, where smell impairment is more often continuous.

Spontaneous improvement in function over time has been reported in patients with smell loss secondary to chronic rhinosinusitis. For example, in a recent longitudinal study of 542 patients presenting to the University of Pennsylvania Smell and Taste Center who were retested, on average, three years after initial presentation, nearly half of those with dysfunction secondary to chronic rhinosinusitis showed statistically significant improvement (i.e., an increase of ≥ 4 in UPSIT score) on the second test occasion. Nearly 25 percent of those who were not initially anosmic improved into the age-adjusted normal range (London *et al.*, 2008), although a significant decline in function occurred in 20 percent of the microsmic patients (Table 3.2).

Viral infections

The olfactory receptor cells are regularly damaged by viruses. Reduction or inhibition of mucociliary transport by disease, drugs, or genetic factors markedly increases susceptibility to viral infection (Bang *et al.*, 1966; Brownstein, 1987). Viruses that gain access to the respiratory tract usually do so in the form of aerosolized droplets. In general, non-enveloped viruses (e.g., adenovirus, rhinovirus, enteroviruses, and poliovirus) are more stable than enveloped viruses (e.g., influenza, parainfluenza, respiratory syncytial, mumps, measles, rubella, and herpes simplex). As noted by Stroop (1995), most viral infections are either entirely asymptomatic or so mildly symptomatic as to go unrecognized. Thus, during seasonal epidemics, the quantity of serologically documented infections of influenza or arboviral encephalitis exceeds the number of acute cases by several hundredfold. Hence, many unexplained cases of smell dysfunction may reflect unrecognized viral infections. On rare occasions, anosmia has been associated with trivalent influenza vaccines whether given intranasally, intramuscularly or intradermally (Doty & Izhar, unpublished; Fiser & Borotski, 1979), perhaps similar to vaccine-associated Guillain–Barré syndrome and Bell's palsy. Such olfactory loss may qualify a patient for compensation in the USA under the National Vaccine Injury Compensation Program, although it may be difficult to eliminate the possibility of anosmia from coincidental viral infection.

It is underappreciated that some viruses that are not ordinarily neurotropic may become so on entering the nose. For example, the NWS strain of influenza virus spreads perivenously when injected into mice intraperitoneally (Reinacher *et al.*, 1983), and viral antigen is restricted to the meninges, choroid plexus, ependymal cells, and perivascular locations within the brain parenchyma. Neurons within the brain parenchyma are unaffected. When this strain of virus is inoculated into the nose, however, it spreads through the olfactory and trigeminal nerves and invades the brainstem nuclei.

In light of such observations, it is not surprising that upper respiratory infections, usually viral in nature, are the most common cause of *chronic* hyposmia or anosmia (Deems *et al.*, 1991; Murphy *et al.*, 2003). Even the common cold may damage olfaction permanently, and this has been

Table 3.2 Percent (number) of anosmic and microsmic patients from four etiological classes with evidence of smell dysfunction on first test occasion that exhibited decline, no change, or improvement in function over time. URTI = upper respiratory tract infection

Etiology	Percent decline (n)[a]	Percent no improvement (n)	Percent some improvement (n)[b]	Percent improvement into absolute normal range (n)[c]	Percent improvement into age-adjusted normal range (n)[d]
Anosmics					
URTI (n=67)	5.97 (4)	37.31 (25)	56.72 (38)	7.46 (5)	14.93 (10)
Head trauma (n=69)	14.49 (10)	40.58 (28)	44.93 (31)	4.35 (3)	7.25 (5)
Nasosinal disease (n=49)	10.20 (5)	32.65 (16)	57.14 (28)	8.16 (4)	14.29 (7)
Idiopathic (n=36)	27.78 (10)	27.78 (10)	44.44 (16)	8.33 (3)	11.11 (4)
Microsmics					
URTI (n=112)	19.64 (22)	37.50 (42)	42.86 (48)	21.43 (24)	25.00 (28)
Head trauma (n=26)	15.38 (4)	42.31 (11)	42.31 (11)	15.38 (2)	26.90 (7)
Nasosinal disease (n=32)	21.89 (7)	40.63 (13)	37.50 (12)	21.88 (7)	25.00 (8)
Idiopathic (n=23)	30.43 (7)	52.17 (12)	17.39 (4)	8.70 (2)	8.70 (2)

Note: Relatively few subjects regained normal function and, in general, more of those with microsmia did so. (From London *et al*, 2008)
[a] Decline denoted by decrease of four or more University of Pennsylvania Smell Identification Test (UPSIT) scale points from test 1 to test 2.
[b] Improvement denoted by increase of four or more UPSIT scale points from test 1 to test 2.
[c] Absolute normal range denoted by UPSIT $\geq$35 for women and $\geq$34 for men. Patients with nonsignificant improvement into the normal range were excluded from consideration.
[d] Age-adjusted normal range denoted by falling at or above the 25th percentile of sex- and age-related norms. Patients with nonsignificant improvement into the normal range were excluded from consideration.

attributed chiefly to parainfluenza type 3 virus – at least in Japan (Sugiura *et al.*, 1998). Hepatitis, flu-like infections, herpes simplex encephalitis, and variant Creutzfeld–Jacob disease are rare causes of olfactory dysfunction and presumably relate to direct viral or prion damage of the olfactory pathways, either peripherally in the olfactory epithelium or more centrally in the olfactory bulb and temporal lobes. Among viruses known to be neurotropic for peripheral olfactory structures in primates or other animals when inhaled or inoculated into the nose are polio, the Indiana strain of wild-type vesicular stomatitis, rabies, herpes simplex types 1 and 2, mouse hepatitis, herpes suis, borna disease, and canine distemper.

Smell loss secondary to viral infection typically does not fluctuate, in contrast to smell loss due to conductive or intranasal inflammatory processes. Patients with the commoner forms of postviral hyposmia may also experience dysosmia or phantosmia – phenomena that usually regress with time. Although most viruses associated with smell loss infect only the olfactory epithelium, more virulent strains can injure central olfactory structures, such as the olfactory bulb. In the latter case, damage can be indirect, e.g., by anterograde degeneration of the affected primary receptors whose axons project into the bulb, or direct, e.g., by invasion of the bulb through intra-cellular transport. In keeping with this, olfactory bulb ablation will prevent the spread of a neurotropic mouse coronavirus into the brain (Perlman *et al.*, 1990). Although olfactory receptor cells, periglomerular cells, and granule cells within the olfactory bulb have retained the capacity to regenerate, animal studies employing toxic agents, such as 3-methyl indole, suggest that only rarely does the number of regenerated receptors return to original levels after insults to the olfactory epithelium (Setzer & Slotnick, 1998). The capacity to die and regenerate may reflect one means by which the olfactory system protects itself from xenobiotics.

Bacterial infections

Like viruses, bacteria can damage the olfactory system, in most cases intra-nasally. Chronic rhinosinusitis is associated with a predominance of anaer-obes, mainly *Prevotella*, *Fusobacterium*, and *Peptostreptococcus*, whereas aerobic bacteria predominate in acute rhinosinusitis (e.g., *Streptococcus pneumoniae*, *Haemophilus influenzae*, and *Moraxella catarrhalis*) (Hamilos, 2000). Although hundreds of species of bacteria can inhabit the oral and nasal passages, to our knowledge no systematic study has sought to identify those forms most likely to damage the olfactory system. Hence, the little we know about bacterial influences on olfaction comes from clinical cases in which smell loss occurs during specific bacteria-related disorders.

Case report 3.1: Postviral anosmia in a previously healthy elderly woman

An 84-year-old woman presented with loss of smell for the preceding six months. The loss was first observed while attending a church social function, when she noted that her sense of smell seemingly "disappeared overnight." She distinctly remembers having contracted a severe upper respiratory infection of three weeks' duration just prior to the smell problem. General health was excellent and the only prescription medication was for esophageal reflux disorder.

The UPSIT score was within the anosmic range (15/40). Performance on the 12-item Odor Memory Test was at chance level (left: 4/12; 10-s delay: 1/4; 30-s delay: 1/4; 60-s delay: 2/4); right: 5/12; 10-s delay: 0/4; 30-s delay: 3/4; 60-s delay: 2/4). Interestingly, the detection threshold values for the rose-like odorant phenyl ethyl alcohol were within normal limits (L: −6.58; R: −6.36; B: −6.75; all values log vol/vol in USP grade light mineral oil). Nasal cross-sectional area, as measured by acoustic rhinometry, and nasal resistance, calculated by anterior rhinomanometry, were normal. The percent correct identification of whole-mouth suprathreshold sweet, sour, bitter, and salty tastant concentrations (sucrose, citric acid, caffeine, and NaCl) was low, reflecting difficulties in identifying nonsweet stimuli (21/40; 53 percent). Intensity and pleasantness ratings given to the five concentrations of each of the test stimuli (citric acid, sodium chloride, sucrose, caffeine) were generally monotonic and unremarkable. Anterior (cranial nerve (CN) VII) and posterior (CN IX) regional tongue tests revealed no marked L:R asymmetries, although performance was depressed for citric acid and caffeine in most quadrants. Electrogustometric thresholds on the anterior left and right sides of the tongue were also normal. At the time of testing, cognitive function was excellent (Mini-Mental Status Examination: 30/30) and she exhibited no significant depression (Beck Depression Inventory Score = 8).

Comment: This woman had experienced considerable loss of smell function, most likely secondary to viral infection. The normal olfactory threshold values are atypical, suggesting that some rudimentary ability to detect low concentrations of the target stimulus remained, or that the trigeminal nerve was sensitized to detecting this agent. The decrease in taste function largely reflected alterations in the ability to differentiate clearly salty, sour, and bitter substances, a common finding in many otherwise healthy elderly people. The prospects of regaining useful smell function in this patient are poor because of her age and the severity of loss when tested six months after the infection.

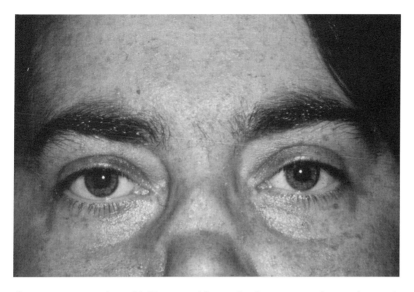

Figure 3.3 Depressed nasal bridge caused by erosion from Wegener's granulomatosis.

Although rare in Europe and North America, leprosy (Hansen's disease) provides a relatively straightforward example of a bacterial-induced chemosensory disturbance. This is a chronic granulomatous infection caused by *Mycobacterium leprae*, a bacterium related to *Mycobacterium tuberculosis*. Although many believe that fewer than 50 percent of people with this disorder have smell dysfunction, a recent study of 77 afflicted patients with mild (tuberculoid, $n = 9$) to severe (borderline, $n = 42$; lepromatous, $n = 26$) forms found all patients exhibited some degree of olfactory dysfunction when tested quantitatively (Mishra *et al.*, 2006). It is unclear how this bacterium alters smell function, although the organism is known to have a predilection for cooler facial areas and the nasal cavity is characteristically $1°C$ below body temperature. Damage to the receptor membrane is a likely mechanism and as the disease advances, intranasal swelling, ulceration, perforation, and cartilaginous collapse occur. A number of other diseases associated with granulomata, such as congenital syphilis, sarcoidosis, lupus, and Wegener's granulomatosis, are associated with decreased smell function (Alobid *et al.*, 2004). Many of the latter granulomatous disorders, but classically congenital syphilis, may produce a characteristic "saddle-nose" deformity (Figure 3.3). In immunocompromised or diabetic patients, fungal infections such as aspergillosis or mucormycosis may grow within the nose or sinuses, sometimes producing ball-like masses within these structures that result in severe olfactory impairment.

By far the most common cause of anosmia from inflammatory disease is pathology in the nose or sinuses as described above, but on rare occasion

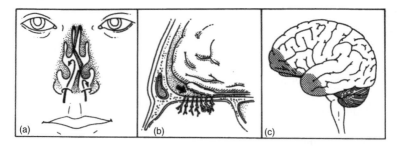

Figure 3.4 Mechanisms of traumatic olfactory dysfunction: (a) Injury to sinonasal tract; (b) tearing of the olfactory nerves; (c) cortical contusions and hemorrhage. (Reproduced from Costanzo *et al.*, 1995. With permission.)

systemic inflammatory disease such as autoimmune vasculitis (e.g., systemic lupus erythematosis (SLE); giant cell arteritis (GCA)) has been linked to smell dysfunction. The mechanism is presumably ischemia in the peripheral olfactory structures, because the vasa nervorum of the olfactory bulb and nasal neuroepithelium derive their blood supply from the anterior and posterior ethmoid arteries, which are tributaries of the ophthalmic branch of the internal carotid artery. There are single-case reports of smell impairment due to Churg–Strauss syndrome (Ros Ruiz *et al.*, 2003), GCA (Schon, 1988), and lymphocytic hypophysitis (Lee *et al.*, 2004). The true frequency of smell impairment in vasculitis is almost certainly underestimated simply because no one bothers to test it. Theoretically hyposmia in someone suspected to suffer from GCA would indicate disease in the ophthalmic artery, and this observation might alert the clinician to pending visual loss.

Head trauma

Head injury is a relatively common cause of smell dysfunction. The various sites of potential damage are shown in Figure 3.4. In neurological practice, the smell loss is usually attributed to shearing of the olfactory nerve fibers as they emerge from the cribriform plate to enter the overlying olfactory bulb (Jafek *et al.*, 1989). In the initial stages there may be temporary anosmia from local trauma (swelling, fracture) of the sinonasal tract. This usually resolves in a few months. To produce posttraumatic anosmia or hyposmia, the skull does not need to be fractured (Delank & Fechner, 1996); a blow to the head or strong acceleration forces, e.g., whiplash (Kramer, 1983), may be sufficient to cause dysfunction – a point of considerable relevance in medicolegal work. According to traditional wisdom, anosmia is most likely to ensue if the front or back or the head is struck rather than the sides (Sumner, 1976), because the opportunity for shearing forces on the frontal lobes is greater with antero-posterior injury. In a detailed study of 179 head-injured patients, occipital and side impact caused most damage and frontal the least (Doty *et al.*, 1997c). Intracranial hemorrhage per se can result in anosmia and, on rare occasions, ageusia (taste loss) or hypogeusia (decreased taste) as well. Beyond lesions of the olfactory receptor cell axons, disorders associated with posttraumatic anosmia are usually located in the temporal lobes. Recent functional imaging studies (single photon emission computer tomography (SPECT) and positron emission tomography (PET)) suggest that in some cases the orbitofrontal cortex is underperfused. A number of such patients exhibit other types of frontal lobe dysfunction, such as changes in executive functioning (Varney & Bushnell, 1998; Varney *et al.*, 2001).

Prevalence estimates of traumatic anosmia or hyposmia vary considerably. If olfactory assessment is undertaken within the first few weeks of injury, local nasal swelling can result in conductive anosmia, a disorder that may reverse when the edema improves. Studies that have not allowed for this may report a falsely high level of posttraumatic anosmia. Where there are large numbers of patients not specifically seeking help for their olfactory condition, the reported prevalence rate ranges from 5 percent to 15 percent. For example, in a study of 355 consecutive, mostly, male head-injured patients (mean age 45 years) presenting mainly because of posttraumatic dizziness, the prevalence rate was 13.7 percent (Ogawa & Rutka, 1999). The majority of these cases were referred from a Workers' Compensation Board and the average time from accident to evaluation was 40 months, so early-stage anosmia was not an issue. When there is cerebrospinal fluid rhinorrhea, typically after skull base injury, the prevalence rises to around 30 percent (Sumner, 1976). Regrettably, most of these surveys have not employed sound quantitative olfactory tests. In the study by Ogawa and Rutka (1999), for example, compounds that may costimulate the trigeminal nerve, such as essence of cloves, camphor, peppermint, and wintergreen, were employed. This could result in an underestimate of the true frequency of odor loss. Studies from clinics that specialize in smell and taste disorders report higher rates of olfactory dysfunction, reflecting in part the greater application of sensitive quantitative tests and the fact that patients who are evaluated come to them specifically seeking medical help and evaluation for their condition (Deems *et al.*, 1991). For these reasons, prevalence estimates from such studies may not apply to the population at large.

As might be expected, the prospect of recovery from posttraumatic anosmia is a function of many variables, including the age of the patient at the time of the insult, severity of trauma, and the elapsed time since injury. When the loss is solely caused by nasal swelling, function returns within a few months at most. Patients amnesic for more than seven days have the poorest outlook according to Sumner (1976). In another study of initial features in 268 head trauma patients presenting to a smell and taste center for evaluation,

67 percent had anosmia, 20 percent microsmia, and only 13 percent had a normal sense of smell (Doty *et al.*, 1997c). The prevalence of parosmia was 41 percent, but it decreased to 15 percent over eight years. Recovery was equally poor: of 66 patients who could be contacted for retesting, 36 percent improved slightly, 45 percent were unchanged, and 18 percent had worsened. Only three patients (5 percent) recovered to normal from initial anosmia. Since this study concerned patients in a specialized referral center, more severe cases were likely to be represented. Recently, it was shown that the prognosis for recovery in anosmic patients depends on the severity rather than the type of initial injury (London *et al.*, 2008). This is probably true in head injury as long as the cortex is not damaged. On basic principles, one would expect a poorer prognosis where there is cortical involvement.

One reason for poor recovery of olfactory function in cases of head trauma relates to the development of scar tissue at the level of the cribriform plate, thereby blocking entry of regenerating olfactory receptor axons into the olfactory bulb (Jafek *et al.*, 1989). In rare cases, traumatic lesions in the frontal and temporal cortices produce centrally based dysfunction; consequently, the prospect of recovery is less (see Figure 3.4). In severe cases, both peripheral and central lesions are present and the olfactory bulbs, devoid of input from olfactory receptor cells, will regress in size over time (Yousem *et al.*, 1996b). Measurement of olfactory bulb volume may be of value in supporting symptom claims of a patient, in particular in cases of litigation, although considerable variation is present in normal bulb volume and the time course of such changes is not well documented. The outlook for patients with head injury and other common disorders of olfaction is summarized in Table 3.2.

If the prefrontal cortex is damaged from head injury, then a dysexecutive syndrome may result and impairment of smell (and taste), which have secondary and tertiary cortical representation in the orbitofrontal region, could provide a marker of such disorder and perhaps offer guidance on the prospect of return to work. If a computed tomography (CT) brain scan or routine magnetic resonance imaging (MRI) is performed, small petechial lesions of the frontal lobes (and temporal polar region) may be overlooked but they may be seen on an MRI gradient echo sequence, which is sensitive to hemosiderin deposits (see Figure 3.5, right). Up to 93 percent of patients with anosmia attributed to closed head injury may be vocationally dysfunctional from orbitofrontal damage, according to two studies (Martzke *et al.*, 1991; Varney, 1988). However, these studies were based on patients referred for cognitive, not olfactory problems, and quantitative olfactory testing was not performed. A quite different result was obtained in 15 patients with documented posttraumatic smell loss secondary to mild–moderate closed head injury who presented to University of Pennsylvania Smell and Taste Center for assessment (Correia *et al.*, 2000). Although about half were upset

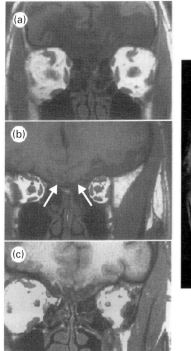 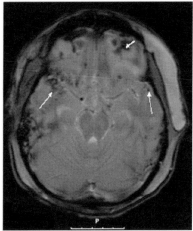

Figure 3.5 *Left images*: Magnetic resonance imaging (MRI) images of posttraumatic injury to the olfactory apparatus. Coronal T1-weighted images in three cases of varying degrees of severity; (a) this shows complete destruction of the inferior frontal lobes, resulting from a major road traffic accident and was associated with anosmia; (b) in this patient there is inferior frontal encephalomalacia, and the patient was microsmic, although the olfactory tracts are visible (arrows); (c) this patient had posttraumatic anosmia with no visible olfactory bulb or tract on the left and just a fragment of a tract on the right (arrowed). Both frontal lobes were sheared. (Reproduced from Yousem *et al.*, 2001. With permission from Elsevier.) *Right image*: Gradient echo axial MRI images from another case of severe head injury that show multiple areas of petechial hemorrhage (small round black areas), mainly in the frontal and temporal poles (long white arrows). The short white arrow in the left frontal region indicates traumatic hemorrhagic contusion in the orbitofrontal cortex, which would probably have damaged the tertiary (orbitofrontal) olfactory cortex. (Copyright © 2007, Christopher Hawkes.)

by the impact of hyposmia on their quality of life, only one had difficulty resuming their former occupation. Thus, smell loss, when taken in isolation, does not appear to be a good predictor of vocational disability. Examples of MRI changes in various degrees of head injury are shown in Figure 3.5.

Case report 3.2: Posttraumatic anosmia

A 56-year-old woman fell on ice in her driveway, striking the back of her head on the ground and suffering brief disorientation but no amnesia. A few days later she discovered smell impairment, and soon thereafter experienced distortions of smell and taste. Routine CT and MRI assessments proved negative. She received a course of systemic steroids without benefit. The UPSIT score was 17/40; bilateral, left, and right detection threshold scores on the phenyl ethyl alcohol detection threshold test were indicative of anosmia, as was the chance performance on the 12-item Odor Memory Test. Nasal airway patency assessed by anterior rhinomanometry and nasal airflow resistance measured by acoustic rhinometry were normal. Scores on a series of taste tests were normal, as were scores on the Mini-Mental State Examination and the Beck Depression Inventory II.

Comment: This is a classical case of trauma-induced bilateral anosmia, unaccompanied by true taste loss. The dysfunction likely reflects contrecoup movement of the brain and the resulting shearing of olfactory filaments at the level of the cribriform plate. The smell and taste "distortions" most likely are due to decreased flavor sensations secondary to lack of retronasal olfactory stimulation and the possible presence of a few aberrant olfactory nerve fibers that are still active.

Case report 3.3: Posttraumatic anosmia in a chef

A 38-year-old chef reported that six months previously he had been knocked to the ground by a van, hitting the back of his head. He was unconscious for one hour, amnesic for two hours, and took one week off work. During this first week he developed headache, positional vertigo, and reduced ability to smell. The smell defect was continuous, with no improvement at any time of the day. On testing, the Mini-Mental State Examination score was normal at 30/30, but the UPSIT score was in the severe microsmic range (21/40). The olfactory event-related potential (OERP) to 2 ppm H_2S was delayed at 1200 ms (position Pz).

Comment: The diagnosis was posttraumatic severe microsmia. The delay on OERP confirms the patient's report and identification test findings, and would provide useful evidence if there was a Court hearing. Given that he worked as a chef, there would likely be litigation and a high compensation fee, depending on the degree of recovery and difficulty at work. Although some return of function may occur over time, it is unlikely that normal smell function would be regained.

Table 3.3 Drugs reported to interfere with olfaction, with some examples

Drug group	Examples
Calcium channel-blocker	Nifedipine, amlodipine, diltiazem
Lipid-lowering	Cholestyramine, clofibrate, statins
Antibiotic and antifungal	Streptomycin, doxycycline, terbinafine
Anti-thyroid	Carbimazole
Opiate	Codeine, morphine, cocaine (snorted)
Antidepressant	Amitriptyline
Sympathomimetic	Dexamphetamine, phenmetrazine
Antiepileptic	Phenytoin
Nasal decongestant	Phenylephrine, pseudoephedrine, oxymetazoline (long-term use probably required for damage)
Miscellaneous	Smoking, argyria (topical application of silver nitrate), cadmium fumes, phenothiazines, pesticides, influenza vaccine, Betnesol-N
Organic solvents	See Table 3.4 (p. 131)

Exposure to medication or airborne toxins

Certain medications, as well as chronic exposure to airborne agents, can result in "toxic anosmia or hyposmia," since these are caused by direct or indirect effects of the environment on an exposed host. They are of considerable relevance to clinical and medicolegal practice as many instances relate to exposure at work or from the unwanted effects of prescribed medication.

Medication

Among the major systemic causes of chemosensory disturbances of which the clinician should be aware are those related to the use of medication (Table 3.3) (for review, see Doty *et al.*, 2008). Many drugs interfere with the ability to smell, although taste is affected more frequently (Doty *et al.*, 2008). Unfortunately, most reports of drug-related alterations are case studies relying on patient self-report with no quantitative testing. Considering how many patients (and clinicians) confuse the two modalities, alleged associations should be viewed with circumspection. It must also be considered that any disease for which a drug is given, e.g., diabetes or hypothyroidism, may be the cause of smell dysfunction, rather than the drug itself.

Drugs known to affect chemosensation (Table 3.3) based on olfactory measurement (rather than anecdotal reporting) include calcium channel-blockers, antibiotics, anti-thyroid drugs, opiates, antidepressants, and sympathomimetics. Some lipid-lowering drugs may cause hyposmia (although taste impairment is more common), possibly acting by altering myelin formation or other lipid-related processes associated with neural transduction in the olfactory pathways (Doty et al., 2003) Antiviral and antifungal drugs may also influence smell in this fashion. Again, they are much more likely to impair the taste than smell (Doty & Haxel, 2005). As mentioned earlier sudden withdrawal of benzodiazepines or antidepressants has been reported to produce hyperosmia (Mourad et al., 1998; Pelissolo & Bisserbe, 1994), although this phenomenon has not been verified by olfactory testing. Several drugs produce volatiles that arise from lung air to stimulate the olfactory receptors, whereas others influence neural or synaptic transmission. Snorted recreational drugs, e.g., cocaine, are sometimes associated with anosmia because of destruction to the olfactory epithelium, although it is likely that the risk for smell loss in this group has been overstated and permanent smell loss is unusual (Gordon et al., 1990). Nasal decongestants and antiviral drugs (e.g., zinc-containing nasal sprays) are alleged on dubious scientific grounds to cause hyposmia, but they have resulted in high-profile lawsuits. It is not clear in most such cases whether the underlying viral infection or the medication is the basis of the problem.

Airborne toxins

Numerous airborne compounds are alleged to cause anosmia. The majority of exposure occurs at work and inevitably promotes lawsuits (for reviews. see Amoore, 1986; Doty & Hastings, 2001). A wide range of agents has been linked to smell loss after acute exposure, with some prospect of recovery. Among such agents are formaldehyde, hydrogen cyanide, hydrogen selenide, hydrogen sulfide, hydrogen selenide, n-methylformimino-methylester, sulfuric acid, and zinc sulfate. Compounds reportedly linked to permanent anosmia following acute exposure include pepper and cresol powder, phosphorus oxychloride, and sulfur dioxide gas.

In common with drug exposure and smell impairment, many alleged instances of olfactory loss due to airborne agents are single-case studies and usually patients' symptomatic reports have been relied on in the absence of formal olfactory testing. However, there is convincing evidence, some of which is quantitative, that chronic exposure to the xenobiotics listed in Table 3.4 has the potential to damage the olfactory system permanently. Certain occupations and manufacturing processes have been associated with loss of smell function, most often those associated with exposure to airborne dusts or aerosolized heavy metals (e.g., welders working without respiratory protection within confined spaces; Antunes et al., 2007).

In an extensive study of occupational exposure to specific volatile chemicals, Schwartz et al. (1989) administered the UPSIT to 731 workers with

Table 3.4 List of compounds alleged to cause some impairment of olfaction

Exposure history		Suspected causal agents
Acute with some prospect of recovery		Formaldehyde, hydrogen cyanide, hydrogen selenide, hydrogen sulfide, hydrogen selenide, n-methylformimino-methyl ester, sulfuric acid, and zinc sulfate
Acute with poor prognosis		Pepper and cresol powder, phosphorus oxychloride, sulfur dioxide gas
Chronic exposure	Metals	Chromium, lead, mercury, nickel, silver, zinc, cadmium, and manganese; either as base metals or salts
	Dusts	Cement, lime, printing powders, and silicon dioxide
	Non-metallic inorganic compounds	Carbon disulfide, carbon monoxide, chlorine hydrazine, nitrogen dioxide, ammonia, sulfur dioxide, and various fluorides
	Organic compounds	Acetophenone, benzene, chloromethane, acrylates, pentachlorophenol, and trichloroethylene

Note: In many instances, the documentation is based on small numbers and the subject's subjective experience has been reported in the absence of formal testing. (Adapted with permission from Amoore, 1986.)

occupational exposure histories at a chemical facility that manufactured acrylates and methacrylates. A nested case–control study designed to evaluate the cumulative effects of exposure revealed elevated crude exposure odds ratios of 2.0 for all workers and 6.0 for workers who never smoked cigarettes, suggesting a protective effect of smoking. Logistic regression, adjusting for multiple confounders, revealed exposure odds ratios of 2.8 and 13.5, respectively, in these same groups. A dose–response relationship between olfactory dysfunction and cumulative exposure scores was observed. Decreasing exposure odds ratios with increasing duration since last exposure suggested that the effects were, to some extent, reversible. Similar observations were made by the same group in a study of olfactory function among paint-manufacturing workers, where once more, nonsmokers paradoxically scored lower on the UPSIT than smokers, suggesting that smoking may be protective (Schwarz *et al.*, 1990).

On occasion, welders develop an extrapyramidal syndrome characterized by rest tremor with some similarity to classical PD. The likely toxin is manganese, and exposure to this in welders involved with maintenance of the San Francisco Bay Bridge was studied recently (Antunes *et al.*, 2007). In 43 bridge welders matched for age, years of education, and smoking, it was found that UPSIT scores were significantly impaired relative to matched control subjects, affecting 37/43 (88 percent) of the exposed group. Paradoxically, blood levels of manganese were inversely associated with the smell deficit, so that those in the highest tertile had lower UPSIT scores than those in the lowest tertile. The reason for this observation is not clear.

Case report 3.4: Loss of smell and taste in an industrial painter

A 48-year-old worker presented with complaint of loss and distortion of smell and taste. This problem occurred after transfer to the painting area of an automobile plant, where he had worked for approximately one year. For most of this time appropriate inhalation protection was not used, and the patient eventually experienced frequent nosebleeds, long bouts of coughing, and flu-like symptoms. The non-chemosensory symptoms resolved when he stayed at home, receiving disability benefit for a broken leg, but smell function never returned, despite treatment with antibiotics, systemic corticosteroids, and antihistamines. The UPSIT score was at chance level (11/40), as were tests of odor detection threshold (bilateral, left or right >−2.00 log vol/vol) and odor memory (8/24). The taste test scores were also diminished slightly, and he exhibited a low score on the Mini-Mental State Examination (25/30). Nasal cross-sectional area, assessed by acoustic rhinometry, and nasal resistance, as measured by anterior rhinomanometry, were within normal limits.

Comment: This patient experienced marked impairment of smell function, and possibly some loss of true taste function, secondary to exposure to paint, solvents, and other volatiles at the workplace. His cognitive function may have been impaired as well, although more sophisticated cognitive testing would be needed to verify this. The complaint of loss and distortion of taste and smell mainly reflects the olfactory deficit, which alters the flavor sensation derived from retronasal stimulation of the olfactory receptors during chewing and swallowing.

Tumors

The ability to smell may be diminished or lost when the nose is invaded by various tumors. Where olfaction is spared prior to surgical treatment or radiotherapy, there is considerable risk of iatrogenic anosmia or hyposmia (Ho *et al.*, 2002). Malignant disease can involve the ethmoid or sphenoid sinuses, and may lead to bacterial infection secondary to poor mucociliary clearance. Lymphoma may also invade the nasal passages or sinuses.

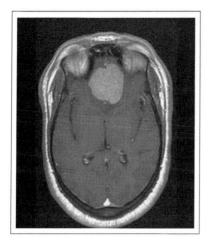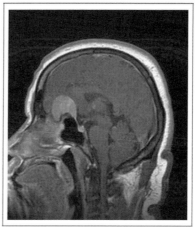

Figure 3.6 Coronal T1-weighted magnetic resonance imaging (MRI) brain scan to show a large olfactory groove meningioma.

Nasopharyngeal carcinoma or adenocystcarcinoma are the more frequent epithelial neoplastic lesions within the nose.

A number of tumors of the CNS also alter smell function. Much of our current knowledge dates back to the classic observations of Elsberg (1935a), who stated, "The olfactory bulbs and tracts lie in a situation in which they can and must be affected by changes in intracranial pressure. Their function must be disturbed early by tumors in their neighborhood. Thus the meningioma which arise from the dura of the cribriform plate and the parts adjacent to it, pituitary growths if they extend above the diaphragm of the sella turcica, and tumors on the floor of or inside the third ventricle must interfere to a greater or less extent with the afferent impulses which pass through the bulbs and tracts. If sufficiently sensitive tests of olfaction were devised, slight disturbances of the functions of the olfactory bulbs and tracts should be recognizable." In fact, Elsberg found that subfrontal meningiomas were recognizable relatively early, by raised threshold to blast injection testing. This involved quantifying the amount of odorized air needed to be injected to produce a smell sensation, a procedure little used nowadays because of potential co-stimulation of the trigeminal nerves.

An olfactory groove meningioma is the most common benign intracranial tumor that impairs the ability to smell, and this is caused by pressure on the olfactory bulb or tract (Figure 3.6). Theoretically an olfactory groove meningioma could damage the overlying orbitofrontal cortex and produce additional central olfactory defects. In the early phase of tumor growth, anosmia, if present, is seldom detected as the patient rarely notices unilateral

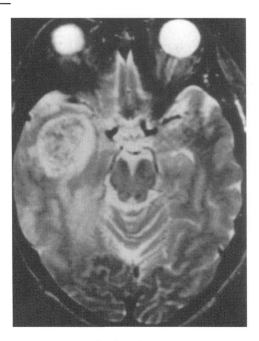

Figure 3.7 T2-weighted axial magnetic resonance imaging (MRI) scan to show a large right temporal pole tumor (glioma) that was causing uncinate attacks.

deficits and the clinician, if he tests smell at all, is unlikely to examine each nostril individually. Smell impairment is also associated with parasellar aneurysms (e.g., internal carotid and anterior communicating), downward expansion of the third ventricle due to hydrocephalus, and meningiomas arising from the anterior clinoid process, sphenoid ridge, or suprasellar region (Murphy *et al.*, 2003). Rarely, inferior frontal malignant tumors produce anosmia from pressure on the bulb or tracts, although such tumors result in prolonged adaptation on the side of the tumor (Elsberg, 1935b). The Foster Kennedy syndrome is characterized by an ipsilateral central scotoma, optic atrophy, and anosmia with contralateral papilledema. If there is a structural cause it is classically a large frontal neoplasm, but other lesions include meningioma of the olfactory groove or the medial third of the sphenoid wing or abscess. In practice, the Foster Kennedy syndrome is rare. It is mimicked sometimes by longstanding anterior ischemic optic atrophy on one side and more recent ischemia on the contralateral side, causing disk swelling suggestive of raised intracranial pressure – the so-called pseudo-Foster Kennedy syndrome.

A major malignancy associated with olfactory dysfunction, notably phantosmia, is the temporal lobe glioma (Figure 3.7) that produces uncinate fits as described earlier. Because the tumor is unilateral and many temporal lobe functions are duplicated contralaterally, it may achieve a large size before clinical presentation, particularly if it involves the side non-dominant for language. Ablation of the right temporal lobe is associated with impaired olfactory discrimination (Zatorre & Jones-Gotman, 1991), and defects in olfactory discrimination occur in subjects with right (smell-dominant) temporal lobe tumors. Such effects are reportedly less obvious in tumors confined to the left temporal lobe (Daniels *et al.*, 2001).

Endocrine disease

Endocrine disorders are rarely responsible for smell dysfunction, but changes have been reported in Addison's disease (where enhancement may occur), Cushing syndrome, diabetes, myxoedema, hypoparathyroidism, pseudo-hypoparathyroidism, and Turner syndrome (for review, see Murphy *et al.*, 2003). In a preliminary survey of nine Turner syndrome patients, abnormal smell function was reported to be present in the mothers (Henkin, 1967), a finding that, if confirmed by others, might assist genetic counseling. Kallman syndrome is typically an X-linked neuronal migration disorder with endocrine deficiency and anosmia, but autosomal dominant and recessive forms are recognized. The gene responsible for the typical X-linked form, KAL1, encodes a protein that plays a key role in the migration of gonadotrophin-releasing hormone (GRH) neurons and olfactory nerves to the hypothalamus (Tsai & Gill, 2006). It is usually associated with complete anosmia owing to aplasia of the olfactory bulb and tracts in association with hypogonadism (Yousem *et al.*, 1996a). Transmitting females often have partial or complete anosmia. In the related condition of congenital maldevelopment of the optic and septal areas (septo-optic aplasia), there is also anosmia and endocrine deficiency (de Morsier, 1962).

Migraine

Sufferers of migraine will occasionally report that an attack is provoked by exposure to certain odors. The triggers are usually of the intense variety, such as gasoline, acetone, or strong perfume (Kelman, 2004a). Olfactory hallucinations, usually unpleasant, may occur as part of the aura, although this is rare, affecting only four of 551 migraineurs in one study (Kelman, 2004a). In this series, osmophobia was a frequent complaint during the attack, involving more than one-quarter of the patients, most of whom were female (Kelman, 2004b). Apart from precipitating migraine, smells may aggravate the headache, a finding that led to the suggestion that odors might be used to distinguish tension from migraine headache (Spierings *et al.*, 2001). Hyperosmia is reported on rare occasions, and claimed to persist in some patients beyond the headache phase (Blau & Solomon, 1985). Interictal hyperosmia, as measured by thresholds to vanillin and acetone, was described in a group of 20 migraine sufferers (Snyder & Drummund, 1997). This finding is in accord with reports that migraine sufferers are hypersensitive to sensory stimuli in general, including smell, taste, light, touch, and sound. In contrast to these observations, Hirsch (1992) found elevated olfactory detection thresholds to pyridine in 12/67 (18 percent) migraineurs, compared with just 1 percent of the general population (Hirsch, 1992), and suggested there was in fact an olfactory defect in migraine. These conflicting results indicate the need for further study, employing strict criteria for the diagnosis of headache and the timing of olfactory assessment in relation to the headache phase.

Epilepsy

Olfactory hallucinations (OHs) may occur at the onset of a seizure, i.e., as an aura, or during the attack itself. Such hallucinations are quite rare in epilepsy as a whole but when epilepsy arises from the temporal lobe, the overall prevalence is about 10 percent (Velakoulis, 2006). One of the earliest descriptions of an OH during an attack, which would now be termed "complex partial seizure" (CPS), was by Hughlings Jackson, who wrote, "In the paroxysm the first thing was tremor of the hands and arms; she saw a little black woman who was always very actively engaged in cooking; the spectre did not speak. The patient had a very horrible smell (so-called subjective sensation of smell) which she could not describe. She had a feeling as if she was shut up in a box with a limited quantity of air . . . she would stand with her eyes fixed . . . and then say 'what a horrible smell!' . . . After leaving her kitchen work she had paroxysms with the smell sensation but no spectre." At autopsy Jackson found a large anterior temporal lobe tumor. Clearly, this growth was irritating the antero-medial temporal lobe and causing the now well-recognized variety of seizure – uncinate epilepsy. In most instances, OHs linked to this condition are unpleasant and difficult to remember or describe in detail. Why this should be is not clear. As explained below, it is thought that most such hallucinations originate in the amygdala rather than the hippocampus (Chen et al., 2003), and that the cause of memory impairment probably results from concurrent disturbance in the nearby hippocampus (Halgren, 1982). Importantly, it is now recognized that the orbitofrontal cortex, an olfactory association area, can also be responsible for seizures that include olfactory illusions, hallucinations, and other autonomic signs or gestural automatisms (Chabolla, 2002).

One of the best-known olfactory disorders for the clinician is the uncinate aura (for review, see West and Doty, 1995). This is an underreported epileptic phenomenon, as patients commonly fail to mention it unless specifically asked, and the nature of the smell is nearly always unpleasant, in keeping with the concept that it is a positive phenomenon resulting from abnormal neuronal discharge rather than a negative phenomenon caused by neuronal inactivity and relative overresponsiveness of adjacent neurons. In one large series of 1423 patients with intractable seizures emanating from the temporal lobe, there were 14 with olfactory auras, lasting 5–30 seconds (Acharya *et al.*, 1998). Five patients had an isolated olfactory aura that did not progress to complex partial seizures (CPS) or generalized attack. The electroencephalogram (EEG) focus was localized to the medial temporal zone in all subjects and more frequently lateralized on the left (9) than on the right (4). Nine patients described the odors as familiar, reporting qualitative sensations of burning, sulfur, alcohol, gas, barbecue, peanut butter, toothpaste, or flowers; five could not identify the smell. Seven thought the odor unpleasant, five were neutral, and two found the smell pleasant and flower-like. Most OHs were associated with other hallucinations: gustatory, epigastric, visual, or psychic (fear, déjà vu). Ten had a medial temporal lobe tumor, of which six involved the amygdala and hippocampus, and two involved the amygdala alone. Thus, OHs probably arise in the amygdala rather than in the uncus, making the term "uncinate attack" a misnomer.

Bilateral amygdala damage results in severe impairment in odor–name matching and odor–odor recognition memory in the absence of impaired auditory verbal learning (Buchanan *et al.*, 2003), confirming that the amygdala plays an important role in odor memory. Irritative processes in this area would therefore cause OHs and this notion is borne out by many reports of such hallucinations from patients with tumors in this area. Conversely, stereotactic lesions of the amygdala alleviate OHs and the accompanying psychiatric disorder (Chitanondh, 1966). Despite this, none of 1132 subjects stimulated by Penfield and Perot (1963), and only one of 75 patients with deep brain electrodes implanted in the temporal or frontal lobes, reported olfactory sensations and that followed left amygdala stimulation (Fish *et al.*, 1993). In general, OHs have good localizing value (to the amygdala), but they are not specific to any particular brain pathology, having been described in medial temporal sclerosis, malignant glioma, and metastatic deposit (Chen *et al.*, 2003). Glioma is probably the most common cause (see Figure 3.7).

Temporal lobe epilepsy is associated with impaired identification, discrimination, and immediate odor memory. Temporal lobe resection studies suggest that such problems are more severe when the lesion is on the right side, although many surgeons remove more right than left temporal lobe tissue for fear of damaging Wernicke's area (Carroll *et al.*, 1993; West & Doty, 1995; Zatorre & Jones-Gotman, 1991). Subjects with CPS have more olfactory impairment than those with generalized epilepsy, and for CPS an olfactory deficit is claimed only when the right (dominant) temporal cortex is affected (Kohler *et al.*, 2001). OERPs show increased latency in those with temporal lesions ipsilateral to the stimulated side (Hummel *et al.*, 1995). Rarely, anticonvulsant drugs such as phenytoin may cause hyposmia (see Table 3.3); conversely, this drug and other antiepileptic medications may be used for treating some cases of dysosmia, phantosmia, and hyperosmia.

An olfactory aura may also result from a lesion in the insular cortex – a brain area also intimately associated with taste function. The hallucination, once more, is usually unpleasant (e.g., gas-like or burning) and may occur in isolation. At other times it is followed by a CPS, a vague dreamy state with disorders of memory and automatic movement. This in turn may progress to a secondary generalized tonic–clonic convulsion.

Although frontal lobe epilepsy may produce hallucinations as described above, it does not appear to cause olfactory impairment, although in theory it might, since resection of the frontal lobes usually impairs odor discrimination, particularly if the excision includes the right orbitofrontal cortex (Jones-Gotman & Zatorre, 1988).

Case report 3.5: Complex partial seizures with olfactory aura

A 59-year-old unemployed man went out drinking heavily one Saturday evening. The next morning, while lying in bed, he experienced a strange smell, like burnt toast. When he looked at the clock, it appeared brighter than normal, he felt slightly dreamy and his right arm began to jerk for a few minutes. There was no loss of consciousness or urinary incontinence. On direct questioning, he recalled there were several isolated episodes of olfactory aura over the preceding six months, but no jerking or loss of consciousness. There were other periods suggestive of déjà vu. He was a nonsmoker but known to abuse alcohol. Physical examination was normal. The UPSIT score was 27/40 (in microsmic range); an MRI brain scan (which included hippocampal views) was unremarkable but the EEG showed intermittent sharp waves and occasional spikes from the left temporal electrodes.

Comment: The history is typical of a CPS with olfactory aura and an epileptic focus in the left temporal zone. It is possible that the main episode was provoked by alcohol withdrawal. The unpleasant smell, which is a positive phenomenon (like the visual enhancement here also), is typical of uncinate attacks – which should be renamed amygdala attacks, as explained. Many patients presenting with a history similar to the above are found to have a temporal lobe glioma or metastasis.

Olfactory reflex epilepsy

This is a rare form of sensory reflex epilepsy, provoked by exposure to strong odors. On EEG it has been demonstrated that the epileptic discharge rate increases in patients with CPS, or that strong odors may induce spike and wave activity in those with absences or tonic–clonic seizures (Stevens, 1962; Takahashi, 1975). Conversely, odorant stimulation has an inhibitory effect on seizure activity in the cat (Ebert & Loscher, 2000), and aromatherapy may help intractable forms of epilepsy (Betts, 2003).

Multiple sclerosis

Initial reports suggested that the olfactory tracts and bulbs were spared in multiple sclerosis (MS), and that this in some way related to the anatomical properties of myelin basic protein (Lumsden, 1983). Early workers were unable to find any plaques in the tract of MS patients (Zimmerman & Netsky, 1950), but subsequently others have shown convincing evidence of demyelination in the olfactory tract (McDonald, 1986; Peters, 1958). Autopsy of the brain in MS characteristically shows widespread demyelination that involves olfactory areas such as the temporal and frontal cortex. Thus it would be amazing if impairment of smell sense were not found – but such defect was not substantiated until relatively recently.

In the first quantitative investigation of 40 MS patients and 24 control subjects there was normal recognition threshold to amyl acetate and nitrobenzene, implying that smell function was spared (Ansari, 1976). Twelve years later Kesslak et al. (1988) reported that both UPSIT values and scores on a match-to-sample discrimination test did not differ significantly between a group of 14 MS patients and 14 control subjects. However, the average age of the MS patients was significantly less than that of control subjects (47 versus 63 years) and there was a preponderance of females in the MS sample – factors that may have contributed to the lack of an effect in this small sample. All other studies using quantitative test procedures have found abnormalities in a significant proportion of patients with MS and, on rare occasion, olfactory dysfunction may be a presenting feature of MS (Bartosik-Psujek et al., 2004; Constantinescu et al., 1994). In an early positive study Pinching (1977) asked 22 MS patients to smell and identify a set of above-threshold odorants, and found that 10 patients (45 percent) exhibited anosmia or hyposmia. An additional five patients (23 percent) had difficulty in describing the odor sensations. Eight of the ten cases with hyposmia or anosmia were only detectable by use of "pure" odorants, which he concluded had minimal or no apparent intranasal trigeminal activity. A subsequent study by Doty et al. (1984) using the UPSIT found microsmia in 7 of 31 (23 percent) MS patients, a ratio not too dissimilar to that reported by Hawkes et al. (1997), who found abnormal UPSIT scores in 11/72 (15 percent) cognitively intact MS patients, as determined by values falling outside the 95 percent confidence interval (95% CI) of their control group.

UPSIT scores fluctuate as a function of the exacerbation and remission of plaque activity (Doty *et al.*, 1998a). Strong inverse correlations between UPSIT scores and the number of MS-related plaques within the frontal and temporal lobes of patients are reported, but not in other brain regions, thus providing a physiological basis for the dysfunction (Doty *et al.*, 1997a, 1998b; Zorzon *et al.*, 2000). Zivadinov *et al.* (1999) assessed B-SIT scores in 40 MS patients and 40 control subjects and found abnormalities in five patients (12.5 percent) and borderline test scores in another four (10 percent). Significant correlations were reported between smell identification test scores and measures of anxiety, depression, and severity of neurological impairment. Only two (5 percent) of the patients were aware of their problem prior to testing.

Abnormal OERPs have also been reported in MS. Using the odorant H_2S, Hawkes *et al.* (1997) found that 6/26 MS patients (23 percent) had a delayed N1 response, and 3 of 26 (12 percent) a delay in the latency of the P2 response. When the largely trigeminal stimulus CO_2 was employed, 5 of 26 patients (19 percent) exhibited latency delays, two for the N1 and three for the P2 responses. Patients with more disability, as measured by the Kurtzke Expanded Disability Status Score, had longer OERP latencies, as well as lower UPSIT scores.

In summary, there is now little doubt that higher-order olfactory processing is altered in a significant number of patients with MS – about 20 percent. Whether odor thresholds are similarly altered is not entirely clear, but given the extent of pathology in advanced cases of MS, elevated thresholds are likely.

Miscellaneous disorders of olfaction

Korsakoff psychosis

This condition is caused by thiamine deficiency usually secondary to malnutrition or chronic alcoholism, and is associated with difficulty in identifying and remembering odors (Gregson *et al.*, 1981; Jones *et al.*, 1975a, b, 1978; Mair *et al.*, 1986). It is possible that olfactory thresholds are unimpaired, although few data are available. How much of their problem relates to cognitive dysfunction (especially memory) is debated; in one study UPSIT scores were impaired, but Picture Identification Test (PIT) scores were normal (Mair *et al.*, 1986). These authors' limited data suggest that the problem may not relate to any defect in olfactory threshold, learning ability, or memory. One possible explanation for this is that the lesions responsible for odor discrimination difficulties lie in the dorsomedial nucleus of the thalamus, an association area for olfactory identification and discrimination with important connections to the orbitofrontal cortex.

Schizophrenia

There are an unusually large number of olfactory studies in schizophrenia (SZ), a situation which has been prompted by the known temporal lobe and limbic system abnormalities, both of which are amenable to smell testing. In brief, the defect is moderate to large with regard to effect size (Cohen's $d = 0.92$), but is less marked than that of Alzheimer's disease (AD) or Parkinson's disease (PD); it occurs relatively early in the illness and is inversely related to duration, raising the possibility that it may be a marker of disease progression (Moberg et al., 1999). This is the case even when allowance is made for variables such as smoking, age, and use of psychotropic medication. UPSIT scores correlate with frontal or temporal dysfunction and negative symptomatology, again reflecting a prefrontal disorder (Moberg et al., 2006). These features were confirmed by functional MRI (fMRI) studies of the peri-rhinal and ento-rhinal cortices (Turetsky et al., 2003a), which also demonstrated reduced olfactory bulb volumes in patients and some outwardly healthy first-degree relatives (Turetsky et al., 2003b).

In general, non-psychotic family members of schizophrenia patients display UPSIT scores intermediate between those from probands and healthy control subjects (Kopala et al., 2001), with over half of the probands and a third of the nonpsychotic family members exhibiting microsmia, in contrast to only about 9 percent of healthy control subjects. In one study of 81 adolescents at high risk of SZ, those who became psychotic exhibited lower baseline UPSIT scores (Brewer et al., 2003). There are unconfirmed reports of olfactory agnosia in male SZ patients (Kopala et al., 1989; Kopala & Clark, 1990), but their reliability is questionable as robust tests of threshold were not undertaken and the word agnosia may have been incorrectly applied.

Miscellaneous causes of anosmia

Superficial siderosis, a chronic basal meningitic process, is caused by recurrent, usually small, hemorrhages on the undersurface of the brain, arising from aneurysms, head injury, or vascular anomalies (Fearnley et al., 1995). Deposition of hemosiderin in the basal meninges most notably damages those cranial nerves with a long glial segment, such as the auditory and olfactory nerves, as well as the olfactory bulbs and tracts. Such patients are often deaf and ataxic, and may be confused with patients showing spino-cerebellar degeneration or mitochondrial disease. The majority have olfactory impairment, a feature that may clinch the diagnosis. In Refsum disease, the typical features are polyneuropathy, ichthyosis, deafness, and retinitis pigmentosa (Wierzbicki et al., 2002). It is less well recognized that most patients with this syndrome are anosmic – thus a patient who presents with impaired vision due to retinitis pigmentosa who is also anosmic most likely has Refsum disease (Gibberd *et al.*, 2004). Impaired smell appreciation is seen on rare occasions as a paraneoplastic disorder in patients with lymphoma or lung cancer (Yu *et al.*, 2001). Lastly, in Sjögren syndrome, where taste disorder is frequent, there may be impairment of smell sense as well (Henkin *et al.*, 1972; Weiffenbach & Fox, 1993). Finally, it has been shown that patients with narcolepsy may have olfactory impairment whether associated with REM-sleep behavior disorder or not. No subject had any extrapyramidal features (Stiasny-Kolster *et al.*, 2007).

Rare genetically determined disorders

In children, there are a variety of rare genetically determined disorders associated with olfactory dysfunction. Among these are Bardet–Biedl syndrome, Aniridia type 2 syndrome, pseudohypoparathyroidism, Kartagener syndrome, DiGeorge syndrome (22q11.2 deletion syndrome), and various forms of congenital anosmia which were described at the beginning of this chapter. *Bardet–Biedl syndrome* is characterized by retinal dystrophy, polydactyly, mental retardation, obesity, and occasionally hyposmia. The condition has several postulated genetic loci, but it is similar to the Laurence–Moon Biedl syndrome. The gene BBS4 may play a role in ciliary motility in the olfactory neuroepithelium (Kulaga *et al.*, 2004) and impaired motility may impair smell function, possibly as the result of bacterial build-up secondary to poor mucociliary clearance (Blacque & Leroux, 2006). *Aniridia type 2*, also a primary visual disorder, is accompanied by the underdevelopment of the iris, usually bilaterally, and severe structural abnormalities of the retina. It has a genetic locus at 11p13. This condition relates to abnormalities in an organizer gene PAX6, but there are less severe forms associated with hyposmia (Sisodiya *et al.*, 2001). *Pseudohypoparathyroidism* is characterized by parathyroid hormone resistance and a paradoxically low blood calcium level. Typical features are short stature, obesity, subcutaneous ossification, and brachydactyly (Spiegel & Weinstein, 2004). It was initially believed that the olfactory dysfunction of pseudohypoparathyroidism was secondary to deficiency in the stimulatory guanine nucleotide-binding protein (Gs-alpha) of adenylcyclase, an enzyme that plays an important role in olfactory transduction. This deficiency is present in the type 1 variety, along with Albright hereditary osteodystrophy, an unusual constellation of skeletal and developmental deficits. However, smell dysfunction was later found in all types of pseudohypoparathyroidism, including those not associated with Gs-alpha deficiency or Albright hereditary osteodystrophy (Doty *et al.*, 1997a). *Kartagener syndrome* comprises bronchiectasis, dextrocardia, infertility, severe headache, and respiratory cilia immotility. Some patients are anosmic, probably because of recurrent sinus infection and olfactory ciliary immotility (Mygind & Pedersen, 1983). The condition is likely to be an incompletely penetrant autosomal recessive disorder. Three loci are known, one of which (9p21-p13) codes for the axonemal dynein complex, a "motor protein" that allows bending movements of cilia. *DiGeorge syndrome* (22q11.2 deletion syndrome) comprises parathyroid and thymic hypoplasia associated with outflow tract defects of the heart, facial dysmorphism, and, in some varieties, velopharyngeal insufficiency. Patients present with neonatal hypocalcemia causing tetany or seizures and susceptibility to infection owing to a deficit of T cells. In the only study of smell function in 62 affected children (Sobin *et al.*, 2006) there was a significant impairment of UPSIT scores compared to controls. Those with velopharyngeal insufficiency did not differ from the classical type of disease. Lastly there is Rett syndrome, an X-linked disorder caused by mutation in the *mecp2* gene that affects mainly females and is characterized, after the age of one year, by loss of speech, stereotyped hand movements, mental retardation, behavioral abnormalities, epilepsy, and episodes of hyperventilation. Olfactory receptor neurons show decreased survival (Ronnett *et al.*, 2003) making it likely such children will have impairment of their sense of smell.

Summary

Olfactory dysfunction manifests in many ways, from mild loss of function to total anosmia, distortion, hallucination or phantosmia, and altered ability to process odorants, including difficulty in smell identification, discrimination, and memory. Excluding neurodegenerative disease (reviewed in Chapter 4), smell loss is most common after exposure to xenobiotics that damage the olfactory membrane, including viruses, bacteria and, less frequently, industrial toxins. A wide range of drugs are alleged to alter smell function, although most impair taste rather than smell. Even minor head injury may cause smell impairment that is usually permanent if present for a long period of time. Variable degrees of smell loss occur in MS, SZ, and a variety of rare genetic disorders. In CPS (temporal lobe epilepsy), there is impairment of identification, discrimination, and immediate odor memory. In about 10 percent of patients with temporal lobe epilepsy, an olfactory aura precedes the attack, the so-called uncinate seizure that is probably a misnomer for amygdala disorder. In migraine, enhancement of olfactory function may develop during the aura and hyperosmia, or at least hyperreactivity, has been reported between episodes.

REFERENCES

Acharya V, Acharya J and Luders H. Olfactory epileptic auras. *Neurology*, 1998, **51**(1), 56–6.

Alobid I, Guilemany JM and Mullol J. Nasal manifestations of systemic illnesses. *Current Allergy and Asthma Reports*, 2004, **4**(3), 208–16.

Amoore JE. Effects of chemical exposure on olfaction in humans. In: CS Barrow, ed., *Toxicology of the Nasal Passages*. Washington, DC: Hemisphere Publishing, 1986, pp. 155–90.

Amoore JE and Steinle S. A graphical history of specific anosmia. In: CJ Wysocki and MR Kare, eds., *Chemical Senses*. Volume 3. *Genetics of Perception and Communications*. New York, NY: Marcel Dekker, Inc., 1991, Chapter 23.

Ansari KA Olfaction in multiple sclerosis. *European Neurology*, 1976, **14**, 138–45.

Antunes M, Bowler RM and Doty RL. San Francisco/Oakland Bay Bridge Welder Study: olfactory function. *Neurology*, 2007, **69**(12), 1278–84.

Bang F, Bang B and Foard M. Responses of upper respiratory mucosa to drugs and viral infections. *American Review of Respiratory Disease*, 1966, **93**, 5142–9.

Bartosik-Psujek H, Psujek M and Stelmasiak Z. Rare first symptoms of multiple sclerosis. *Annales Universitatis Mariae Curie-Sklodowska, Sectio D, Medicina*, 2004, **59**(1), 242–4.

Betts T. Use of aromatherapy (with or without hypnosis) in the treatment of intractable epilepsy – a two-year follow-up study. *Seizure*, 2003, **12**(8), 534–8.

Blacque OE and Leroux MR. Bardet–Biedl syndrome: an emerging pathomechanism of intracellular transport. *Cellular and Molecular Life Sciences*, 2006, **63**(18), 2145–61.

Blau JN and Solomon F. Smell and other sensory disturbances in migraine. *Journal of Neurology*, 1985, **232**(5), 275–6.

Brewer WJ, Wood SJ, McGorry PD *et al.* Impairment of olfactory identification ability in individuals at ultra-high risk for psychosis who later develop schizophrenia. *American Journal of Psychiatry*, 2003, **160**(10), 1790–4.

Brownstein D. Resistance/susceptibility to lethal Sendai virus infection generally linked to a mucociliary transport polymorphism. *Journal of Virology*, 1987, **61**, 1670–1.

Buchanan TW, Tranel D and Adolphs R. A specific role for the human amygdala in olfactory memory. *Learning and Memory*, 2003, **10**(5), 319–25.

Cameron EL. Measures of human olfactory perception during pregnancy. *Chemical Senses*, 2007, **32**, 775–82.

Carroll B, Richardson JT and Thompson P. Olfactory information processing and temporal lobe epilepsy. *Brain and Cognition*, 1993, **22**(2), 230–43.

Chabolla DR. Characteristics of the epilepsies. *Mayo Clinic Proceedings*, 2002, **77**, 981–90.

Chen C, Shih YH, Yen DJ *et al.* Olfactory auras in patients with temporal lobe epilepsy. *Epilepsia*, 2003, **44**(2), 257–60.

Chitanondh H. Stereotaxic amygdalotomy in the treatment of olfactory seizures and psychiatric disorders with olfactory hallucination. *Confinia Neurologica*, 1966, **27**(1), 181–96.

Constantinescu CS, Raps EC, Cohen JA, West SE and Doty RL. Olfactory disturbances as the initial or most prominent symptom of multiple sclerosis. *Journal of Neurology, Neurosurgery, and Psychiatry*, 1994, **57**(8), 1011–2.

Correia S, Faust D and Doty RL. A re-examination of the rate of vocational dysfunction among patients with anosmia and mild/moderate closed head injury. *Journal of Clinical and Experimental Neuropsychology*, 2000, **15**, 1–12.

Costanzo RM, DiNardo LJ and Zasler ND. Head injury and olfaction. In: RL Doty, ed., *Handbook of Olfaction and Gustation*. New York, NY: Marcel Dekker, Inc., 1995, pp. 629–38.

Daniels C, Gottwald B, Pause BM, Sojka B, Mehdorn HM and Ferstl R. Olfactory event-related potentials in patients with brain tumors. *Clinical Neurophysiology*, 2001, **112**(8), 1523–30.

Deems DA, Doty RL and Settle RG *et al.* Smell and taste disorders, a study of 750 patients from the University of Pennsylvania Smell and Taste Center. *Archives of Otolaryngology, Head, and Neck Surgery*, 1991, **117**(5), 519–28.

Delank KW and Fechner G. Pathophysiology of post-traumatic anosmia. *Laryngorhinootologie*, 1996, **75**(3), 154–9.

de Morsier, G. Median cranioencephalic dysraphias and olfactogenital dysplasia. *World Neurology*, 1962, **3**, 485–506.

Doty RL and Bromley SM. Effects of drugs on olfaction and taste. *Otolaryngologic Clinics of North America*, 2004, **37**(6), 1229–54.

Doty RL and Frye R. Influence of nasal obstruction on smell function. *Otolaryngologic Clinics of North America*, 1989, **22**(2), 397–411.

Doty RL and Hastings L. Neurotoxic exposure and olfactory impairment. *Clinics in Occupational and Environmental Medicine*, 2001, **1**, 547–75.

Doty RL and Haxel BR. Objective assessment of terbinafine-induced taste loss. *Laryngoscope*, 2005, **115**, 2035–7.

Doty RL and Izhar M. Can influence vaccinations after smell function? Unpublished manuscript.

Doty RL, Snyder PJ, Huggins GR and Lowry LD. Endocrine, cardiovascular, and psychological correlates of olfactory sensitivity changes during the human menstrual cycle. *Journal of Comparative Physiology and Psychology*, 1981, **95**(1), 45–60.

Doty RL, Shaman P and Dann M. Development of the University of Pennsylvania Smell Identification Test: A standardized microencapsulated test olfactory function. *Physiology and Behavior*, 1984; **32**, 489–502 (monograph).

Doty RL, Deems DA, Frye RE, Pelberg R and Shapiro A. Olfactory sensitivity nasal resistance and autonomic function in patients with multiple chemical sensitivities. *Archives of Otolaryngology, Head, and Neck Surgery*, 1988, **114**, 1422–7.

Doty RL, Li C, Mannon LJ and Yousem DM. Olfactory dysfunction in multiple sclerosis. *New England Journal of Medicine*, 1997a, **336**(26), 1918–19.

Doty RL, Yousem DM, Pham LT, Kreshak AA, Geckle R and Lee WW. Olfactory dysfunction in patients with head trauma. *Archives of Neurology*, 1997b, **54**, 1131–40.

Doty RL, Fernandez AD, Levine MA, Moses A and McKeown DA. Olfactory dysfunction in type I pseudohypoparathyroidism: dissociation from Gs alpha protein deficiency. *Journal of Clinical Endocrinology and Metabolism*, 1997c, **82**(1), 247–50.

Doty RL, Li C, Mannon LJ and Yousem DM. Olfactory dysfunction in multiple sclerosis: relation to longitudinal changes in plaque numbers in central olfactory structures. *Neurology*, 1998a, **53**(4), 880–2.

Doty RL, Li C, Mannon LJ and Yousem DM. Olfactory dysfunction in multiple sclerosis. Relation to plaque load in inferior frontal and temporal lobes. *Annals of the New York Academy of Sciences*, 1998b, **30**(855), 781–6.

Doty RL, Philip S, Reddy K and Kerr K-L. Influences of antihypertensive and antihyperlipid-emic drugs on the senses of taste and smell: a review. *Journal of Hypertension*, 2003, **21**, 1805–13.

Doty RL, Shah M and Bromley SM. Drug-induced taste disorders: incidence, prevention and management. Drug Safety, 2008, 31, 199–215.

Duncan HJ and Smith DV. Clinical disorders of olfaction. In: RL Doty, ed., *Handbook of Olfaction and Gustation*. New York, NY: Marcel Dekker Inc., 1995, pp. 345–66.

Ebert U and Loscher W. Strong olfactory stimulation reduces seizure susceptibility in amygdala-kindled rats. *Neuroscience Letters*, 2000, **287**(3), 199–202.

Elsberg CA. XI. The value of quantitative olfactory tests for the localization of supratentorial tumors of the brain. A preliminary report. *Bulletin of the Neurological Institute of New York*, 1935a, **4**, 511–22.

Elsberg CA. The sense of smell XII. The localization of tumors of the frontal lobe of the brain by quantitative olfactory tests. *Bulletin of the Neurological Institute of New York*, 1935b, **4**, 535–43.

Fadool DA, Tucker K, Perkins R *et al.* Kv1.3 channel gene-targeted deletion produces "Super-Smeller Mice" with altered glomeruli, interacting scaffolding proteins, and biophysics. *Neuron*, 2004, **41**(3), 389–404.

Fearnley JM, Stevens JM and Rudge P. Superficial siderosis of the central nervous system. *Brain*, 1995, **118**(Pt 4), 1051–66.

Fiser Dj and Borotski L. Anosmia after administration of influenza vaccine. *Medicinski Pregled*, 1979, **32**(9–10), 455–7.

Fish DR, Gloor P, Quesney FL and Olivier A. Clinical responses to electrical brain stimulation of the temporal and frontal lobes in patients with epilepsy. Pathophysiological implications. *Brain*, 1993, **116**(Pt 2), 397–414.

Fuller GN and Guiloff RJ. Migrainous olfactory hallucinations. *Journal of Neurology, Neurosurgery, and Psychiatry*, 1987, **50**(12), 1688–90.

Gauntlett-Gilbert J and Kuipers E. Phenomenology of visual hallucinations in psychiatric conditions. *Journal of Nervous and Mental Disease*, 2003, **191**(3), 203–5.

Ghadami M, Morovvati S, Majidzadeh AK *et al.* Isolated congenital anosmia locus maps to 18p11.23-q12.2. *Journal of Medical Genetics* 2004, **41**, 299–303.

Gibberd FB, Feher MD, Sidey MC and Wierzbicki AS. Smell testing: an additional tool for identification of adult Refsum's disease. *Journal of Neurology, Neurosurgery, and Psychiatry*, 2004, **75**(9), 1334–6.

Goetz CG, Vogel C, Tanner CM and Stebbins GT. Early dopaminergic drug-induced hallucinations in parkinsonian patients. *Neurology*, 1998, **51**(3), 811–14.

Gordon AS, Moran DT, Jafek BW, Eller PM and Strahan RC. The effect of chronic cocaine abuse on human olfaction. *Archives of Otolaryngology, Head, and Neck Surgery*, 1990, **116**(12), 1415–18.

Gregson RA, Free ML and Abbott MW. Olfaction in Korsakoffs, alcoholics and normals. *British Journal of Clinical Psychology*, 1981, **20**(Pt 1), 3–10.

Halgren E. Mental phenomena induced by stimulation in the limbic system. *Human Neurobiology*, 1982, **1**(4), 251–60.

Hamilos DL. Chronic sinusitis. *The Journal of Allergy and Clinical Immunology*, 2000, **106**, 213–27.

Hawkes CH and Shephard BC. Selective anosmia in Parkinson's disease? *Lancet*, 1993, **341** (8842), 435–6.

Hawkes CH, Shephard BC and Kobal G. Assessment of olfaction in multiple sclerosis: evidence of dysfunction by olfactory evoked response and identification tests. *Journal of Neurology, Neurosurgery, and Psychiatry*, 1997, **63**(2), 145–51.

Heinrichs L. Linking olfaction with nausea and vomiting of pregnancy recurrent abortion hyperemesis gravidarum and migraine headache. *American Journal of Obstetrics and Gynecology*, 2002, **186**(5 Suppl.), S215–19.

Henkin RI. Abnormalities of taste and olfaction in patients with chromatin negative gonadal dysgenesis. *Journal of Clinical Endocrinology and Metabolism*, 1967, **27**(10), 1436–40.

Henkin RI, Talal N, Larson AL and Mattern CF. Abnormalities of taste and smell in Sjogren's syndrome. *Annals of Internal Medicine*, 1972, **76**(3), 375–83.

Hirsch AR. Olfaction in migraineurs. *Headache*, 1992, **32**(5), 233–6.

Ho WK, Kwong DL, Wei WI and Sham JS. Change in olfaction after radiotherapy for nasopharyngeal cancer – a prospective study. *American Journal of Otolaryngology*, 2002, **23**(4), 209–14.

Hockaday TDR. Hypogonadism and life-long anosmia. *Postgraduate Medical Journal*, 1966, **42**, 572–4.

Hummel T, Pauli E, Schuler P, Kettenmann B, Stefan H and Kobal G. Chemosensory event-related potentials in patients with temporal lobe epilepsy. *Epilepsia*, 1995, **36**(1), 79–85.

Hummel T, Roscher S, Jaumann MP and Kobal G. Intranasal chemoreception in patients with multiple chemical sensitivities: a double-blind investigation. *Regulatory Toxicology and Pharmacology*, 1996, **24**(1 Pt 2), S79–86.

Jafek BW, Eller PM, Esses BA and Moran DT. Post-traumatic anosmia. Ultrastructural correlates. *Archives of Neurology* 1989, **46**(3), 300–4.

Jones BP, Moskowitz RH and Butters N. Olfactory discrimination in alcoholic Korsakoff patients. *Neuropsychologia*, 1975a, **13**(2), 173–9.

Jones BP, Moskowitz HR, Butters N and Glosser G. Psychophysical scaling of olfactory, visual, and auditory stimuli by alchoholic Korsakoff patients. *Neuropsychologia*, 1975b, **13**, 387–93.

Jones BP, Butters N, Moskowitz HR and Montgomery K. Olfactory and gustatory capacities of alcoholic Korsakoff patients. *Neuropsychologia*, 1978, **16**, 323–37.

Jones-Gotman M and Zatorre RJ. Olfactory identification deficits in patients with focal cerebral excision. *Neuropsychologia*, 1988, **26**(3), 387–400.

Joyner RE. Olfactory acuity in an industrial population. *Journal of Occupational Medicine*, 1963, **5**, 37–42.

Kelman L. The premonitory symptoms (prodrome): a tertiary care study of 893 migraineurs. *Headache*, 2004a, **44**(9), 865–72.

Kelman L. Osmophobia and taste abnormality in migraineurs: a tertiary care study. *Headache*, 2004b, **44**(10), 1019–23.

Kern RC. Chronic sinusitis and anosmia: pathologic changes in the olfactory mucosa. *Laryngoscope*, 2000, **110**(7), 1071–7.

Kesslak JP, Cotman CW, Chui HC *et al*. Olfactory tests as possible probes for detecting and monitoring Alzheimer's disease. *Neurobiology of Aging*, 1988, **9**, 399–403.

Kohler CG Moberg PJ Gur RE O'Connor MJ Sperling MR and Doty RL. Olfactory dysfunction in schizophrenia and temporal lobe epilepsy. *Neuropsychiatry, Neuropsychology, and Behavioral Neurology*, 2001, **14**(2), 83–8.

Kopala L and Clark C. Implications of olfactory agnosia for understanding sex differences in schizophrenia. *Schizophrenia Bulletin*, 1990, **16**(2), 255–61.

Kopala L, Clark C and Hurwitz TA. Sex differences in olfactory function in schizophrenia. *American Journal of Psychiatry*, 1989, **146**(10), 1320–2.

Kopala LC, Good KP, Morrison K, Bassett AS, Alda M and Honer WG. Impaired olfactory identification in relatives of patients with familial schizophrenia. *American Journal of Psychiatry*, 2001, **158**(8), 1286–90.

Kramer G. Diagnosis of neurologic disorders after whiplash injuries of the cervical spine. *Deutsche Medizinische Wochenschrrift*, 1983, **108**(15), 586–8.

Kulaga HM, Leitch CC, Eichers ER *et al.* Loss of BBS proteins causes anosmia in humans and defects in olfactory cilia structure and function in the mouse. *Nature Genetics*, 2004, **36**, 994–8.

Lee SJ, Yoo HJ, Park SW and Choi MG. A case of cystic lymphocytic hypophysitis with cacosmia and hypopituitarism. *Endocrine Journal*, 2004, **51**(3), 375–80.

Lehrner J, Baumgartner C, Serles W *et al.* Olfactory prodromal symptoms and unilateral olfactory dysfunction are associated in patients with right mesial temporal lobe epilepsy. *Epilepsia*, 1997, **38**(9), 1042–4.

London B, Nabet B, Fisher AR, White B, Sammel MD and Doty RL. Predictors of prognosis in patients with olfactory disturbance. *Annals of Neurology*, 2008, **63**, 159–66.

Lumsden CE. The neuropathology of multiple sclerosis. In: PJ Vinken and GW Bruyn, eds, *Handbook of Clinical Neurology*. New York, NY: Elsevier, 1983, p. 217.

Lundstrom JN, Hummel T and Olsson MJ. Individual differences in sensitivity to the odor of 4 16-androstadien-3-one. *Chemical Senses*, 2003, **28**(7), 643–50.

Luzzi S, Snowden JS, Neary D, Coccia M, Provinciali L and Lambon Ralph MA. Distinct patterns of olfactory impairment in Alzheimer's disease, semantic dementia, frontotemporal dementia, and corticobasal degeneration. *Neuropsychologia*, 2007, **45**(8), 1823–31.

Lygonis CS. Familiar absence of olfaction. *Hereditas*, 1969, **61**(3), 413–6.

Mainland RC. Absence of olfactory sensation. *Journal of Heredity*, 1945, **36**, 143–4.

Mair RG, Doty RL, Kelly KM *et al.* Multimodal sensory discrimination deficits in Korsakoff's psychosis. *Neuropsychologia*, 1986, **24**(6), 831–9.

Martzke JE, Swan CS and Varney NR. Posttraumatic anosmia and orbital frontal damage: neuropsychological and neuropsychiatric correlates. *Neuropsychology*, 1991, **5**, 213–25.

McDonald WI. The mystery of the origin of multiple sclerosis. *Journal of Neurology, Neurosurgery, and Psychiatry*, 1986, **49**, 113–23.

Mendez MF and Ghajarnia M. Agnosia for familiar faces and odors in a patient with right temporal lobe dysfunction. *Neurology*, 2001, **57**(3), 519–21.

Mishra A, Saito K, Barbash SE, Mishra N and Doty RL. Olfactory dysfunction in leprosy. *Laryngoscope*, 2006, **116**, 413–16.

Moberg PJ, Agrin R, Gur RE, Gur RC, Turetsky BI and Doty RL Olfactory dysfunction in schizophrenia: a qualitative and quantitative review. *Neuropsychopharmacology*, 1999, **21**(3), 325–40.

Moberg PJ, Arnold SE, Doty RL *et al.* Olfactory functioning in schizophrenia: relationship to clinical, neuropsychological, and volumetric MRI measures. *Journal of Clinical and Experimental Neuropsychology*, 2006, **28**, 1444–61.

Mourad I, Lejoyeux M and Ades J. Prospective evaluation of antidepressant discontinuation *Encephale*, 1998, **24**(3), 215–22.

Murphy M, Doty RL and Duncan HJ. Clinical disorders of olfaction. In: RL Doty, ed., *Handbook of Olfaction and Gustation* (2nd edition). New York, NY: Marcel Dekker, 2003, Chapter 22, pp. 461–78.

Mygind N and Pedersen M. Nose- sinus- and ear-symptoms in 27 patients with primary ciliary dyskinesia. *European Journal of Respiratory Diseases*, 1983, **127**(Suppl.), 96–101.

Nordin S, Almkvist O, Berglund B and Wahlund LO. Olfactory dysfunction for pyridine and dementia progression in Alzheimer disease. *Archives of Neurology*, 1997, **54**(8), 993–8.

Ogawa T and Rutka J. Olfactory dysfunction in head injured workers. *Acta Otolaryngologica*, 1999; **540**(Suppl.), 50–7.

Pelissolo A and Bisserbe JC. Dependence on benzodiazepines. Clinical and biological aspects *Encephale*, 1994, **20**(2), 147–57.

Penfield W and Perot P. The brain's record of auditory and visual experience. A final summary and discussion. *Brain*, 1963, **86**, 595–696.

Perlman S, Evans G and Afifi A. Effect of olfactory bulb ablation on spread of a neurotropic coronavirus into the mouse brain. *Journal of Experimental Medicine*, 1990, **172**(4), 1127–32.

Peters G. Multiple sklerose. In: O Lubarsche, F Henke and R Rossle, eds, *Handbuch der Speziellen Pathologischen Anatomie und IIistologie*, Vol XIII. Erkrankungen des Zentralen Nerven Systems. II. Bandtiel A. IV 525–590, 1958.

Pinching AJ. Clinical testing of olfaction reassessed. *Brain*, 1977, **100**, 377–88.

Pryse-Phillips W. An olfactory reference syndrome. *Acta Psychiatrica Scandinavica*, 1971, **47**(4), 484–509.

Pryse-Phillips W. Disturbance in the sense of smell in psychiatric patients. *Proceedings of the Royal Society of Medicine*, 1975, **68**, 472–4.

Reinacher M, Bonin J, Narayan O and Scholtissek C. Pathogenesis of neurovirulent influenza – a virus infection of mice. *Laboratory Investigation*, 1983, **49**, 686–92.

Roalf DR, Turetsky BI, Owzar K *et al.* Unirhinal olfactory function in schizophrenia patients and first-degree relatives. *Journal of Neuropsychiatry and Clinical Neurosciences*, 2006, **18**, 389–96.

Ronnett GV, Leopold D, Cai X *et al.* Olfactory biopsies demonstrate a defect in neuronal development in Rett's syndrome. *Annals of Neurology*, 2003, **54**(2), 206–18.

Ros Ruiz S, Bernardino de la Serna JI, Peiteado Lopez D and Garcia Puig J. Anosmia as presenting symptom of Churg–Strauss syndrome. *Revista Clínica Española*, 2003, **203**(5), 263–4.

Sandyk R. Olfactory hallucinations in Parkinson's disease. *South African Medical Journal*, 1981, **60**(25), 950.

Sayek I. The incidence of the inability to smell solutions of potassium cyanide in the rural health center of Ortabereket. *Turkish Journal of Pediatrics*, 1970, **12**(3), 72–5.

Schon F. Involvement of smell and taste in giant cell arteritis. *Journal of Neurology, Neurosurgery, and Psychiatry*, 1988, **51**(12), 1594.

Schwartz BS, Doty RL, Monroe C, Frye R and Barker S. Olfactory function in chemical workers exposed to acrylate and methacrylates vapors. *American Journal of Public Health*, 1989, **79**(5), 613–18.

Schwartz BS, Ford DP, Bolla KI, Agnew J, Rothman N and Bleecker ML. Solvent-associated decrements in olfactory function in paint manufacturing workers. *American Journal of Industrial Medicine*, 1990, **18**(6), 697–706.

Setzer AK and Slotnick B. Odor detection in rats with 3-methylindole-induced reduction of sensory input. *Physiology and Behavior*, 1998, **65**(3), 489–96.

Sherman AH, Amoore JE and Weigel V. The pyridine scale for clinical measurement of olfactory threshold: a quantitative re-evaluation. *Otolaryngology, Head, and Neck Surgery*, 1979, **87**(6), 717–33.

Siegel RK. Cocaine hallucinations. *American Journal of Psychiatry*, 1978, **135**(3), 309–14.

Silberstein SD, Niknam R, Rozen TD and Young WB. Cluster headache with aura. *Neurology*, 2000, **11**, 54(1), 219–21.

Silveira-Moriyama L, Williams D, Katzenschlager R and Lees AJ. Pizza, mint and licorice: smell testing in Parkinson's disease in a UK population. *Movement Disorders*, 2005, **20**(Suppl. 10), P471 (abstract).

Singh N, Grewal MS and Austin JH. Familial anosmia. *Archives of Neurology*, 1970, **22**, 40–4.

Sisodiya SM, Free SL, Williamson KA *et al.* PAX6 haploinsufficiency causes cerebral malformation and olfactory dysfunction in humans. *Nature Genetics*, 2001, **28**(3), 214–16.

Slotnick B and Bodyak N. Odor discrimination and odor quality perception in rats with disruption of connections between the olfactory epithelium and olfactory bulbs. *Journal of Neuroscience*, 2002, **22**(10), 4205–16.

Snyder RD and Drummond PD. Olfaction in migraine. *Cephalalgia*, 1997, **17**(7), 729–32.

Sobel N, Khan RM, Saltman A, Sullivan EV and Gabrieli JD. The world smells different to each nostril. *Nature*, 1999, **402**(6757), 35.

Sobin C, Kiley-Brabeck K, Dale K, Monk SH, Khuri J and Karayiorgou M. Olfactory disorder in children with 22q11 deletion syndrome. *Pediatrics*, 2006, **118**(3), e697–703.

Spiegel AM and Weinstein LS. Inherited diseases involving g proteins and g protein-coupled receptors. *Annual Review of Medicine*, 2004, **55**, 27–39.

Spierings EL, Ranke AH and Honkoop PC. Precipitating and aggravating factors of migraine versus tension-type headache. *Headache*, 2001, **41**(6), 554–8.

Stevens JR. Central and peripheral factors in epileptic discharge. Clinical studies. *Archives of Neurology*, 1962, **7**, 330–8.

Stiasny-Kolster K, Clever SC, Möller JC, Oertel WH, Mayer G. Olfactory dysfunction in patients with narcolepsy with and without REM sleep behaviour disorder. *Brain*, 2007, **130**(Pt 2), 442–9.

Stroop WG. Viruses and the olfactory system. In: RL Doty, ed. *Handbook of Olfaction and Gustation* (1st edition). New York, NY: Marcel Dekker, 1995, pp. 367–93.

Sugiura M, Aiba T, Mori J and Nakai Y. An epidemiological study of postviral olfactory disorder. *Acta Otolaryngologica*, 1998, **538**(Suppl.), 191–6.

Sumner D. Disturbances of the senses of smell and taste after head injuries. In PJ Vinken and GW Bruyn, eds, *Handbook of Clinical Neurology*, Vol. 24 Injuries of the Brain and Skull Part II. Amsterdam: Elsevier Press, 1976, pp. 1–25.

Takahashi T. Seizures induced by odorous stimuli. *Clinical Electroencephalography*, 1975, **17**, 769.

Tsai PS and Gill JC. Mechanisms of disease: insights into X-linked and autosomal-dominant Kallman syndrome. *National Clinics in Practical Endocrinology and Metabolism*, 2006, **2**(3), 160–71.

Turetsky BI, Moberg PJ, Roalf DR, Arnold SE and Gur RE. Decrements in volume of anterior ventromedial temporal lobe and olfactory dysfunction in schizophrenia. *Archives of General Psychiatry*, 2003a, **60**(12), 1193–200.

Turetsky BI, Moberg PJ, Arnold SE, Doty RL and Gur RE. Low olfactory bulb volume in first-degree relatives of patients with schizophrenia. *American Journal of Psychiatry*, 2003b, **160**(4), 703–8.

Varney NR. Prognostic significance of anosmia in patients with closed-head trauma. *Journal of Clinical and Experimental Neuropsychology*, 1988, **10**, 250–4.

Varney NR and Bushnell D. NeuroSPECT findings in patients with posttraumatic anosmia: a quantitative analysis. *Journal of Head Trauma Rehabilitation*, 1998, **13**(3), 63–72.

Varney NR, Pinkston JB and Wu JC. Quantitative PET findings in patients with posttraumatic anosmia. *Journal of Head Trauma Rehabilitation*, 2001, **16**(3), 253–9.

Velakoulis D. Olfactory hallucinations. In: W Brewer, D Castle and C Pantelis, eds, *Olfaction and the Brain*. Cambridge, UK: Cambridge University Press, 2006, pp. 322–33.

Weiffenbach JM and Fox PC. Odor identification ability among patients with Sjogren's syndrome. *Arthritis and Rheumatism*, 1993, **36**(12), 1752–4.

West SE and Doty RL. Influence of epilepsy and temporal lobe resection on olfactory function. *Epilepsia*, 1995, **36**(6), 531–42.

Wierzbicki AS, Lloyd MD, Schofield CJ, Feher MD and Gibberd FB. Refsum's disease: a peroxisomal disorder affecting phytanic acid alpha-oxidation. *Journal of Neurochemistry*, 2002, **80**(5), 727–35.

Yamamoto K, Ito K and Yamaguchi, M. A family showing smell disturbance and tremor. *Japanese Journal of Human Genetics*, 1966, **11**, 36–8.

Yousem DM, Geckle RJ, Bilker WB, McKeown DA and Doty RL. Posttraumatic olfactory dysfunction: MR and clinical evaluation. *American Journal of Neuroradiology*, 1996a, **17**(6), 1171–9.

Yousem DM, Geckle RJ, Bilker W, McKeown DA and Doty RL. MR evaluation of patients with congenital hyposmia or anosmia. *American Journal of Roentgenology*, 1996b, **166**(2), 439–43.

Yousem DM, Oguz KK and Li C. Imaging of the olfactory system. *Seminars in Ultrasound CT and MR*, 2001, **22**(6), 456–72.

Yu Z, Kryzer TJ, Griesmann GE, Kim K, Benarroch EE and Lennon VA. CRMP-5 neuronal autoantibody: marker of lung cancer and thymoma-related autoimmunity. *Annals of Neurology*, 2001, **49**(2), 146–54.

Zatorre RJ and Jones-Gotman M. Human olfactory discrimination after unilateral frontal or temporal lobectomy. *Brain*, 1991, **114**(Pt 1A), 71–84.

Zhao K, Pribitkin EA, Cowart BJ, Rosen D, Scherer PW and Dalton P. Numerical modeling of nasal obstruction and endoscopic surgical intervention: outcome to airflow and olfaction. *American Journal of Rhinology*. 2006, **20**(3), 308–16.

Zimmerman HM and Netsky MG. Pathology of multiple sclerosis. *Research Publications Association for Research in Nervous and Mental Disease*, 1950, **28**, 271–312.

Zivadinov R, Zorzon M, Monti Bragadin L, Pagliaro G and Cazzato G. Olfactory loss in multiple sclerosis. *Journal of Neurological Science*, 1999, **168**(2), 127–30.

Zorzon M, Ukmar M and Bragadin LM et al. Olfactory dysfunction and extent of white matter abnormalities in multiple sclerosis: a clinical and MR study. *Multiple Sclerosis*, 2000, **6**(6), 386–9.

4

Neurodegenerative diseases that affect olfaction

Of great interest to the neuroscientist is the fact that a number of neurological diseases associated with non-inflammatory neuronal cell loss such as Alzheimer's disease and various forms of Parkinson's disease are accompanied, at their earliest stages, by olfactory disturbances (see later in Figure 4.1 and Figure 4.4, Table 4.1 and Table 4.2). Some other neurodegenerative diseases, such as progressive supranuclear palsy (PSP), are not similarly associated with smell dysfunction, suggesting that olfactory testing may be of value in differential diagnosis. A wide variety of xenobiotic agents, including viruses, pesticides, and heavy metals, can damage the olfactory epithelium and, in some instances, may enter the brain via the olfactory pathways. This fact, along with patterns of developmental brain pathology, has led to the hypothesis that some neurodegenerative diseases may be caused or catalyzed by xenobiotics that damage the olfactory system and enter the brain via the nose, possibly by acting upon genetically determined substrates. The strengths and weakness of this hypothesis – termed the "olfactory vector hypothesis" (OVH) – are discussed in detail later in the chapter.

It is debatable whether aging and neurodegeneration are the same process, but it is essential to be aware that aging itself is the most important variable affecting olfaction (Doty *et al.*, 1984). After the age of 80 years, about 70 percent of individuals have marked impairment of olfaction, and between 65 and 80 years, 50 percent have a demonstrable deficit (Doty *et al.*, 1984; Murphy *et al.*, 2002). In one study of 211 healthy control subjects in the UK, it was shown that identification ability begins to decline significantly as early as 36 years of age and thereafter more steeply (Hawkes *et al.*, 2005) (Figure 4.2). In keeping with other studies, females performed better with scores of 1–2 University of Pennsylvania Smell Indentification Test (UPSIT) points higher than men at all ages. The female rate of decline was not noticeably different from that of males.

Alzheimer's disease

Pathological studies of the olfactory system

There was considerable excitement when it was suggested that Alzheimer's disease could be diagnosed from post-mortem samples of nasal olfactory neuroepithelium (Talamo *et al.*, 1989) and the clear consequence that an accurate diagnosis could be made via biopsy of the olfactory epithelium (Lovell *et al.*, 1982). Although changes in morphology, distribution, and immunoreactivity of neuronal structures typical of Alzheimer's disease were noted, subsequent studies have cast doubt on the general finding, partly because the control subjects were significantly younger than the cases and because the changes were not specific for Alzheimer's disease, being similar to those seen in other neurodegenerative diseases and even in some healthy elderly control subjects (Kishikawa *et al.*, 1994; Trojanowski *et al.*, 1991). Nevertheless, it is still possible that the apparently healthy elderly control subjects were in the preclinical phase of Alzheimer's disease and that olfactory or cognitive measurement before death may have detected early changes of Alzheimer's disease.

A number of other attempts to diagnose Alzheimer's disease from nasal biopsy samples have been made. However, nasal biopsies have limitations, in particular sampling issues. Apart from lack of specific changes it can be

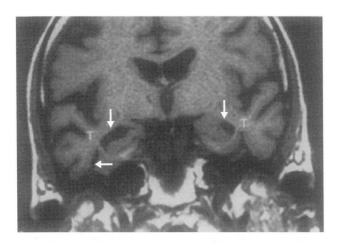

Figure 4.1 Coronal T1-weighted MRI scan of a patient with probable Alzheimer's disease. The temporal horns are markedly enlarged (down-pointing arrows) and the temporal lobes (T) are atrophic. The parahippocampal fissures are atrophic also (horizontal white arrow). (Modified and reproduced from Yousem *et al.*, 2001. With permission from Elsevier.)

difficult to identify olfactory neurons even with the specific olfactory marker protein stain. With advancing years the neuroepithelium is replaced progressively by respiratory epithelium; for example, in one biopsy study (Yamagishi *et al.*, 1994), only 6/13 samples contained olfactory neurons. Furthermore, it is not known whether the progressive deterioration occurs more rapidly in patients with Alzheimer's disease than in normal people of similar age. The reader is referred to Smutzer *et al.* (2003) for an in-depth review of this complex topic.

Despite the controversies of olfactory nasal epithelial involvement, olfactory bulb changes in Alzheimer's disease are well recognized and probably universal (Kovacs *et al.*, 2001). Neurofibrillary tangles (NFTs) and amyloid deposits – the hallmarks of Alzheimer's disease – are found in all cell layers of the olfactory bulb, as well as in the anterior olfactory nucleus. It is not yet known whether the earliest pathological changes occur in the nasal mucosa, bulb, or more centrally in the temporal cortex. Studies by Braak and Braak (1998) suggest that the earliest area of central damage is in the transentorhinal cortex, a bottleneck zone for cortical sensory afferents to the hippocampus (see Chapter 2, Figure 2.20). Abnormalities in this region are followed by changes in the adjacent entorhinal cortex – an area concerned with memory, emotion, and olfaction. In a study by Kovacs *et al.* (2001), NFTs occurred in the anterior olfactory nucleus (AON) of some Alzheimer's disease cases before any change was seen in the entorhinal cortex. The primary olfactory cortex was less severely affected than the medial orbitofrontal cortex (an olfactory association area) and there was a correlation between the pathology of the olfactory bulb and some non-olfactory areas. This led to the suggestion that NFT formation developed independently of synaptic connections, i.e., it was not a process that advanced along established fiber pathways, in contrast to Braak's observations.

In a study of elderly community-dwelling subjects who died and underwent autopsy, odor identification test scores prior to death were inversely related to the level of Alzheimer's disease pathology, principally NFT in the entorhinal cortex and CA1/subiculum area of the hippocampus (Wilson *et al.*, 2007b). This association remained after controlling for dementia or semantic memory, leading to the suggestion that impaired odor identification in old age is partly due to accumulation of NFT in the primary olfactory cortex. As the authors note, their study conflicts with two other post-mortem-based studies: McShane *et al.* (2001), where the perception of the odor of lavender water was assessed, and Olichney *et al.* (2005), who used butanol. Neither of these two studies found an association between smell measurement and Alzheimer's disease pathology, but there was a good correlation between smell impairment and the presence of Lewy bodies (dementia with Lewy bodies or Lewy body variant). The importance of the study by Wilson and colleagues (2007a) is that it used validated olfactory testing and provided a

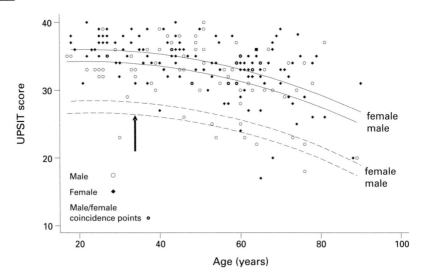

Figure 4.2 Correlation of University of Pennsylvania Smell Identification Test (UPSIT) scores and age in 211 healthy males and females. The top two continuous lines are the female/male mean regression lines, which show superiority of females at all ages. The lower pair of dotted lines represents their lower 95 percent reference ranges. Note the superior performance of females at all ages. In this model using a quadratic term in age, UPSIT score begins to deviate from horizontal at the age of 36 years, as shown by the vertical arrow. (From Hawkes *et al.*, 2005. With permission from Wiley.)

sound pathological substrate for the clinical and epidemiological studies described later in this chapter.

Clinical evidence for olfactory dysfunction in Alzheimer's disease

Over 50 psychophysical studies employing quantitative tests in clinically diagnosed cases of Alzheimer's disease have shown olfactory abnormalities, often at an early stage of disease (for review, see Doty, 2003a). The majority of such studies have used clinical criteria for diagnosis as only rarely have autopsy data been available. Severe abnormalities were documented in most instances for identification, recognition, and threshold detection. In a meta-analysis, Mesholam *et al.* (1998) found that the Alzheimer's disease- and Parkinson's disease-related defects in olfaction were relatively uniform, although there was a non-significant trend toward better performance on threshold tests than recognition and identification tests. Unfortunately, no measure distinguished Alzheimer's disease from Parkinson's disease. A recent study of 90 patients with Alzheimer's disease (Westervelt *et al.*, 2007) found that some had normal, or near normal, scores on the Brief Smell Identification Test (B-SIT). It was suggested that there might be a subgroup of patients with apparently typical Alzheimer's disease who were male, without a family history of dementia, and performed less well on visuospatial tests. The deficit in Alzheimer's disease reportedly progresses with time (Nordin *et al.*, 1997), although the validity of psychophysical test results from more demented individuals is questionable. The majority (>90 percent) of Alzheimer's disease patients seem unaware of their defective smell sense until they are formally tested (Doty *et al.*, 1987), probably reflecting the fact that total anosmia is relatively rare or that it relates to the dementia itself. Such lack of awareness of less-than-total smell loss is a general phenomenon, since it is observed in other, non-demented, patient groups (Nordin *et al.*, 1995a).

While it has not been established exactly when the olfactory deficit observed in Alzheimer's disease first arises, it is clear that it is an early and consistent element of Alzheimer's disease that precedes its clinical diagnosis. In one prospective population-based study, 1836 healthy people were tested at baseline using the B-SIT and a cognitive screening procedure (Graves *et al.*, 1999). Reduced smell identification ability, in particular anosmia, was significantly associated with an increased risk of cognitive dysfunction several years later. At baseline, anosmics who had at least one ApoE-4 allele had nearly five times the risk of developing subsequent cognitive decline. A more recent study has shown that B-SIT scores predict the onset of mild cognitive impairment in patients with no measurable cognitive dysfunction (Wilson *et al.*, 2007b). Another group examined UPSIT scores in older patients with mild cognitive impairment (Devanand *et al.*, 2000). Those scoring 34 or less who were unaware of their defect were more at risk of developing Alzheimer's disease within two years. In theory lack of awareness may have been a manifestation of their cognitive impairment, but insight is usually well preserved in the early stages of Alzheimer's disease and, as mentioned, lack of knowledge of microsmia is common in non-demented people. Essentially similar olfactory findings have been documented by others on the basis of longitudinal studies of older subjects with minimal or no cognitive defect on initial assessment (Bacon *et al.*, 1998; Royall *et al.*, 2002; Swan & Carmelli, 2002). Schiffman *et al.* (2002) found at-risk relatives of Alzheimer's disease patients had higher phenyl ethyl alcohol detection thresholds than control subjects, as well as decreased ability to remember smells, tastes, and narrative information. In this instance, ApoE-4 status was not associated with at-risk status.

One study potentially at variance with the aforementioned studies examined the predictive value of the UPSIT in Alzheimer's disease patients with the autosomal dominant presenilin-1 mutation (Nee & Lippa, 2001). The test was administered to 18 at-risk family members 10 years previously and although four individuals subsequently developed dementia, the UPSIT did not foretell this. There were two patients who showed abnormal UPSIT scores at the onset of dementia; the remaining two were unable to cooperate with testing. The reason for this anomalous finding is unclear, but it is possible that the smell loss occurs with a latency of less than 10 years before the clinical manifestations of the disease. It is also possible that smell impairment is predictive only for the sporadic form of Alzheimer's disease.

Further controversy concerns the influence of Alzheimer's disease on event-related potentials. In a study of eight non-depressed patients with Alzheimer's disease, all of whom had mild or moderately severe forms of the disease, age-matched UPSIT scores were all abnormal (Hawkes & Shephard, 1998). However, the H_2S olfactory event-related potential (OERP) was normal in the four subjects who could be tested. In contrast, research from a different group found significant delay in the OERP to amyl acetate in all of 12 Alzheimer's disease cases (Morgan & Murphy, 2002). The same group found that healthy individuals, positive for the ApoE4 allele, exhibited a more delayed OERP than healthy, negative, people (Wetter & Murphy, 2001). The basis for the differing OERP findings is not clear. It is generally accepted, however, that odor identification tests are more sensitive and specific than OERPs in distinguishing Alzheimer's disease from control subjects (Hawkes & Shephard, 1998). These physiological observations are complemented by functional imaging, which shows decreased activation of central olfactory structures, principally on the right side (Kareken *et al.*, 2001), as well as hippocampal atrophy (see Figure 4.1).

Despite the presence of clear olfactory abnormalities in Alzheimer-type dementia, relatively little is known about other varieties of dementia, such as fronto-temporal dementia (Pick disease), semantic dementia, vascular dementia, and normal pressure hydrocephalus. One study examined olfaction in mild semantic dementia (8 cases), frontotemporal dementia (11 cases), corticobasal degeneration (7 cases), and mild Alzheimer's disease (14 cases) – all defined by clinical criteria (Luzzi *et al.*, 2007). As expected, the Alzheimer's disease group did poorly on odor discrimination, naming, and odor picture-matching tasks. The semantic dementia group had particularly low scores on odor-naming in the presence of normal discrimination, in keeping with the concept of olfactory agnosia. In fronto-temporal dementia and corticobasal degeneration there was mild impairment of olfactory naming and discrimination. The marked impairment of naming in the presence of normal discrimination in semantic dementia might permit differentiation from other dementias.

A recent study sought to find which subset of UPSIT items predicts best the conversion to dementia in people with minimal cognitive impairment (Tabert *et al.*, 2005). The authors identified 10 items (leather, clove, menthol, strawberry, pineapple, natural gas, lemon, lilac, soap, and smoke) that had high predictive power after a mean follow-up of 42 months, but as they point out, the odors may not be able to predict Alzheimer's disease specifically and could indicate other dementias or Parkinson's disease. Importantly, the focus on odor qualities, per se, may be misleading, since each UPSIT item is a complex odor mix. For example, just the oregano component of pizza contains at least 22 volatile agents (Diaz-Maroto *et al.*, 2002) and the odors are not equally intense.

Olfactory testing has potential value in distinguishing dementia from depression (Duff *et al.*, 2002), as patients with uncomplicated depression usually have little or no olfactory impairment (Amsterdam *et al.*, 1987).

Case report 4.1: Early probable Alzheimer's disease

A 62-year-old taxi driver presented with a two-year history of progressive failure of short-term memory and bouts of confusion. He had been driving until one year previously but gave up after a minor road traffic accident that was probably caused by poor concentration or lack of visuo-spatial awareness (Balint syndrome). There was no family history of dementia and according to his wife his general health was good apart from difficulties with smelling since the age of 50 years. Examination revealed weakly positive grasp and pout reflexes. Blood pressure was 155/95 mmHg. The Mini-Mental State Examination (MMSE) score was 27/30 (normal/borderline). The UPSIT score was in the anosmic range (13/40). OERP showed a normal response to H_2S at 700 ms. Psychometric evaluation revealed a mild degree of general intellectual decline. A magnetic resonance imaging (MRI) brain scan was normal, including views of the sinuses. A brain single photon emission computed tomography (SPECT) scan with Ceretec® showed reduced perfusion in both temporal lobes, more pronounced on the left. There was slight improvement in cognitive function with rivastigmine (Exelon®), the centrally acting anticholinesterase drug.

Comment: The most likely diagnosis is early Alzheimer's disease, in which there is often a long prior history of anosmia. It is interesting that the OERP is within normal limits, despite anosmia on identification testing. This could mean that signals arrive at the central processing areas (temporal lobes), thus eliciting an evoked response, but cognitive difficulty impairs the ability to identify smells on the UPSIT. Olfactory tests are useful in this situation as many who present with memory problems have pseudo-dementia secondary to depression. As long as a patient has depression uncomplicated by dementia, the smell tests should be normal.

In summary, there is abundant evidence of early olfactory impairment in typical Alzheimer's disease. It still has to be determined whether olfactory pathology appears first in the nasal receptor zone, bulb, or temporal cortex. Although olfactory dysfunction appears to be a marker of future cognitive decline, prior smell loss is not specific for Alzheimer's disease and could reflect the early development of other dementias or Parkinsonian syndromes. Although knowledge of the site of initial pathology, if peripheral, may help establish the etiology and implicate an environmental cause (e.g., toxin or virus) this is not always the case. Thus, the olfactory neuroepithelium can be the major invasion route of blood- or airborne viruses into the central nervous system (CNS) (Charles et al., 1995; Doty, 2008). Moreover, some viruses may be transported from the olfactory epithelium to the olfactory bulb without imparting major damage to the epithelium, despite using this route of entry into the brain (Youngentoub et al., 2001), and different CNS cell types may be preferentially infected by certain viruses, depending, for example, on the presence or absence of receptors to which a given virus binds (Schlitt et al., 1991).

Down syndrome

Down syndrome carries a high risk of subsequent Alzheimer's disease and is more likely to occur in people with a family history of Alzheimer's disease (Katzman, 1986). Alzheimer-type neuropathology is observed inevitably in patients with Down syndrome who live to the fourth decade, and worsens with advancing years (Ball & Nuttall, 1980; Berger & Vogel 1973; Mann, 1988; Wisniewski et al., 1985). Neurons in layer II of the entorhinal cortex and the CA1/subiculum field of the hippocampus are first to be affected by tangle formation, suggesting early involvement of structures critical to olfactory processing (Oliver & Holland, 1986).

Early clinical observations suggested that Down syndrome is accompanied by smell dysfunction (Brousseau & Brainerd, 1928). Subsequent empirical studies have confirmed this, showing deficits on tests of identification, detection, and memory, as well as OERP (Hemdal et al., 1993; McKeown et al., 1996; Murphy & Jinich, 1996; Warner et al., 1988; Wetter & Murphy, 1999; Zucco & Negrin, 1994). It has been suggested that the olfactory defect is progressive (Nijjar & Murphy, 2002). In general, the average degree of smell loss observed in Down syndrome is very close to that observed in Alzheimer's disease, i.e., mean UPSIT scores around 20 (McKeown et al., 1996; Warner et al., 1988).

It is not clear when individuals with Down syndrome first exhibit olfactory loss. In the sole study designed to shed light on this question, McKeown et al. (1996) administered the UPSIT and a 16-item odor discrimination test to 20 adolescents with Down syndrome and to 20 non-Down syndrome retarded children matched on the basis of mental age using the *Peabody Picture Vocabulary Test – Revised* (PPVT-R) (Dunn, 1981). Twenty non-retarded children similarly matched on mental age were also tested. Although no meaningful differences in olfactory function were found among the three study groups, the test scores of both the Down syndrome and non-Down syndrome retarded subjects were lower than non-retarded, age-matched children and of similar magnitude to those of adult Down syndrome subjects.

Hyposmia may precede the Alzheimer's disease-type dementia of Down syndrome (as in Alzheimer's disease and Parkinson's disease), but the lower scores may simply reflect greater ease of demonstrating smell impairment compared with subtle Alzheimer's disease-related pathology. Characteristic Alzheimer's disease pathology may be present in relatively silent cortical areas, which are difficult to probe by current techniques. Given such observations and the fact that olfactory test scores of individuals with Down syndrome may not differ from those of individuals with other forms of cognitive retardation, preclinical olfactory testing for predicting future cognitive decline in Down syndrome may prove unfruitful.

Parkinson's disease

Pathological studies of the olfactory system

Olfactory epithelium

Dystrophic neurites without Lewy bodies have been found in the olfactory epithelium in autopsies from individuals with Parkinson's disease. Several patients also display accumulation of amyloid precursor protein fragments apparently equivalent to those observed in Alzheimer's disease (Crino et al., 1995). All varieties of synuclein (α, β, γ) are expressed in olfactory receptor neurons, in particular α-synuclein, which, when misfolded, becomes highly insoluble and forms the hallmark pathology of Parkinson's disease. The expression of abnormal α-synuclein within the olfactory mucosa has been found to be no different from that expressed in Lewy body disease, Alzheimer's disease, multiple system atrophy, and seemingly healthy older control subjects (Duda et al., 1999). More recently, nasal biopsy specimens from seven patients with symptomatic Parkinson's disease were compared with nasal biopsies from four anosmic control subjects using antibodies against olfactory marker protein (OMP; Witt et al., 2006), neurotubulin, protein gene product 9.5 (PGP 9.5; a specific stain for olfactory receptor neurons), and mRNA for OMP. Irregular areas of olfactory epithelium were positive for PGP 9.5 and neurotubulin, but mostly negative for OMP even though mRNA for OMP was found in the olfactory cleft and respiratory mucosa. In this small series there was no clear difference between Parkinson's disease and anosmic control subjects. It appears that sections were not examined for the presence of Lewy bodies or Lewy neurites, and it might be argued that those with anosmia may have been in the presymptomatic phase of Parkinson's disease. It is still possible that those healthy subjects coincidentally found to have α-synuclein-containing dystrophic neurites in the nasal receptor zone (Duda et al., 1999) may have been in the preclinical stage of Parkinson's disease and that the changes actually represent a disease-related, if not disease-specific, finding.

Olfactory bulbs

There have been few studies of the olfactory bulbs in Parkinson's disease beyond anatomical description, but it is clear that there is considerable cell loss, particularly in the more posteriorly located anterior olfactory nucleus (AON). Daniel and Hawkes (1992) examined olfactory bulbs and tracts from formalin-fixed brains of eight control subjects and eight patients with a clinical and pathological diagnosis of Parkinson's disease taken from the UK Parkinson's disease brain bank. All eight Parkinson's disease cases contained Lewy bodies, which were most numerous in the AON but also present in mitral cells, the first cells to receive input from the bipolar olfactory cells. The morphology of Lewy bodies at this site resembled their cortical counterparts but inclusions showing a classical trilaminar structure were rare. It was subsequently shown that loss of AON neurons correlated with disease duration (Pearce *et al.*, 1995). Braak and colleagues (2003a) (Figure 4.3 and Figure 4.4) confirmed the presence of Parkinson's disease-related lesions in mitral

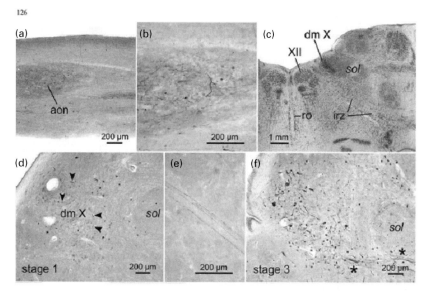

Figure 4.3 (See also Figure 4.3 in the color plate section, p. 82–3.) (a) and (b) show Lewy pathology in the anterior olfactory nucleus in stage 1; aon, anterior olfactory nucleus. (c) is a low- power view of the dorsal medulla in a normal control to show the main structures involved in Parkinson's disease: dm X, dorsal motor nuclear complex of X; irz, intermediate reticular zone; sol, nucleus of the solitary tract; XII, hypoglossal nucleus. (d) to (f) show increasing Lewy pathology with advancing stages. (e) shows Lewy neurites in the vagus as it crosses the medulla. (Reproduced from Braak *et al.*, 2004. With permission from Springer Science and Business Media.)

and tufted neurons of the olfactory bulb and in projection neurons of the AON – lesions that were dispersed throughout the olfactory tract. A tightly woven network of Lewy neurites was noted to develop within the AON over the successive stages of the Braak classification system, as described in the next section. The pathology extended from the AON into more remote olfactory sites (olfactory tubercle, piriform and periamygdalar cortex, entorhinal cortex of the ambient gyrus) without advancing into non-olfactory cortical areas (Braak *et al.*, 2003a, 2004; Del Tredici & Braak, 2004).

The human olfactory bulb contains at least 20 different neurotransmitters, including dopamine (see Figure 1.13). Simple dopamine replacement, however, does not improve smell function in Parkinson's disease patients (Doty *et al.*, 1992a), and dopamine deficiency within the bulb does not appear to be present in Parkinson's disease. Indeed, one report found that expression of tyrosine hydroxylase in the olfactory bulb of patients with Parkinson's disease is *increased* 100-fold, possibly explaining the hyposmia of Parkinson's disease by a toxic gain of function (Huisman *et al.*, 2004). In a mouse methylphenyltetrahydropyridine (MPTP) model of Parkinson's disease, a fourfold *increase* of dopamine expression in the olfactory bulb has been reported (Yamada *et al.*, 2004). This increase in dopamine may reflect migration into the olfactory bulb of dopamine-secreting cells from the subventricular zone/ rostral migratory stream, as shown in humans (Bedard & Parent, 2004). This experiment implies that ongoing compensation is taking place in the adult brain and infers that only when the process fails do the symptoms of disease become apparent.

Central olfactory changes

In 2003 Braak and colleagues performed a detailed neuropathological analysis of 41 cases of Parkinson's disease by immunostaining the autopsied brains with α-synuclein, the aggregated protein found in Lewy neurites and Lewy bodies (Braak *et al.*, 2003a). A similar approach was taken in 69 autopsy "incidental" cases that displayed no extrapyramidal signs in life but were found to have Lewy neurites or Lewy bodies, or both. A third group assessed in this study comprised 58 age- and gender-matched cases that had no Lewy bodies or Lewy neurites, and no history of neurological or psychiatric illness. Their data suggested that the pathological process advances in a predictable sequence, with the earliest changes (which develop before any motor components appeared in life) occurring within the olfactory bulb, the associated AON (Figures 4.3 and 4.4), and the dorsal motor nuclear complex (DMC) of the glossopharyngeal and vagus nerves. Where Lewy bodies could be found in the substantia nigra, invariably there were similar and more severe changes in the olfactory bulb, the anterior olfactory nucleus, and the dorsal medulla. Interestingly, the involvement of DMC led to the proposal that Parkinson's disease starts in the enteric plexus (Auerbach's submucosal plexus) and that a pathogen, possibly viral or

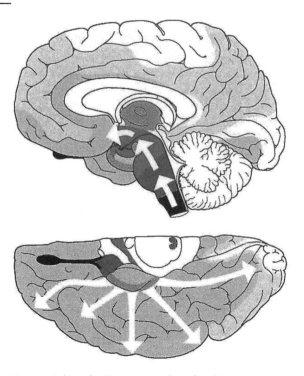

Figure 4.4 (See also Figure 4.4 in the color plate section, p. 82–3.) Braak stages 1–6 in idiopathic Parkinson's disease. In Stage 1 there is simultaneous involvement of the brain in olfactory and medullary regions (colored black). In Stage 4 (colored red) the two processes converge on the medial temporal lobes and then spread widely into the neocortex. (Reproduced from Braak *et al.*, 2003a. With permission from Elsevier.)

chemical, ascends the motor vagal fibers in retrograde fashion to the dorsal medulla (Braak *et al.*, 2006). This theory, whilst appealing because it explains the presence of abnormal α-synuclein deposits in the enteric plexus, does not explain the olfactory bulb changes or the probable early deposits in sympathetic ganglia (Kaufmann *et al.*, 2004). An alternative explanation is that a "dual hit" occurs where a pathogen simultaneously enters the olfactory bulb and enteric plexus (Hawkes *et al.*, 2007). This concept is elaborated later in this chapter under the olfactory vector hypothesis.

Given that at least 50 percent of substantia nigra cells have to die before there are clinical symptoms (Fearnley & Lees, 1991; Ross *et al.*, 2004), it is clear that the clinical motor manifestations of Parkinson's disease must represent the late stage of a pathological process that probably started many years previously. This point is borne out by anecdotal clinical observations from patients with Parkinson's disease who report regularly that smell impairment occurred several years before their first motor symptoms. According to the study by Braak *et al.* (2003a), Lewy pathology in central olfactory areas such as the entorhinal cortex develops much later – in the fourth of six phases, implying that olfactory dysfunction in Parkinson's disease starts peripherally.

The proposed sequential development of Parkinson's disease as formulated by Braak and colleagues (2003a) has been challenged recently. For example, Parkkinen *et al.* (2005) conducted post-mortem assessment of 904 brains that had α-synuclein pathology in the dorsal motor nucleus of the vagus, substantia nigra, and/or basal forebrain nuclei. Retrospective assessment showed that only 32 (30 percent) of 106 alpha-synuclein-positive cases were diagnosed with a neurodegenerative disorder in life, and that the distribution of α-synuclein pathology did not allow a reliable diagnosis of an extrapyramidal syndrome. Some neurologically unimpaired cases had a moderate burden of α-synuclein pathology in both brainstem and cortical areas, suggesting that α-synuclein-positive structures outside olfactory system-related structures are not unequivocal markers of neuronal dysfunction. Kalaitzakis *et al.* (2008) examined the topography of α-synuclein pathology in 57 Parkinson's disease brains, excluding the olfactory bulb. There were 4/57 (7 percent) cases of Parkinson's disease without medullary involvement, which led these authors to conclude that the medulla is not always the induction site of pathology in sporadic Parkinson's disease. Another study used Braak staging to group an autopsy cohort into *preclinical* (stages 1–2); *early* (stages 3–4; 35 percent with clinical Parkinson's disease), and *late* (stages 5–6; 86 percent with clinical Parkinson's disease) cases (Halliday *et al.*, 2006). Preclinical compared with early- or late-stage cases should progressively be more elderly at the time of sampling, but this feature was not observed. Other studies support the proposed Braak sequential changes. In a preliminary report, Duda *et al.* (2007) examined 126 brains taken from the Honolulu Asia Aging Study (HAAS), of whom 23 had clinically diagnosed Parkinson's disease and 35 had incidental Lewy bodies. The vast majority of cases were consistent with the Braak classification. Furthermore, the reliability of the findings by Braak and coworkers was demonstrated in a study in which six observers from five different institutions were asked to classify 21 cases of the original pathological material upon which the Braak staging was based. A near perfect correlation was obtained for inter- and intra-rater reliability (Muller *et al.*, 2005). Braak staging concurs well with "premotor" symptoms (Hawkes & Deeb, 2006), but further proof will hinge upon detailed analysis based on separate pathological material.

Clinical evidence for olfactory dysfunction in Parkinson's disease

The first study reporting olfactory loss in Parkinson's disease was that of Ansari and Johnson (1975). They described 22 patients with a clinical diagnosis of Parkinson's disease who, relative to control subjects, had elevated thresholds to the banana-smelling substance amyl acetate. They noted an association between the higher threshold scores (i.e., greater olfactory dysfunction) and more rapid disease progression. There appeared to be no influence from medication (levodopa, anticholinergic drugs) or smoking behavior. In a study of 78 Parkinson's disease patients and 40 control subjects, Quinn *et al.* (1987) similarly found elevated amyl acetate thresholds. However, no influence from age, sex, on–off state, or use of levodopa on the threshold measures was found. Unlike the findings of Ansari and Johnson (1975), there was no association with disease severity, assuming that severity is associated with disease duration.

Subsequent studies suggested that olfactory dysfunction, as measured by the UPSIT and the detection threshold for phenyl ethyl alcohol, is independent of disease duration or disability, and not meaningfully correlated with measures of motor function, tremor, or cognition (Doty *et al.*, 1988, 1989, 1992a). It was also demonstrated that the olfactory deficit was typically bilateral and uninfluenced by anti-Parkinsonian medication. A more recent evaluation of clinically defined Parkinson's disease subtypes showed that females with mild disability and tremor-dominant disease had slightly better UPSIT scores than males with moderate to severe disability and little or no tremor; age at disease onset was not a factor (Stern *et al.*, 1994). A comparable survey was undertaken by Hawkes *et al.* (1997) in 155 cognitively normal, depression-free Parkinson's disease patients and 156 age-matched controls. UPSIT scores for the Parkinson's disease patients were dramatically lower than the UPSIT scores of the age-matched controls. Only 19 percent (30/155) of the Parkinson's disease patients had a score within the normal range defined by 95 percent population limits. Sixty-five (42 percent) were classified as anosmic, i.e., scoring less than 17/40. There was no correlation between disease duration and UPSIT score ($r = 0.074$). A somewhat lower prevalence of abnormality (64 percent) was obtained for odor identification in 380 Dutch Parkinson's disease patients assessed by the extended version of Sniffin' Sticks test (Boesveldt *et al.*, 2007). The reason for this lower percentage is not clear but there may be some reduction of sensitivity through use of just 16 odors in the Sniffin' Sticks test compared with 40 in the UPSIT.

In the first study to address sniffing behavior in Parkinson's disease, Sobel and colleagues (2001) found sniffing to be impaired in Parkinson's disease, resulting in a slight reduction in their performance on identification and detection threshold tests. In the case of the UPSIT, this reduction was about 2–3 UPSIT points (see below). Increasing sniff vigor improved olfactory scores. Investigations that have not allowed for this effect (which includes most) may tend to exaggerate slightly the severity of any defect, especially where the disease is known to involve bulbar function.

Altered chemosensory ERPs (Kobal & Plattig, 1978) are found in Parkinson's disease. Hawkes and Shepard (1992) and Hawkes *et al.* 1997) evaluated OERP in 73 non-depressed, cognitively normal patients with Parkinson's disease and in 47 control subjects of similar age and sex. In 36 of 73 patients (49 percent), responses were either absent or unsatisfactory for technical reasons. Regression analysis on the 37 individuals with a measurable trace showed a highly significant latency difference between Parkinson's disease patients and control subjects for the odorant hydrogen sulfide (H_2S). Similar results were reported in 31 Parkinson's disease patients using vanillin and H_2S (Barz *et al.*, 1997). Prolonged latencies were observed whether or not medication was being taken for the condition. However, more marked change was evident for those receiving treatment, conceivably reflecting greater Parkinson's disease-related disability. A correlation between disability, as measured by Webster score, and latency to the H_2S derived OERP was noted. Increased latency typically indicates demyelination, but in Parkinson's disease there is no evidence of this and a satisfactory explanation for such prolongation has not been found.

There is debate about the temporal characteristics of the olfactory defect in Parkinson's disease, i.e., whether it is stable or progressive and whether it correlates with indicators of disease severity. A slight decline in smell function with age is unavoidable even in healthy people, but the critical issue is whether there is additional impairment from Parkinson's disease superimposed on aging effects. Several studies of smell identification or detection threshold sensitivity found no correlation with disease duration (Doty *et al.*, 1988; Hawkes *et al.*, 1997; Quinn *et al.*, 1987). This contrasts with the early observations of Ansari and Johnson (1975), who reported an association between olfactory thresholds and rapid progression. Others describe an association between disability and olfactory event related potentials (Barz *et al.*, 1997). Support for the concept of pathological progression within the olfactory system derives from studies that show neuronal loss in the AON, along with progressive development of Lewy bodies and neurites which advance with disease duration (Pearce *et al.*, 1995) and increasing Braak stage (Braak *et al.*, 2003a). The concept of functional progression receives tangential support from the finding of a significant correlation ($r = 0.66$) between dopamine transporter uptake, as measured by [^{99m}Tc]TRODAT–SPECT, and UPSIT scores (Siderowf *et al.*, 2005), but not with symptom duration or disability, as measured by the Unified Parkinson's Disease Rating Scale (UPDRS). Using Sniffin' Sticks in 40 non-demented Parkinson's disease subjects, Daum *et al.* (2000) found a significant negative correlation between odor discrimination and disease severity. Similar results were reported by Tissingh and colleagues (2001), who documented a negative correlation between olfactory discrimination and both the UPDRS motor score and Hoehn

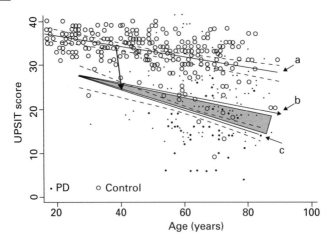

Figure 4.5 Decline of University of Pennsylvania Smell Identification Test (UPSIT) scores in control subjects (a) and patients (c), assuming linear regression on age for both groups. Black dots represent Parkinson's disease patients and open circles are control subjects. The large down-sloping arrow indicates a proposed acute event causing a decline in olfaction from the healthy control level. Stability of the defect, which would be represented by a horizontal line, is improbable as it equates to progressive *improvement* in UPSIT score with aging. The hypothetical regression line (b) represents the effect of aging alone in the Parkinson's disease group. If there is accelerated deterioration of smell function with age in Parkinson's disease patients (as proposed here), this additional component corresponds to the gray shaded area between lines b and c. (Hawkes, 2007.)

and Yahr stage. Hawkes (2007) compared the UPSIT scores of 266 patients with Parkinson's disease with those of 263 healthy control subjects. The linear regression lines on age, apart from showing a lower mean UPSIT score at all ages, diverged with age (Figure 4.5). Although this is a cross-sectional rather than a longitudinal study, it implies that the olfactory disorder reflects the combined effect of aging and Parkinson's disease itself. Finally, Deeb *et al.* (2006) reported a significant correlation between UPSIT and motor scores in *early* cases of Parkinson's disease. This observation, along with the recent findings of others, reopens the question of an association between olfactory function and the motor deficit of Parkinson's disease.

Selective anosmia in sporadic Parkinson's disease?
If a small number of odors could be found which distinguish reliably between Parkinson's disease patients and healthy control subjects then a brief test based on these would have clinical utility. In the first formal study to address this issue, two UPSIT odors, pizza and wintergreen, were found to best discriminate between British Parkinson's disease patients and control subjects, with a

sensitivity of 90 percent and specificity of 86 percent (Hawkes & Shephard, 1993). Other investigations using UPSIT or B-SIT items have found different sets of odors to be the best discriminators. Thus, Silveira-Moriyama (2005a) found pizza, mint, and licorice to be optimal in another British sample; Double *et al.* (2003) found banana, licorice, and dill pickle to be most favorable in Australians, and Bohnen *et al.* (2007) found banana, gasoline, pineapple, smoke, and cinnamon to be most selective in an American population. The latter odors correlated better with striatal dopamine transporter imaging (DATScan) activity than the total UPSIT score (Bohnen *et al.*, 2007). A German study implementing the 12-odor Sniffin' Sticks test reported that licorice, followed by aniseed, pineapple, apple, turpentine, and banana, separated Parkinson's disease patients from control subjects (Daum *et al.*, 2000), and a Dutch study using the 16-odor Sniffin' Sticks found aniseed to be the best discriminator (Boesveldt *et al.*, 2007). Even though there is some overlap among studies (e.g., banana, pizza, licorice), this is not consistent. Although it is conceivable that genetically based specific anosmias are present in Parkinson's disease, the use of complex odorants such as those indicated above, which are not equally intense, would be unlikely to identify them. As mentioned earlier, even oregano, a major component of pizza, is composed of multiple volatile components (Diaz-Maroto *et al.*, 2002). Moreover, different response alternatives are present for a variety of odor items in the currently employed tests, making the stimulus–response complexes even more multifaceted. Cultural or socio-economic factors may play a role, bringing forth issues related to familiarity or frequency of interactions with specific odors. If progress is to be made in this area, a dedicated test battery will most likely be needed to include odors that are less complex and of equal intensity.

In summary, the available data suggest that smell impairment is a frequent (80–90 percent) and early sign of Parkinson's disease that is independent of cognitive function. This suggests that olfactory test information may be used to identify apparently healthy people who are at risk of future disease. Moreover, such investigations may permit early neuroprotective therapy if this becomes available.

Familial and presymptomatic Parkinson's disease

Preliminary data are now emerging about smell dysfunction in families and individuals with known monogenetic disorder, but all observations are based on small numbers and must be regarded as provisional. In the initial Michigan study of familial parkinsonism (Markopoulou *et al.*, 1997), the UPSIT was administered to six kindreds, three of whom had typical Parkinson's disease and three a "parkinsonism-plus" syndrome. In the typical families there were four apparently healthy individuals at 50 percent risk, of whom

---

Case report 4.2: Parkinson's disease with longstanding prior anosmia

A 63-year-old retired male electrical engineer presented with a three-year history of slight impairment of walking and tendency to stumble. Relatives remarked that he had become more stooped and did not swing the arms on walking. His handwriting had become smaller and there was increased fatigue when playing a round of golf. Twenty years previously he developed what was thought to be Bornholm's disease (intercostal myalgia) and shortly after that it was noticed that he could not detect the smell of gas. Examination, including cognitive tests, was unremarkable apart from reduced arm-swing and minimal increase of arm tone on reinforcement. The provisional diagnosis was early classical Parkinson's disease corresponding to Hoehn and Yahr Stage I. An MRI brain scan showed no abnormality and there were no significant inflammatory changes in the paranasal sinuses, implying that local nasal disease did not contribute to the smell deficit. The olfactory bulbs and tracts appeared normal. The UPSIT score was 16/40 (anosmic range) and there was delay on OERP at 1120 ms (normal less than 937 ms). Electrogustometry showed a markedly raised threshold over the fungiform and circumvallate papillae. The DATScan showed significant loss of dopamine transporter uptake in the putamen of both sides. One year later there was slight progression of disability and he was placed on levodopa (Sinemet® CR), to which he made an excellent response.

Comment: This patient had signs of early Parkinson's disease, which was confirmed by the DATScan and his excellent response to levodopa on follow-up. The prior history of anosmia in the absence of local nasal disease is in keeping with the proposal that smell impairment is an early warning sign of Parkinson's disease – here by as much as 20 years.

The taste involvement is an intriguing aspect here. Initial reports suggested that taste is unaffected in Parkinson's disease (Sienkiewicz-Jarosz et al., 2005) but this has now been challenged (Shah et al., 2008) and is thought to involve about 28 percent of subjects with established disease.

---

three were microsmic. In the Parkinson's disease-plus families there were eight at-risk subjects, two of whom had abnormal UPSIT scores. It has now been shown that the typical Parkinson's disease families had the PARK 1, 3, and 8 mutations (Hentschel et al., 2005). The single case of PARK 1 was anosmic and the two PARK 3 families had variable findings but were mostly normal. There were seven cases of genetically confirmed pallidopontonigral degeneration in the atypical group and their mean UPSIT score was indicative

Case report 4.3: Anosmia and ageusia with unclear diagnosis

A 61-year-old man presented initially with a two-year history of difficulty in appreciating the smell or taste of food. The problem appeared to have evolved over a few days in the absence of local nasal infection. The smell symptoms showed no tendency to fluctuate, as might be expected if there was an element of obstructive anosmia. Strong perfume made him sneeze but he could not smell the fragrance. He thought that his appreciation of food flavor was impaired – for example, salted potato crisps tasted completely bland. Physical examination, including nasal endoscopy, was normal. The UPSIT score was 19/40 (severe microsmic range) and he was unable to detect bitter, sweet, sour, or salt liquids on whole-mouth testing. MRI brain scan showed minor vascular changes in keeping with his age and blood pressure (167/89 mm Hg). Three years later he was referred because of involuntary kicking movements in bed, suggestive of restless legs syndrome – an occasional precursor of Parkinson's disease. A DATScan showed reduced uptake in the left putamen, confirming the possibility of preclinical Parkinson's disease. Routine clinical examination showed no obvious sign of Parkinson's disease, but he was advised that he might develop this disorder over the next 5–10 years.

   Comment: The patient's history suggests that the olfactory impairment might be a precursor of Parkinsonism – but the coexistence of taste impairment is not typical of classical Parkinson's disease which, if it occurs at all, is probably a late feature (Fernando *et al.*, 2005). The abnormal DATScan gives objective confirmation of a Parkinsonian syndrome, but time will tell whether this patient will turn out to have classical Parkinson's disease.

of anosmia (mean = 10.5). Four cases with the PARK 8 mutation scored an average of 29.7 on the UPSIT, which appeared lower than those at risk, whose mean score was 34. There was no clear relationship between olfaction and parkinsonian phenotype.

   Since these observations were made, it has become clear that the PARK 8 mutation (LRRK2/Dardarin) is currently the most prevalent cause of familial Parkinson's disease, accounting for 2–5 percent of all Parkinson's disease in Europe with a much higher level in Spain, Portugal, and North Africa (Ferreira *et al.*, 2007). Khan *et al.* (2005) reported a Lincolnshire (UK) kindred with the PARK 8 mutation and found slight olfactory impairment in 2/4 individuals. More recently, olfaction in PARK 8 families was assessed by UPSIT in 5 patients from London and 16 from Lisbon (Ferreira *et al.*, 2007; Silveira-Moriyama *et al.*, 2007). There was severe impairment in

Table 4.1 Relative degree of olfactory dysfunction in various "neurodegenerative" conditions on an arbitrary scale

Disease	Relative severity of smell loss
Idiopathic Parkinson's disease, Alzheimer's disease, dementia with Lewy bodies, Guam Parkinson's disease–dementia complex	++++
Huntington's disease, Down syndrome, PARK 8?	+++
Multiple system atrophy (type-P), PARK 1, pallidopontonigral degeneration, drug-induced Parkinson's disease? Schizophrenia. Semantic dementia? X-linked dystonia-parkinsonism (Lubag)	++
Motor neuron disease, SCA2, Friedreich's ataxia	+
PARK 3, Essential tremor? Corticobasal degeneration? Fronto-temporal dementia	+
Vascular parkinsonism, MPTP parkinsonism, idiopathic dystonia, SCA3, progressive supranuclear palsy, PARK 2?	0

Key: ++++ marked damage; + mild; 0 normal. SCA = spinocerebellar atrophy.
Note: Most of these scores, except for idiopathic Parkinson's disease, are based on relatively small patient numbers and should be interpreted conservatively.

both the London and Lisbon populations, and the UPSIT scores and clinical phenotype were indistinguishable from their idiopathic Parkinson's disease subjects. In PARK 2 (Parkin disease), a dominant form of parkinsonism, the sense of smell appeared relatively preserved on a culturally modified UPSIT in 27 subjects, an observation that would be in keeping with the absence of Lewy bodies in this condition (Khan *et al.*, 2004). In a study of PARK 1, two of seven patients from separate families were found to be anosmic (Bostantjopoulou *et al.*, 2001). Table 4.1 summarizes these findings and places them into perspective relative to the smell loss observed in other neurodegenerative diseases.

Another approach to assessing familial Parkinson's disease has been to administer tests of motor function, olfaction (UPSIT), and mood in first-degree relatives of Parkinson's disease patients (Montgomery *et al.*, 1999, 2000). Using this procedure, significant differences were found in first-degree relatives (both sons and daughters), in particular where the affected parent was the father. Ponsen *et al.* (2004) raised the possibility that the results of these studies may be influenced by self-selection in allegedly unaffected relatives who may have had some undisclosed motor complaints. This would explain the unusually high two-year positive prediction rate in 40 out of the 59 subjects. Ponsen *et al.* (2004) evaluated olfactory function and dopamine striatal transporter activity (DATScan) in a prospective study of 78 asymptomatic first-degree relatives of non-familial Parkinson's disease patients. Forty relatives were hyposmic at baseline. When evaluated two years later, four had abnormal DATScans and displayed clinical evidence of Parkinson's disease. In the remaining 36 individuals with hyposmia who displayed no sign of Parkinson's disease, the rate of decline of dopamine transporter binding was higher than in normosmic relatives.

Sommer and colleagues (2004) tested 30 patients with unexplained smell impairment to determine whether any might be in the premotor phase of Parkinson's disease. Apart from detailed olfactory testing, subjects were evaluated by DATScan and transcranial sonography (TCS) of the substantia nigra. Eleven displayed increased (abnormal) echogenicity on TCS. Ten subjects volunteered for DATScan, and of these five were abnormal and a further two were borderline, suggesting they might be in a presymptomatic phase of parkinsonism. At follow-up four years later two had developed Parkinson's disease (Haehner *et al.*, 2007).

In one large study of olfaction and sleep, nearly all of 30 patients with rapid eye movement (REM) sleep behavioral disorder (RBD) had significantly increased olfactory threshold and there was evidence of parkinsonism in eight, implying that olfaction and RBD are early features of Parkinson's disease (Stiasny-Kolster *et al.*, 2005). Similar findings were documented by Iranzo *et al.* (2006). In keeping with most such sleep studies no pathological confirmation was available, and where such confirmation has been done (e.g., Boeve *et al.*, 2003) the changes in RBD were more in keeping with parkinsonism than classical Parkinson's disease. Recent observations indicate that acute sleep deprivation per se has a specific but mild adverse influence on the ability to identify odors – an influence that cannot be explained on the basis of task difficulty (Killgore & McBride, 2006). As yet, it is not clear whether this phenomenon compromises the RBD findings described above.

The first long-term, community-based prospective study of the development of Parkinson's disease has now been published (Ross *et al.*, 2008). Smell function was tested using the 12-item B-SIT in 2263 healthy Japanese-American males aged 71–95 years who participated in the HAAS. After seven years of follow-up, 19 individuals developed Parkinson's disease at an average latency of 2.7 years from baseline assessment. Adjustment for multiple confounders gave relative odds for Parkinson's disease in the lowest B-SIT score tertile of 4.3 (95 percent confidence interval 1.1–16.1; $p = 0.02$) compared with those in the highest tertile, thus indicating the moderately strong predictive power of olfactory testing. In the same cohort, those who later died underwent autopsy of the brainstem to identify Lewy bodies in the substantia nigra and locus coeruleus (Ross *et al.*, 2006). Of 163 autopsied men without clinical

Parkinson's disease or dementia, there were 17 with incidental Lewy bodies. Those who scored in the lowest tertile of the B-SIT were significantly more likely to have Lewy body changes at autopsy.

Findings that potentially conflict with the studies of Ross and colleagues (Ross *et al.*, 2008) were reported by Marras *et al.* (2005) in a study of 62 male twin pairs discordant for Parkinson's disease. At baseline, these authors found impaired UPSIT scores in the affected twins, but not in their brothers who were rated normal by clinical examination. After a mean of 7.3 years, 28 brothers were still alive and, of these, 19 were retested using the B-SIT. Two of the 28 brothers had developed Parkinson's disease. Neither of the two had impaired UPSIT scores at baseline, but the average decline in their UPSIT scores was greater than that of the remaining 17 brothers who had not developed the disease. Although it was suggested that smell testing may not be a reliable predictor of Parkinson's disease, the dropout rate was unusually high and smell was reassessed by two different methods (UPSIT and then B-SIT).

If we assume that the staging of Parkinson's disease by Braak *et al.* (2003a) is correct, and that there is a prodromal phase, then it is possible to estimate the duration of this presymptomatic period. Approximations based on patients' reports of olfactory loss are less robust, as most Parkinson's disease patients rarely report abnormalities in smelling, and we must rely on baseline measurement derived from apparently healthy people, as undertaken in the HAAS. The latent period of development of Parkinson's disease from the onset of a smell problem according to the study by Ponsen *et al.* (2004) was about two years; in the clinically and pathologically based study by Ross *et al.* (2008), the mean latency was 2.7 years, although the range was wide. The latter study was based on only 19 cases of Parkinson's disease in 2263 subjects. Anecdotal reports from patients make it likely that longer follow-up in the HAAS might reveal a considerably greater latent period, and, of course, the onset of smell impairment in those who subsequently develop Parkinson's disease clearly *would be some time before* the date of testing.

In a recently published follow-up study of 30 subjects with idiopathic anosmia, two developed Parkinson's disease after a four-year interval (Haehner *et al.*, 2007). According to the Braak staging of Parkinson's disease, olfactory and vagal pathology develop synchronously. Constipation, in part, reflects vagal dysfunction and this can be evaluated by measurement of bowel habit. The Honolulu Heart Program collected bowel data on 6790 healthy males from 1971 to 1974, of whom 96 developed Parkinson's disease at an average latent period of 12 years (range: 2 months to 24 years). After adjustment for multiple variables it was shown that those at baseline with less than one bowel movement per day suffered a fourfold increased risk of subsequent Parkinson's disease. The investigation by Iranzo *et al.* (2006) confirms the suspected status of RBD as a precursor of Parkinson's disease. According to their table, the time interval between onset of RBD and clinically manifest sporadic Parkinson's disease in seven patients was, on average, 12 years (range: 3–17 years). RBD indicates among other areas, damage to the pons, in particular the locus coeruleus, reticular and pedunculopontine nuclei, and corresponds to Braak stage 2. Much of the reasoning here assumes the accuracy of the Braak staging, which has yet to achieve universal acceptance although it corresponds remarkably well with many clinical and epidemiological studies. Provisionally it may be concluded that the latent period for typical features of Parkinson's disease has a wide range, but the mean interval from symptom-onset to clinically manifest disease approximates to at least 12 years. Personal observations of one of the authors (CHH) from patients who have been aware of their smell loss suggest that many have a much longer latent period – in some cases over 30 years.

A major question is whether the olfactory deficit represents an epiphenomenon that is just easy to measure, or whether it reflects some underlying predilection of the basic pathological process for olfactory neurons. Is there, for example, some underlying neurochemical or metabolic common susceptibility in olfactory and vagal neurons? Both regions utilize dopamine, but this transmitter is widely distributed throughout the nervous system. According to Braak *et al.* (2003b), the selective pathological change may be explained by preferential damage to fibers with long, thin, incompletely myelinated axons. Nevertheless, it has yet to be shown beyond reasonable doubt whether olfactory dysfunction precedes or develops synchronously with changes in the nigro-striatal system as measured, for example, by DATScan. Other issues to be resolved are why some patients with apparently typical Parkinson's disease have normal olfaction and why patients at risk who display smell impairment do not all develop the disease. All of these issues are discussed in more detail later in the olfactory vector hypothesis section later in this chapter.

Parkinsonism

Parkinsonism ("Parkinson plus" syndromes) refers to those diseases that resemble Parkinson's disease but differ on pathological, clinical, or genetic grounds. Among such disorders are Lewy body disease, multiple system atrophy, progressive supranuclear palsy, corticobasal degeneration, drug-induced Parkinson's disease, the Parkinson's disease–dementia complex of Guam, X-linked dystonia–parkinsonism ("Lubag"), and vascular parkinsonism. All of the olfactory data in this group have been obtained by psychophysical measurement. Since pathological verification has rarely been made, and the number of patients studied has been small, most observations should be regarded as provisional. These diseases are described separately below.

Lewy body disease

Classical Parkinson's disease is a disorder associated with widespread deposition of Lewy bodies; thus, Parkinson's disease may be considered a major variety of Lewy body disease. It is well recognized that many patients with typical Parkinson's disease develop dementia after 10 or more years – a process that most would interpret to mean spread of pathology into the cerebral hemispheres as defined by Braak stages 4–6. There are several subtypes of Lewy body disease that show variable degrees of dementia which develop before, synchronously or at varying intervals after the onset of parkinsonism. If dementia comes on before, at the same time, or at the latest within one year of the motor symptom onset then it is called dementia with Lewy bodies (McKeith, 2006). If dementia develops *more than* a year after well established Parkinson's disease, it is called Parkinson disease dementia. Pathologically, many consider that dementia with Lewy bodies, Parkinson disease dementia, and Parkinson's disease are indistinguishable (Ballard *et al.*, 2006; Galvin *et al.*, 2006). In the clinical setting it may also be difficult to distinguish Parkinson disease dementia from dementia with Lewy bodies;, hence the generic term "Lewy body disease" is often used. Many alternative names have been applied, leading to further confusion. Thus, dementia with Lewy bodies has been termed "diffuse Lewy body disease," "Lewy body dementia," "Lewy body variant of Alzheimer's disease," "senile dementia of Lewy body type," and "dementia associated with cortical Lewy bodies" (Geser *et al.*, 2005). The sole histological study of olfactory bulbs from patients with dementia with Lewy bodies (Tsuboi *et al.*, 2003) found 9 of 10 cases with tau pathology, Lewy bodies, and α-synuclein deposits, suggesting it would be difficult to distinguish from Parkinson's disease on pathological grounds alone.

Table 4.2 Comparison of pathology and smell impairment in three related disorders

Diagnosis	Lewy bodies	Alzheimer's pathology	Severity of smell loss
Parkinson's disease	++++	+	++++
Dementia with Lewy bodies	++++	++	++++
Alzheimer's disease	+	++++	++++

The number of "+" signs is an arbitrary measure of severity. These observations are preliminary and many await pathological correlation.
Note: Dementia with Lewy bodies has also been termed "diffuse Lewy body disease," Lewy body dementia," "Lewy body variant of Alzheimer's disease;" "senile dementia of Lewy body type," and "dementia associated with cortical Lewy bodies."

In a study of clinically defined dementia with Lewy bodies, but without pathological verification, severe impairment of olfactory identification and detection was observed, and test scores were independent of disease stage and duration (Liberini *et al.*, 2000). In another investigation, McShane *et al.* (2001) examined simple smell perception to one odor (lavender water) in 92 patients with autopsy-confirmed dementia, of whom 22 had dementia with Lewy bodies and 43 had only Alzheimer's disease pathology. They were compared with 94 age-matched controls. The main finding consisted of impaired smell perception in the dementia with Lewy bodies group, but little or no defect in patients with Alzheimer's disease. Despite the lack of robust smell testing, this study affords pathological confirmation for the clinically based conclusion of Liberini *et al.* (2000) that impairment of smell is significant in dementia with Lewy bodies, given that we are dealing with a disorder separate from Parkinson's disease. In a study of what was termed "Lewy body variant of Alzheimer's disease" (equivalent to dementia with Lewy bodies) with autopsy confirmation, smell dysfunction was common and its presence was thought useful to improve the sensitivity for detecting Lewy body variant of Alzheimer's disease, but it did not improve discrimination between Alzheimer's disease and its Lewy body variant because of false positives (Olichney *et al.*, 2005). The overall picture awaits considerable clarification, but a "best-guess" was given earlier in Table 4.2.

Multiple system atrophy

There are two major varieties of multiple system atrophy (MSA). A common, predominantly parkinsonian variety in which akinesia and rigidity predominate, comprises 80 percent of the total cases (MSA-P, Shy–Drager syndrome). In the remaining 20 percent, cerebellar ataxia prevails (MSA-C). Both varieties display comparatively rapidly evolving parkinsonism with dysautonomia that affects principally bladder and orthostatic blood pressure control.

Pathological changes of MSA may be seen in the olfactory bulbs and are characterized by cytoplasmic inclusions in oligodendrocytes, sometimes called Papp–Lantos filaments (Kovacs *et al.*, 2003). In an initial study of odor identification in 29 patients with a *clinical* diagnosis of MSA-P, mild impairment of odor identification ability was noted, with a mean UPSIT score of 26.7 compared with the control mean of 33.5 (Wenning *et al.*, 1993). There were no UPSIT differences between the parkinsonian and cerebellar types. Nee *et al.* (1993) and Muller *et al.* (2002) each found reduced smell function in seven of eight patients (in both publications), although neither distinguished between the parkinsonian and cerebellar varieties. More recently, Abele *et al.* (2003) focused particularly on MSA-C in comparison to other ataxias of unknown etiology and found no useful difference in olfactory

---

Case report 4.4: Dementia with Lewy bodies?

An 82-year-old woman complained of loss of taste and smell function for the previous five years. She recalled no upper respiratory infection or other specific incident associated at the outset of the symptoms. About two years after the onset of the smell loss, she was diagnosed with Parkinson's disease. Olfactory testing revealed a marked inability to identify odors (UPSIT score of 9/40) and markedly elevated phenyl ethyl alcohol odor detection threshold values both bilaterally and unilaterally. Performance on the 12-item Odor Memory Test was at chance level. Nasal cross-sectional area, by acoustic rhinometry, and nasal airway resistance, measured by anterior rhinomanometry, were normal. Whole-mouth and regional taste test results were unremarkable, as were scores on the *Beck Depression Inventory* (4), the *Picture Identification Test* (40/40), and the *Mini-Mental State Examination* (30/30). On follow-up approximately two years later, the patient was admitted to a nursing home with a revised diagnosis of Alzheimer's disease.

Comment: This lady's complaint of taste dysfunction was most likely secondary to loss of smell. The subjective olfactory impairment that occurred approximately two years previously was probably a precursor of the parkinsonian syndrome. In the absence of further details on examination and brain imaging, it is difficult to be certain of the disease label. Assuming the initial diagnosis of "Parkinson's disease" was correct and that this was revised to Alzheimer's disease of sufficient severity to warrant nursing home care, a clinical diagnosis of dementia with Lewy bodies would seem likely. As described, these patients present with characteristic features of Parkinson's disease but within one year show cognitive decline typical of Alzheimer's disease. In this context smell testing is of value in separating other parkinsonian syndromes associated with dementia, such as corticobasal degeneration and progressive supranuclear palsy, where the sense of smell sense is usually preserved.

---

test scores between the two categories. Taken together, the aforementioned studies suggest that mild to moderate olfactory impairment is present in MSA-P, but the overall severity of the defect is less than that of Parkinson's disease.

Corticobasal degeneration

In corticobasal degeneration (CBD), parkinsonian features are compounded by limb dystonia, ideomotor apraxia, myoclonus, and ultimately, cognitive

---

Case report 4.5: Parkinson disease dementia

A 66-year-old male former insurance worker had noted that for three years his golf handicap was worsening progressively. Six months previously he became aware of mild symmetrical hand tremor. He reckoned his sense of smell had been poor for 40 years at least. More recently there was some clumsiness on eating, slowing of walking speed, and reduction of speech volume. Examination showed an expressionless face and quiet monotonous speech. Upgaze was slightly impaired and ocular saccades were jerky. There was marked axial rigidity, failure of arm-swing on walking, and mild hand tremor at rest. An MRI brain scan showed multiple small ischemic lesions mostly in the subcortical white matter but not in the deep white matter or basal ganglia regions. His UPSIT score was 18 (severe microsmia) and there was significant asymmetric reduction of tracer uptake on DATScan in keeping with a parkinsonian syndrome. This patient responded moderately well to levodopa and his golf handicap improved. However, four years later (which would be after seven years of symptoms), he developed visual hallucinations, further cognitive decline, and levodopa-related involuntary movements.

Comment: The initial presentation was compatible with classical Parkinson's disease except for the possibility of cognitive decline during the second or third years of illness.

The abnormalities on olfactory tests and DATScan would be in keeping with typical Parkinson's disease. Development of hallucinations and cognitive decline within the first year of presentation is characteristic of dementia with Lewy bodies, but in this instance the symptoms occurred later. According to many, dementia with Lewy bodies is pathologically indistinguishable from classical Parkinson's disease (Ballard *et al.*, 2006), suggesting that there is a continuous spectrum from typical Parkinson's disease to dementia with Lewy bodies. Olfactory testing cannot distinguish these varieties since olfaction is probably severely affected in both (see Table 4.2). The most likely clinical diagnosis here is Parkinson disease–dementia – an Alzheimer-like disorder that develops in Parkinson's disease, typically 10 or more years after its onset.

---

decline. The disorder is thought to result from accumulation of tau protein typically in the fronto-parietal cortex and basal ganglia. In a large pathological survey of 93 olfactory bulbs there were three cases of CBD (Tsuboi *et al.*, 2003) but none displayed tau pathology. The last observation may explain in part why smell tests in CBD are normal or nearly so. Thus, in one survey of seven patients with clinically suspected CBD (Wenning *et al.*, 1995b),

UPSIT scores were in the low normal range with a mean of 27, a value not significantly different from their age-matched controls. A more recent study of another seven patients with clinically defined CBD showed mild impairment of odor-naming and odor picture-matching in the presence of normal discrimination (Luzzi *et al.*, 2007). Provisionally, the finding of normal or near-normal smell function in suspected CBD may permit differentiation from typical Parkinson's disease and Alzheimer's disease.

Progressive supranuclear palsy

In progressive supranuclear palsy (PSP), also known as the Steele–Richardson syndrome, there is failure of voluntary vertical gaze, progression of motor dysfunction at a rate more rapid than that seen in Parkinson's disease, marked imbalance, and advancing cognitive decline. The characteristic pathology in PSP consists of widespread deposits of tau protein in degenerating neurons, but (like CBD) tau and α-synuclein pathology was absent in the olfactory bulbs of 27 patients studied by Tsuboi *et al.* (2003). On the basis of a large clinicopathological study of 103 cases, Williams *et al.* (2005) proposed a new classification to distinguish two major varieties. The first, which these authors termed the "Richardson syndrome," accounted for 54 percent of their patients and was characterized by early onset of postural instability and falls, supranuclear vertical gaze palsy, and cognitive dysfunction. The second, entitled PSP-P, applied to 32 percent of the patients who exhibited asymmetrical onset tremor with moderate initial therapeutic response to levodopa. Patients were frequently misdiagnosed as classical Parkinson's disease. The remaining 14 percent of the patients were difficult to classify. In the first substantial olfactory study on PSP, no significant difference was observed, either in UPSIT scores or phenyl ethyl alcohol threshold values, between 21 patients and matched control subjects, although there was a trend toward higher threshold values ($p = 0.09$) which may have failed to reach significance because of the somewhat small number of patients (Doty *et al.*, 1993). Similar results were found in 15 cases of PSP that were also tested by use of the UPSIT (Wenning *et al.*, 1995a). In all instances, the diagnosis was clinically, not autopsy, based. The relative absence of tau or α-synuclein pathology in the olfactory bulb of these patients gives some support to the clinically based observation of preserved olfactory function.

A more complex picture has been found in relatives of patients with PSP (Baker & Montgomery, 2001). These workers used the same test battery as in their Parkinson's disease study, i.e., measures of motor function, odor identification, and mood. In 23 first-degree relatives, nine (39 percent) scored in the abnormal range, which is a remarkably high value. As noted earlier, this study may be confounded by self-selection of at-risk relatives, as the familial risk of PSP is nowhere near this magnitude. While there is clearly a need for pathologically confirmed studies, evidence at present suggests that olfaction is normal or nearly so in the Richardson syndrome, which is the easier of the two syndromes to diagnose. The existence of the newly identified PSP-P variety, which may simulate Parkinson's disease, might explain why some patients with apparent classical Parkinson's disease have normal olfactory function.

Vascular parkinsonism

Some patients with extensive cerebrovascular disease involving the basal ganglia, in particular the putamen and striatum, may develop a syndrome that mimics Parkinson's disease, but the response to levodopa is variable. If someone has significant cerebrovascular disease and unilateral parkinsonism develops acutely, then the diagnosis is relatively straightforward. The diagnosis is more difficult when the onset is insidious or stepwise. Although brain MRI may show extensive vascular lesions, it can be tricky to know whether this is coincidental, especially in the presence of known cerebrovascular disease. In one study, those with acute onset vascular parkinsonism (VP) had lesions located in the subcortical grey nuclei (striatum, globus pallidus, and thalamus), whereas those with insidious onset displayed lesions distributed diffusely in watershed areas (Zijlmans et al., 1995). Dopamine transporter imaging in the striatal region is usually normal in VP (Tzen et al., 2001), although it may show a "punched out" appearance reflecting local ischemia. One study of 14 patients fulfilling strictly defined clinical criteria for VP showed their UPSIT scores did not differ significantly from those of controls (respective means 25.5 and 27.5), suggesting that identification tests may aid differentiation from idiopathic Parkinson's disease (Katzenschlager et al., 2004). Theoretically this information may be of value in identifying the parkinsonian syndrome that is seen occasionally after head trauma and may present a difficult diagnosis, especially if there is litigation. Normal smell function in this context would support a vascular process rather than true Parkinson's disease.

Case report 4.6: Probable Parkinson disease with a vascular component

A 62-year-old housewife found that for one year previously her automatic watch kept stopping. This was an old-fashioned analogue watch that was worn on the left wrist. It had been checked over by her jeweler several times, but no fault was discovered. Over the same period it was found that, on swimming, the left lower limb felt peculiar – like a balloon and that it

Case report 4.6: (cont.)

was starting to drag when walking. She reported that for 20 years her sense of smell had been poor for no obvious reason. She had mild untreated hypertension, with systolic pressures around 180 mmHg. Examination showed a staring facial expression with a brisk, non-fatiguing glabella tap reflex. There was moderate rigidity of the trunk and neck muscles and limbs, more pronounced on the left side, and no arm-swing on walking. The blood pressure was 190/110 mmHg. Her UPSIT score was 27/40, which is just below the local 95 percent population limit (28/40) for a female of her age. OERP latency to P2 was 1120 ms, which is above the 2 standard deviation (SD) limit for control subjects (937 ms). DATScan imaging was not performed. An MRI brain scan showed multiple small white matter high signal changes in the right supraventricular and sub-cortical white matter, in keeping with small-vessel disease. The basal ganglia were normal and so were the sinuses. There was a good response to levodopa, confirming the diagnosis of classical Parkinson's disease of the akinetic rigid type.

Comment: The presentation because of recurrent stopping of an automatic watch is well recognized among neurologists and is sometimes known as the "Marsden sign" after the late Queen Square neurologist, David Marsden, who contributed enormously to the field of movement disorders. This sign reflects the relative immobility of the arm on which the watch is worn. Other limb features are in keeping, with rigidity in the limbs more marked on the left side. The longstanding hypertension would explain the MRI changes but their distribution is not suggestive of vascular Parkinson's disease. Furthermore, smell function is usually normal in vascular Parkinson's disease. A DATScan would have clinched the diagnosis but this is still an expensive investigation, not undertaken routinely. Smell testing showed clear abnormalities reflecting microsmia. The likely onset of smell impairment 20 years prior to the initial signs of Parkinson's disease is in keeping with the concept that smell dysfunction along with vagal motor disorder are among the earliest features of Parkinson's disease.

Drug-induced Parkinson's disease

This disorder can be clinically indistinguishable from Parkinson's disease and it was common when broad-spectrum dopamine antagonists were used widely for psychotic disorders. With the advent of selective D2 blockers (e.g., clozapine, olanzepine, quetiapine), the prevalence has subsided dramatically. A small study of drug-induced Parkinson's disease (DPD) was undertaken in 10 patients (Hensiek *et al.*, 2000), all of whom scored normally (27/30 or more) on the Mini-Mental State Examination. Parkinsonism had developed in response to a variety of phenothiazine preparations that were administered for at least two weeks. Of the 10 patients, five had an abnormal age-matched UPSIT score and none made a complete recovery from DPD even when the offending medication was changed or stopped. Of the remaining five who did regain motor function after their treatment was adjusted, all but one had normal smell function. Unfortunately, a number of these patients had a psychotic disorder which may have contributed or even caused their smell problem. Nonetheless, it is possible that some individuals with DPD are predisposed to develop Parkinson's disease and that exposure to a dopamine-depleting drug unmasks underlying disease and its associated olfactory dysfunction.

In parkinsonism induced by methylphenyltetrahydropyridine (MPTP), all six of the young drug addicts exhibited normal values on both the UPSIT and a phenyl ethyl alcohol detection threshold test (Doty *et al.*, 1992b). However, there was a trend toward higher threshold values in the exposed group relative to age-matched controls and there is some evidence that MPTP may produce damage to the olfactory system in monkeys. Thus, three common marmosets injected with MPTP reportedly had difficulty locating bananas by smell, and were not averse to eating bananas odorized with skatole (putrid, fecal) or isovaleric acid (dirty socks, rancid cheese), which was not the case in two controls or prior to the MPTP treatment (Miwa *et al.*, 2004). The reason for the differences between humans and monkeys is not clear, but could reflect differences in age, species, or drug concentrations. Rotenone, the pesticide and complex I inhibitor, reproduces features of Parkinson's disease in animals, including selective nigrostriatal dopaminergic degeneration and α-synuclein-positive cytoplasmic inclusions (Betarbet *et al.*, 2000; Sherer *et al.*, 2003). Brains from rotenone-treated animals demonstrate oxidative damage, notably in the same midbrain and olfactory bulb dopaminergic regions that are affected by Parkinson's disease (Sherer *et al.*, 2003). There are no reported human cases of rotenone-induced Parkinson's disease, but it is freely available and certainly has the potential to cause a form of parkinsonism.

Guam Parkinson's disease–dementia complex

The Guam Parkinson's disease–dementia complex (PDC) is largely confined to the Chamorro population that inhabits the Pacific Island of Guam and is typified by coexistence of Alzheimer-type dementia, parkinsonism, and motor neuron disease (amyotrophic lateral sclerosis; ALS), either alone or in combination. The cause of the disorder is still debated, i.e., whether mainly environmental or genetic, but the marked decline in prevalence since 1970 favors an environmental toxin such as the plant excitotoxin derived from Cycad nuts, high aluminium, or low calcium and magnesium levels in drinking water

(Oyanagi, 2005). Pathologically, the presence of NFTs and the absence of Lewy bodies place this disorder well apart from idiopathic Parkinson's disease. Like Parkinson's disease, the numbers of cells within the AON are significantly decreased (Doty *et al.*, 1991). Administration of the UPSIT to 24 patients with PDC revealed severe olfactory dysfunction of magnitude similar to that seen in idiopathic Parkinson's disease, although a few had additional cognitive impairment which could have lowered the scores slightly (Doty *et al.*, 1991). These observations were confirmed subsequently by Ahlskog and colleagues (1998) in Chamorro with ALS, pure parkinsonism, pure dementia, or PDC.

X-linked recessive dystonia–parkinsonism ("Lubag")

This X-linked disorder, also termed "Lubag," affects Filipino male adults with maternal roots from the Philippine Island of Panay. A single study of 20 affected males, using a culturally modified UPSIT, showed that olfaction was moderately impaired in Lubag (mean score of 18 of 25 items compared with a control score of 20), even early on in the disorder. The smell loss was independent of the degree of dystonia, rigidity, severity, and disease duration (Evidente *et al.*, 2004).

Essential tremor

Classical essential tremor (ET), especially where there is a strong family history, is often diagnosed without difficulty. There may be problems in a minority of cases when the tremor appears to be dystonic or there is coexisting rigidity. Also, there may be confusion between ET and benign tremulous Parkinson's disease where cogwheeling is absent or equivocal. There are no published studies of the olfactory pathology in ET, and only a few on the rest of the brain (Louis *et al.*, 2006). The first appraisal of identification ability, which was completed in 15 subjects with benign ET, found all to be normal on the UPSIT (Busenbark *et al.*, 1992). This study was subsequently challenged by Louis and colleagues (2002), who reported that a significant proportion of ET patients had mild impairment, prompting the suggestion that this defect may relate to the postulated olfactory function of the cerebellum. In a subsequent study of ET patients with isolated rest tremor (Louis & Jurewicz, 2003), the UPSIT score was no different from typical ET patients, suggesting that involvement of the basal ganglia is part of the ET syndrome. Recent olfactory findings using the UPSIT in ET (Adler *et al.*, 2005; Shah *et al.*, 2005) are normal overall, but errors may creep in if a patient with apparent ET is confused with benign tremulous Parkinson's disease, a condition where olfactory function is usually impaired. Clearly it would help diagnostically if all ET subjects had normal olfactory function, as this would allow better distinction of ET from Parkinson's disease subjects with tremor. A recent study has addressed this problem by comparing ET in 59 healthy

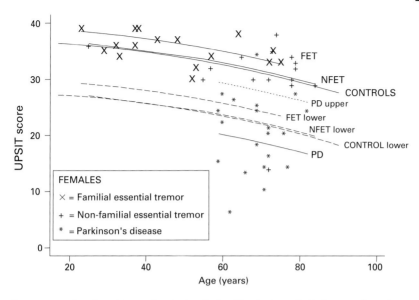

Figure 4.6 University of Pennsylvania Smell Identification Test (UPSIT) score plotted against age in females for familial (FET) and non-familial essential tremor (NFET) using a quadratic regression model. Lines for males are similar except they are about 2 UPSIT points below females at all ages. Solid lines are model-fitted values assuming a common slope in all groups. Dashed lines are limits of 95 percent reference ranges. The graph shows the slight superiority of familial essential tremor patients compared with the non-familial group. The regression line for Parkinson's disease is well below that for control subjects and essential tremor groups. (Reproduced from Shah *et al.*, 2008.)

control subjects with 64 subjects suffering from tremor-dominant Parkinson's disease (Shah *et al.*, 2008). There was almost complete separation of the two groups on the basis of UPSIT scores and to a lesser degree on the OERP. When ET subjects were separated by family history of tremor in a first-degree relative (FET), this group scored significantly better than age- and gender-matched control subjects (Figure 4.6). There was a suggestion of resistance to the effects of olfactory aging in FET as well. These unexpected findings need to be verified but it is likely that patients with ET have no important disorder of olfaction.

In practical terms, the expectation of normal olfactory function in ET (whether familial or not) could be used diagnostically: if a patient with suspected ET has abnormal olfactory test scores, when allowing for age and gender, then the diagnosis would merit review. If the patient is thought to have tremor-dominant Parkinson's disease then olfaction should be abnormal. At present it would be unwise to use a smell test in isolation, but olfactory testing may provide a useful initial guide to the diagnosis.

Case report 4.7: Benign tremulous Parkinson's disease with positive family history

A 64-year-old former engineer presented on account of left-sided tremor for the preceding two years. It started in the foot and spread to the hand, and was diminished slightly by alcohol. He was unaware of any problem with the sense of smell. Both parents developed tremor late in life, neither of whom were significantly disabled. Examination showed a moderately severe rest tremor on the left with slight cogwheel rigidity on that side. There was mild postural tremor and increased fatigue on repeated hand movement. The provisional diagnosis was either benign tremulous Parkinson's disease with a positive family history of the same condition or familial ET. The UPSIT score was in the severe microsmic range (23/40) and OERP was delayed at 1116 ms (normal less than 937 ms). The MRI brain scan was normal but there was mild mucosal prominence in the sphenoid air sinus. DATScan showed bilateral reduction of transporter uptake in the putamen. Response to levodopa was good and the final clinical diagnosis was benign tremulous Parkinson's disease.

Comment: The clinical assessment here pointed to tremulous Parkinson's disease with a family history of tremor, which is unusual, although it is increasingly recognized. The fact that neither parent was disabled suggests that they had essential tremor or benign tremulous Parkinson's disease, neither of which is characterized by severe disability.

In some families with typical Parkinson's disease in one generation, there may be others with typical essential tremor (Yahr *et al.*, 2003). The diagnosis of Parkinson's disease in our case is confirmed by clinical examination, abnormality of smell identification, good response to levodopa, delayed OERP and by an abnormal DATScan. If this patient had essential tremor the smell tests should be normal (Shah *et al.*, 2008).

Cerebellar ataxia

If the cerebellum is concerned with olfaction, either through control of sniffing or actual identification, then abnormalities might be present in some ataxias. Given the possibility of confusion between cerebellar tremor and parkinsonism, olfactory tests might aid the differential diagnosis. In one study, mild abnormalities in UPSIT scores were found in Friedreich's ataxia (Connelly *et al.*, 2003). No correlation was seen between the UPSIT scores and trinucleotide repeat length, disease duration, or walking disability. Other patients with a variety of ataxic disorders, as a whole, did not differ from the Friedreich's patients. Fernandez-Ruis *et al.* (2003) examined olfactory function in an assortment of ataxic subjects. Mild olfactory impairment was found in autosomal dominant spinocerebellar ataxia type 2 (SCA2), but not in Machado–Joseph syndrome (SCA3). In contrast, Hentschel et al. (2005) found normal UPSIT scores in seven individuals with the SCA2 mutation. Patients with SCA2 or SCA3 mutations may have parkinsonian tremor or dystonia (SCA3), which can cause diagnostic difficulty; hence, the finding of normal olfaction in suspected Parkinson's disease could indicate an inherited cerebellar syndrome. It is important to note that all these observations have been based on small numbers of patients and should be interpreted conservatively. Clearly it would be premature to suggest that the cerebellum is responsible for the smell defect in ataxic disorder until there has been pathological examination of the classical olfactory pathways.

Motor neuron disease (amyotrophic lateral sclerosis)

Nomenclature varies worldwide, but here "motor neuron disease" (MND) will be used as a generic term for all varieties affecting motor neurons of which amyotrophic lateral sclerosis (ALS) is the most common, followed by bulbar forms and then the mildest form – progressive muscular atrophy (PMA). In the North American literature, ALS approximates to MND in the UK. Pathologically there has been just one olfactory study and that examined the olfactory bulb. In eight autopsy cases of MND which were compared to age-matched controls, Hawkes et al. (1998) found marked accumulation of lipofuscin in both the neurons of the AON and other neuronal types of the olfactory bulb, suggesting increased lipid peroxidation.

An initial clinically based pilot study examined 15 patients with MND, of whom eight had moderate or severe bulbar involvement and eight were chair-bound (Elian, 1991). No test for dementia was administered but a significant lowering of the UPSIT score was documented. In another study of 37 patients with ALS (Sajjadian et al., 1994), 28 (75.7 percent) had significantly lower scores on UPSIT compared with age-matched controls. Four of these 28 (i.e., 11 percent) had near or total anosmia. Hawkes et al. (1998) examined UPSIT scores in 58 cognitively normal patients with an established diagnosis of MND. Seven had PMA, 34 typical ALS, and 17 had bulbar disease. Overall, 9 of 58 patients (16 percent) displayed UPSIT scores that were significantly below those of age-matched controls. The effect of group status overall (i.e., MND versus control) was statistically significant ($p = 0.02$). However, analysis among the patient groups found that only bulbar patients differed meaningfully from control subjects. OERPs were performed in 15 patients: in nine the responses were normal for latency and amplitude measurements; one was delayed; in two the response was absent; and in three the recording could not be obtained. In this study, the reason for a proportionately larger number of patients with normal olfactory function is not clear, but it could reflect case selection effects or diagnostic bias. Also there is a possibility of falsely lowered identification scores from reduced sniffing, as seen in Parkinson's disease (Sobel *et al.*, 2001), since many bulbar MND patients are likely to have respiratory weakness. The OERP findings, which circumvent the need to inhale actively, suggest that olfaction is affected in MND, although to a mild degree.

Huntington's disease (Huntington's chorea)

This is a late-presenting autosomal dominant disorder of basal ganglia function typified by choreic movement, dementia, and, in rare cases, muscular rigidity similar to that of Parkinson's disease (Westphal variant). An initial study of 38 Huntington's disease subjects reported early defective odor memory in some cases prior to the expression of cognitive or marked involuntary movement (Moberg *et al.*, 1987). Subsequent analysis, using tests of odor identification and detection, confirmed the presence of moderate olfactory impairment in Huntington's disease patients with established disease, but of less severity than Parkinson's disease (Bylsma *et al.*, 1997; Hamilton *et al.*, 1999; Moberg & Doty, 1997; Nordin *et al.*, 1995b). According to one study (Hamilton *et al.*, 1999), n-butanol threshold measurement in early-stage Huntington's disease provided good classification of sensitivity and specificity between the patients (7) and matched control subjects (7), suggesting that olfactory testing may provide a sensitive measure of disease onset. Two studies have explored smell function in relatives at 50 percent risk of Huntington's disease. In one, UPSIT scores and phenyl ethyl alcohol thresholds were normal in 12 at-risk relatives, but abnormal in 25 probands (Moberg & Doty, 1997). In the other, 20 healthy subjects known to have the Huntington's disease mutation exhibited normal UPSIT scores, whereas the Huntington's disease group (20) were mildly abnormal (Bylsma *et al.*, 1997). Just one study explored the value of OERP in eight subjects with established Huntington's disease, showing that the late positive (cognitive) component "P3" was significantly delayed (Wetter *et al.*, 2005). The aforementioned studies, while demonstrating that smell loss is present at the time of HD phenotypic expression, do not explain when the olfactory loss first appears. A provocative recent report suggests that subtle smell dysfunction may occur, along with mild cognitive and motor changes, in HD gene carriers 10–15 years before HD is clinically manifest (Paulsen *et al.*, 2008).

Patients with Huntington's disease may show deficits in recognizing disgust in the facial expressions and vocal intonations of others (Gray *et al.*, 1997), and this may relate to dysfunction in the amygdala. These difficulties with facial expression recognition were also seen in otherwise healthy Huntington's disease gene carriers. Extending this principle, it has been suggested that disgust-related deficits may apply to foul-smelling olfactory stimuli and inappropriate combinations of taste stimuli (Mitchell *et al.*, 2005). Subjects at 50 percent risk of future disease were not tested, but this would be an obvious extension of such work. The utility of this observation, and indeed all olfactory assessments so far, is offset by the widely available and specific DNA test for Huntington's chorea. Even if smell impairment does develop very early in the clinical phase of disease, there are usually subtle signs of involuntary movement, cognitive, or personality changes. In any event, neuroprotective therapy, if it becomes available, will be most beneficial if it is administered long before the stage of manifest symptoms (Pavese *et al.*, 2006).

Several other conditions are now recognized that can simulate the Huntington's disease phenotype: spinocerebellar atrophy type 17 (SCA-17), neuroacanthocytosis, benign hereditary chorea, and Huntington disease-like disorder (HDL1 and HDL2). In all of these, a molecular diagnosis can be made, but so far there are no published studies on olfactory function. This would clearly be an interesting line of research.

Diagnostic implications for neurodegenerative disorders

It is well established that the olfactory system is damaged to varying degree in clinically evident parkinsonism (see Table 4.1). Most severe changes are seen in the idiopathic, Guamanian, and Lewy body varieties. Least involvement is found in CBD and PSP, and intermediate involvement in MSA. However, there is considerable variability and overlap of smell dysfunction in these syndromes, limiting the diagnostic value of smell testing. Broadly speaking, where the pathological features are those of tauopathy, olfaction is probably normal (e.g., PSP, CBD); if the pathology is an α-synucleinopathy (Parkinson's disease, Lewy body disease, dementia with Lewy bodies), abnormal olfaction is to be expected. However, such pathological diagnoses must be conservatively interpreted, since tau and α-synuclein may be differentially expressed in diverse brain regions within these disorders. At present there are too few studies on familial parkinsonism to state whether smell testing will be helpful, but there is clearly considerable potential for olfactory testing in subjects at risk of familial Parkinson's disease.

With these caveats, differences in smell function can aid diagnosis. For example, if a patient is suspected to have Parkinson's disease, especially of the akinetic rigid variety, the presence of normal olfaction *on testing* should prompt review of the diagnosis. Abnormal smell function in presumed CBD or PSP would also be unexpected. Normal olfaction in alleged Parkinson's disease would imply six alternative diagnoses: vascular parkinsonism; the parkinsonian variant of PSP (PSP-P); spinocerebellar ataxia type 3 (and perhaps SCA2); corticobasal degeneration; ET and benign tremulous Parkinson's disease, particularly in females. DATScan is useful in confirming a suspected diagnosis of Parkinson's disease, but it is not specific and cannot distinguish Parkinson's disease from parkinsonian syndromes. Its diagnostic utility is comparable to olfactory testing (Deeb *et al.*, 2006), although at much greater expense and it is not yet known which test – DATScan, olfactory, or now, transcranial sonography – is best able to detect presymptomatic Parkinson's disease (Sommer *et al.*, 2004).

Olfactory testing in Huntington's disease and ALS shows abnormalities relatively early, but it is likely to prove less rewarding both for diagnostic and presymptomatic testing. It is apparent that olfaction is severely impaired in the majority of cases with Alzheimer's disease, probably reflecting more central than peripheral pathology. Although early-stage Alzheimer's disease may be assessed validly using psychophysical procedures, the results of such testing in later stages are questionable, because of confounding by cognitive issues. Hence, there is need for studies using test measures less dependent upon cognitive responses, such as OERPs. Although many investigations suggest that olfactory dysfunction is a pre-cognitive abnormality in Alzheimer's disease, it might be argued that olfaction is just easier to measure than early cognitive decline. A parallel argument may be applied to Parkinson's disease, although the studies of Braak and those now emerging from the HAAS make this unlikely. Olfactory testing in asymptomatic relatives of those with Parkinson' disease or Alzheimer's disease could act as a useful biomarker for those at risk of subsequent disease. Further long-term prospective studies in families with Alzheimer's disease and Parkinson's disease containing substantial members at 50 percent risk will help solve this problem.

The olfactory vector hypothesis

Although the olfactory pathways are among the first to exhibit Alzheimer's disease- and Parkinson's disease-related neuropathology, the underlying reason for such olfactory dysfunction is obscure. Viruses and toxins have been implicated, but their specific role, if any, in disease pathology has not been established.

It has long been known that foreign agents are able to move from the nasal cavity to the brain via the olfactory nerves or surrounding mucosa. In the second century AD, Claudius Galen alluded to the permeability of the dura mater around the cribriform plate to both water and air, and propagated the theory, which was widely accepted until the early nineteenth century, that agents responsible for olfactory sensation pass into the ventricles of the brain through the foramina of the cribriform plate (Doty, 2003b; Wright, 1914). In the early twentieth century it was demonstrated conclusively that olfactory nerve cells are a major route for viruses from the nasal cavity to the brain. By 1912, Flexner and his collaborators had shown that polio virus could enter the simian central nervous system via the olfactory neuroepithelium (Flexner & Lewis, 1910; Flexner & Clark, 1912). Sabin and Olitsky (1936) found olfactory bulb pathology in monkeys that had received the virus intranasally, but not in those that had been exposed intracerebrally, subcutaneously, or via the sciatic nerve (Doty, 2008; Sabin & Olitsky, 1936). In children who had succumbed to the disease, similar olfactory bulb pathology was noted independently by two groups, implicating the olfactory system as the most common, if not sole, pathway of the virus into the brain under normal circumstances (Robertson, 1940; Sabin, 1940). Cauterization of the olfactory neuroepithelium with zinc sulfate had been shown to be protective against poliomyelitis when the virus was instilled intranasally in primates (Schultz & Gebhardt, 1936). The evidence for olfactory nerve transmission of the polio virus was then so strong that in the late 1930s Canadian public health officials used zinc sulfate cauterization during poliomyelitis epidemics in an attempt to stem the disease (Schultz & Gebhardt, 1937; Tisdall *et al.*, 1937).

One of the more interesting and controversial theories proposed to explain the olfactory loss and the etiology of some neurodegenerative diseases is the "olfactory vector hypothesis" (OVH) (Doty, 1991, 2008; Ferreyra-Moyano & Barragan, 1989; Harrison, 1990; Pearson *et al.*, 1985). Hawkes *et al.* (1999) elaborated this theory further, suggesting that classical Parkinson's disease was a primary disorder of olfaction. A major component of the hypothesis implies that the olfactory deficit reflects, directly or indirectly, damage to the olfactory system from an environmental agent that enters the brain via the olfactory fila, subsequently inducing disease (Doty, 1991; Ferreyra-Moyano & Barragan, 1989; Roberts, 1986). This concept stems from the fact that the olfactory receptor cells (ORC), whose cilia and dendritic knobs in the human have an extensive combined surface area of ~23 cm^2 (Doty, 2001), are in relatively direct contact with the potentially hostile external environment. As noted in Chapter 1 these cells act as both receptor and first-order neurons, projecting an axon directly from the nasal cavity into the olfactory bulb without an intervening synapse. The ORCs can transport viruses, ionized metals (e.g., cadmium, gold, and manganese), nano-particles, and other environmental agents, including non-volatile compounds which become incorporated into aerosols and dusts, at rates higher than 2 mm/h (Baker & Genter, 2003; Gottofrey & Tjalve, 1991; Tjalve *et al.*, 1996; Tjalve & Henriksson, 1999). Although some xenobiotics are actively detoxified in the epithelium by nasal enzyme systems, including P450-dependent mono-oxygenase, others are metabolized into *more* neurotoxic or carcinogenic compounds (Bond, 1986; Dahl, 1986). Interestingly, herbicides, such as the dioxins (Gillner *et al.*, 1987) or chlorthiamid (Brittebo *et al.*, 1991), are selectively taken up by, and are harmful to, the olfactory epithelium, even when administered systemically (Doty, 2008).

A wealth of data from animal studies shows that many xenobiotics can be transported beyond the olfactory system to multiple brain regions, including sites in common with the neuropathology of Alzheimer's disease and Parkinson's disease. For example, Herpes simplex virus type I, placed intranasally in six-week-old mice, is detected in the olfactory bulbs after four days and subsequently spreads as far as the temporal lobe, hippocampus, and cingulate cortex (Tomlinson & Esiri, 1983). Horseradish peroxidase (HRP), when applied intranasally, is transported to the bulb, anterior olfactory nucleus, transmitter-specific projection neurons of the diagonal band (cholinergic), raphe nucleus (serotonergic), and locus coeruleus (noradrenergic) (Shipley, 1985). This is of particular relevance as the locus coeruleus and raphe nuclei are involved in the premotor phase of Parkinson's disease – Braak stage 2 (Braak et al., 2003a). HRP, when injected into the olfactory tubercle, results in *retrograde* labeling of the ipsilateral olfactory bulb, AON, and other primary olfactory areas, as well as *anterograde* labeling of the ipsilateral ventral tegmental area, substantia nigra, (pars reticulata), and ventral pallidum (Newman & Winans, 1980), emphasizing the existence of direct connections between primary olfactory areas and the substantia nigra. Many viruses, such as the Epstein–Barr virus, encode proteins that exploit the ubiquitin–proteasome system to regulate latency and allow the persistence of infected cells in immunocompetent hosts (Masucci, 2004; Shackelford & Pagano, 2005). Importantly, some inhaled neurotoxins may activate latent viruses; for example, trichloroethylene may reactivate herpes simplex 1 infection within the trigeminal nerve (Buxton & Hayward, 1967).

In light of such observations, is there any convincing evidence that neurodegenerative diseases are caused or catalyzed by agents that enter the brain via the olfactory receptor cells? In this section we address major arguments for and against the OVH (see summary in Table 4.3). The areas of focus are: (1) the degree to which environmental and genetic factors are implicated in most forms of Alzheimer's disease and Parkinson's disease; (2) the types of xenobiotic agents implicated as risk factors for Alzheimer's disease and Parkinson's disease which may enter the brain via the olfactory pathways; and (3) the pattern of direction, i.e., peripheral to central versus central to peripheral, of neurodegenerative pathology within the CNS.

Environmental versus genetic determinants

Although an increasing number of abnormal genes have been identified in Alzheimer's disease and Parkinson's disease, at present they account for a small percentage of apparently sporadic cases. This would imply that heritability is low and that environmental agents may be critically involved in their etiology. Given that smell loss is an early sign of such disorders, it would seem possible that such loss signifies the early pathology relating to an offending xenobiotic agent, as implied by the OVH. Conversely, and as discussed earlier in this chapter, patients with an early-onset familial form of Alzheimer's disease who express the presenilin-1 mutation may not have pre-symptomatic smell impairment (Nee & Lippa, 2001), and some with apparent Alzheimer's disease have normal smell function (McShane *et al.*, 2001; Westervelt *et al.*, 2007). The fact that Alzheimer's disease-like pathology occurs inevitably in

Table 4.3 Arguments for and against the olfactory vector hypothesis in Alzheimer's disease and Parkinson's disease

Proposal	For	Against
Low rate of inheritance	Less than 10 percent of sporadic cases are inherited and most have less smell loss than classical Parkinson's disease. Genetic forms may represent different diseases. Mutations may still produce susceptibility to environmental agents rather than directly cause disease	More mutations are being discovered. Down syndrome progresses to Alzheimer's disease. Transgenic mice can be induced to overexpress Parkinson's disease and Alzheimer's disease pathology. Families with α-synuclein triplication always suffer a form of Parkinson's disease
Transport of agents into brain from nose	Known to occur for herbicides, pesticides, toxins, heavy metals, viruses	Epidemiological data inconclusive. One case of Alzheimer's disease in someone with imperforate cribriform plate
Clinical evidence of early olfactory involvement	Long-term prospective studies, family surveys. 80–90 percent of patients with Parkinson's disease are microsmic. Those who are not may be misclassified	10–20 percent patients with Parkinson's disease apparently have normal sense of smell. Not all surveys that show microsmia have pathological confirmation. Patients with presenilin-1 mutation did not have prior olfactory loss, nor do all cases of apparently typical Alzheimer's disease
Pathological findings	Pathology in Braak Parkinson's disease stage 1 involves olfactory bulb and medullary vagal nucleus only. Honolulu-Asia Aging Study (HAAS) showed pre-symptomatic microsmia was predictive of later Lewy pathology. The pattern of movement of xenobiotic does not have to reflect direction of movement of pathogen	No typical changes are seen in the olfactory epithelium, only in bulb which is one synapse away. Not yet clear whether Alzheimer's disease starts in the bulb or more centrally. In Parkinson's disease, some find no Lewy pathology in medulla or pons when the substantia nigra is involved

Table 4.3 (*cont.*)

Proposal	For	Against
Herbicide use and Parkinson's disease	Epidemiology suggests link with farming. Rotenone causes typical changes of Parkinson's disease in animals	Epidemiological data mostly inconclusive and often retrospective
Olfactory epithelium is metabolically highly active	Possibly a defective cytochrome system permits entry of neurotoxin	Not much direct evidence in humans apart from disordered debrisoquine metabolism (P450-dependant)
Allergic rhinitis	Prevalence raised in Parkinson's disease. Suggests there may be reduced nasal protection that might facilitate entry of pathogen	Single retrospective case-note-based study. Needs replication

older people with Down syndrome implies genetic causation for Alzheimer's disease (Rebeck & Hyman, 1993). Olfactory impairment is probably minimal in PARK 2 and PARK 3 (but not in PARK 1 and PARK 8; see Table 4.1) and while the phenotype may be similar to classical Parkinson's disease, the olfactory features suggest that at least some may represent a different disease. According to Hardy (2005) the majority of Parkinson's disease cases are genetically based and the key factor is the degree of genetic loading. For example, where there is triplication of normal α-synuclein the disease is always expressed and at an earlier age (Singleton *et al.*, 2004). Although genetic predisposition is undoubtedly relevant in Alzheimer's disease and Parkinson's disease, multiple etiologies are likely and the contribution from environmental protection or facilitation cannot be ignored. Not all cases of Alzheimer's disease or Parkinson's disease need be explained by the OVH, including the Alzheimer-type pathology associated with Down syndrome. Importantly, the OVH does not necessarily exclude other determinants within the same individual.

Environmental agents known to be transported into the brain through the nose

Several environmental agents suspected to be risk factors for Alzheimer's disease and Parkinson's disease can theoretically enter the brain via the olfactory route. Among such agents are viruses, toxic metals, air pollutants, herbicides, and defoliants (Ascherio *et al.*, 2006; Itzhaki & Itzhaki, 2004; Li *et al.*, 2005; Liou *et al.*, 1997; Semchuk *et al.*, 1992; Tyas *et al.*, 2001). Calderon-Garciduenas *et al.* (2004) measured the expression of the inflammatory mediator cyclo-oxygenase-2 (COX2) and the 42-amino acid form of beta-amyloid (Abeta42) in autopsy brain tissues of cognitively and neurologically intact lifelong residents of cities having low or high levels of air pollution. Residents of a city with severe air pollution had significantly higher COX2 expression in the olfactory bulb, frontal cortex, and hippocampus, and greater neuronal and astrocytic accumulation of Abeta42 compared with residents in a low-air-pollution city. Brain inflammation and Abeta42 accumulation are believed to precede the appearance of neuritic plaques and NFTs. Interestingly, UPSIT scores are lower in the high-pollution-city cohort than in the low-air-pollution-city cohort (Calderón-Garcidueñas et al., in press).

Several large epidemiological studies have found occupational herbicide or defoliant use in association with Alzheimer's disease and Parkinson's disease (Ascherio *et al.*, 2006; Li *et al.*, 2005; Liou *et al.*, 1997; Semchuk *et al.*, 1992; Tyas *et al.*, 2001). Such agents may be inhaled and enter the brain via the lungs and bloodstream; alternatively, they might accumulate initially within the olfactory neuroepithelium and then migrate to the olfactory bulb. Indeed, there is evidence that this occurs for rotenone (Sherer *et al.*, 2003), a widely available herbicide. This toxin, which acts by complex I inhibition, causes selective nigrostriatal dopaminergic degeneration, Lewy body formation, and damage to areas typically associated with Parkinson's disease, including the olfactory bulbs (Betarbet *et al.*, 2000; Sherer *et al.*, 2003). In light of such observations, as well as the aforementioned study by Calderon-Garcidueñas *et al.* (2004), it may not be coincidental that a disproportionate number of Parkinson's disease patients have significantly increased prevalence of intermediate-type hypersensitivity disorder, in particular allergic rhinitis (Bower *et al.*, 2006), a disorder with compromised olfactory function (Klimek, 1998).

Recently, it was found that 88 percent of 43 confined-space workers exposed to airborne metals such as cadmium, iron, manganese, and lead for standard shift periods over the course of one to two years exhibited olfactory dysfunction and 28 percent developed signs of parkinsonism (Antunes *et al.*, 2007). Whether this reflects movement of such metals into the brain via the olfactory receptors is unknown, but clearly a possibility.

An argument leveled at the OVH for Alzheimer's disease concerns a 65-year-old anosmic non-demented woman who displayed plaques and tangles in typical Alzheimer's disease distribution. The cribriform plate was imperforate, the olfactory bulbs and tracts were rudimentary, and there were sulcal abnormalities of the orbitofrontal region (Arriagada *et al.*, 1991). However, it is possible that in this single case a pathogen entered the olfactory system several years prior to occlusion of the cribriform plate foramina. Indeed, such occlusion occurs in many elderly people (Kalmey *et al.*, 1998).

Primacy of olfactory involvement

As detailed above, numerous behavioral and pathological studies indicate compromise of the olfactory system in Alzheimer's disease and Parkinson's disease, and suggest that, in some, this may take place several years before the expression of typical signs of disease. According to the Braak staging of Parkinson's disease, Lewy pathology is found first within the olfactory bulb and dorsal motor nuclear complex of cranial nerves IX and X (Braak *et al.*, 2003a). From here it is proposed that the disease simultaneously ascends the brainstem to the substantia nigra and travels along the olfactory tracts to the temporal lobes. However, as described earlier in this chapter, not all pathologists concur with this progressive staging (Halliday *et al.*, 2006; Kalaitzakis *et al.*, 2008; Parkkinen *et al.*, 2005).

In Alzheimer's disease, the evidence for a peripheral origin of olfactory damage is less robust than in Parkinson's disease. Thus, Vogt *et al.* (1990) pointed out that sectors of the amygdala which receive olfactory projections are not those most reliably laden with plaques and tangles, and Mann (1989) proposed that Alzheimer's disease-related degeneration begins in cortical, not subcortical, brain regions. He pointed out that the major subcortical nuclei damaged in Alzheimer's disease (i.e., nucleus basalis, locus coeruleus, and dorsal raphe) project to the same cortical areas, whereas subcortical nuclei that do not project to such areas are not similarly damaged. Elsewhere he argued that, because the frequency of plaques and tangles is lower in the olfactory bulbs and tracts than in the amygdala and hippocampus, the direction of damage must be centrifugal (Mann, 1989). A similar argument was made by Okamoto *et al.* (1990) in a study of 100 Alzheimer's disease patients who exhibited plaques in the olfactory bulbs only when greater numbers were present in the cerebral cortex. More recently, Braak and Braak (1998) inferred from pathological studies that the transentorhinal cortex is the first site of injury. This brain region is a narrow area involved with transmission of information from the major cortical sensory areas to the entorhinal cortex and hippocampus (see Chapter 1, Figure 1.20 and in color section).

Despite this, not all pathological studies support the notion of centrifugal spread. For example, Kovacs *et al.* (2001), who examined 15 brains from patients with Alzheimer's disease, discovered early involvement of the olfactory bulbs, sometimes before other brain structures. Moreover, it is possible that formation of senile plaques (SP) and NFTs within the amygdala and hippocampus results from other processes (e.g., a defect in blood–brain barrier function) in which areas "triggered off" by a pathogenic agent spread via the olfactory pathways. If so, formation of Alzheimer's disease pathology in olfactory nuclei would not necessarily occur during orthograde transport of such an agent, but could result from later retrograde spread. Consequently, less severe changes in the bulb and tracts would be expected. Thus the pattern of Alzheimer's disease pathology need not necessarily reflect the direction of movement of a xenobiotic in the CNS. Viruses or other pathogens that enter the CNS via the olfactory fila could selectively damage more central regions of the limbic system, beginning with the most vulnerable areas and subsequently produce centrifugal propagation of damage (Mann, 1988). Indeed, neurovirulent viral and toxin selectivity is well documented. For example, Barnett *et al.* (1993) employed in situ hybridization to compare the spread of two viruses, herpes simplex virus type I and a mouse hepatitis virus strain (JHM), through the olfactory pathways of the mouse. While both viruses entered the brain via the olfactory system, only herpes-simplex-infected noradrenergic neurons in the locus coeruleus. Although both viruses infected dopaminergic neurons in the ventral tegmental area, mouse hepatitis virus produced much more widespread infection. These arguments are somewhat circular, but it is safe to conclude that the site of initial damage in Alzheimer's disease is not yet established.

Nasal metabolism of xenobiotics

As a first line of defense against xenobiotics, several studies imply that the nasal cytochrome system is probably as important as the liver. Microsomes in the olfactory epithelium have, in some cases, higher levels of cytochrome P450 and other detoxification enzymes than are found in the liver (Ding & Coon, 1990; Hext & Lock, 1992). In the monkey, P450 levels are higher in the olfactory bulb than other brain structures (Iscan *et al.*, 1990). Compounds shown to be metabolized *in vitro* by the nasal P450-dependent mono-oxygenase system include nasal decongestants, essences, anesthetics, alcohols, nicotine, cocaine, and many nasal carcinogens (Dahl, 1988). Importantly, individuals with a mutation in the P450 cytochrome CYP2D6-debrisoquine hydroxylase gene appear to have increased risk for Parkinson's disease (Elbaz *et al.*, 2004; Smith *et al.*, 1992), raising the possibility that a compromised P450 enzyme system may facilitate the penetration of xenobiotics into brain tissue, thereby producing neural damage. The existence of familial forms of Alzheimer's disease or Parkinson's disease does not exclude the possibility that a breakdown occurs in metabolic pathways at some stage (such as cytochrome P450 within the olfactory mucosa), rendering such individuals more susceptible to neurotoxic environmental agents. In accord with this are studies suggesting that tobacco smokers have reduced risk of contracting Parkinson's disease but not Alzheimer's disease (Aggarwal *et al.*, 2006; Tanner *et al.*, 2002), and that smoking may protect the olfactory system from damage by industrial exposure to methacrylates, acrylates, and acetone (Schwartz *et al.*, 1989, 1990). Cigarette smoke contains high levels (100–250 ng/cigarette) of polyaromatic hydrocarbons which are known to induce cytochrome P450 enzyme activity. Stimulation of such enzymes leads to increased metabolism of xenobiotics in the olfactory epithelium (as well as the liver), conceivably preventing environmental neurotoxins from reaching their target organs (Gresham *et al.*, 1993). Of possible relevance, although speculative, is the fact that elderly dogs may spontaneously display Alzheimer-type pathology (Papaioannou *et al.*, 2001), but they do not develop Parkinson's disease spontaneously nor do they show Lewy pathology in the substantia nigra (Uchida *et al.*, 2003). This may relate to their highly developed nasal detoxification system, which protects their brain against Parkinson's disease. If this preliminary observation is confirmed, it lends support to the OVH for Parkinson's disease but not for Alzheimer's disease.

In summary, the evidence for nasal entry of a pathogen that might cause Alzheimer's disease is less persuasive than for Parkinson's disease. If such an Alzheimer's disease-related pathogen does enter the brain via the olfactory fila, it probably influences central more than peripheral brain structures. In Parkinson's disease, the argument is more believable but the presence of early CN IX and CN X pathology in the medulla presents a potential barrier to acceptance. It could be argued that a pathogen such as a neurotropic virus enters the nose, damages the sense of smell, and then travels along sensory fibers of CN IX and CN X in the pharynx to reach the medulla. However, the medullary nuclei of these cranial nerves are spared in the early stages of Parkinson's disease (Braak *et al.*, 2003b). Wakabayashi *et al.* (1990) and Braak *et al.* (2006) showed Lewy pathology in Auerbach's and Meissner's plexus in the stomach wall (Figure 4.7), which led to the proposal that the pathogen ascends retrogradely

central nervous system   **enteric nervous system**

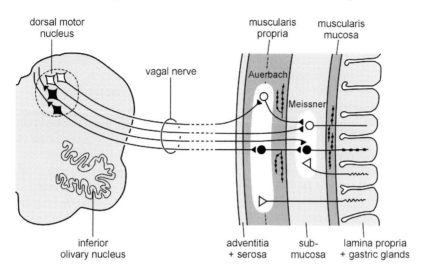

Figure 4.7 Schematic diagram showing the interconnections between the enteric nervous system and brain. A neurotropic agent that succeeded in passing the mucosal epithelial barrier of the stomach could enter terminal axons of postganglionic VIPergic neurons (black, rounded cell somata) in the submucosal Meissner's plexus and via retrograde axonal and transneuronal transport (black, rounded cell somata in Auerbach's plexus), reaching the preganglionic cholinergic neurons (black, diamond-shaped cell somata) of the dorsal motor nucleus of the vagus. Two triangular-shaped cells (white) represent primary viscerosensory neurons. Two white, rounded cells represent cholinergic excitatory visceromotor neurons. (Reproduced from Braak *et al.*, 2006. With permission from Elsevier.)

in the motor fibers of the vagus to its medullary nucleus (Braak *et al.*, 2006). Retrograde vagal entry into the CNS, of course, will not explain the early peripheral olfactory changes. To explain such initial pathology, a pathogen would need concurrently to enter and damage the olfactory pathway via the nose, be swallowed in nasal secretions, invade the enteric plexus of the stomach, and ascend in motor vagal fibers. This sequence of somewhat tortuous events has been termed the "dual hit" hypothesis because of the simultaneous entry of pathogen via the nose and stomach (Hawkes *et al.*, 2007). Further studies, now underway, may clarify this interesting concept.

Summary

Altered olfactory function is common, to a variable degree, in a wide range of neurodegenerative diseases. To what extent such changes reflect accelerated aging is not known. In the typical forms of both Alzheimer's disease and Parkinson's disease there is abundant anatomical and physiological evidence of olfactory impairment early in the disease process. Indeed, a number of prospective community-based studies make it likely that an attenuated sense of smell is a precursor of the classical disease features. Pending further verification from large, ongoing prospective studies, olfactory testing may prove to be of value in genetic counseling and highlighting the best time for initiating neuroprotective therapy.

It may be argued that hyposmia is simply a readily detectable epiphenomenon of no real or additional diagnostic value for detecting the preclinical stage of Parkinson's disease compared with imaging striatal dopamine by DATScan, FluoroDopa PET, or iron content by transcranial sonography (TCS). However, there is little support for such arguments. Thus, odor identification, as measured by the UPSIT, and DATScan imaging exhibit similar sensitivity (Deeb *et al.*, 2006), and correlations between DAT imaging in the striatum and UPSIT scores are strong (Siderowf *et al.*, 2005). To date, the correlation between TCS measures and DATScan images is weak, making it questionable whether TCS contributes additional diagnostic information (Spiegel *et al.*, 2006), although it may be argued that TCS measures a different pathological process.

There is considerable evidence that olfactory testing may be of use in differential diagnosis. Such testing may differentiate between Alzheimer's disease and major affective disorders, as well as distinguishing Parkinson's disease from progressive supranuclear palsy, with reasonable sensitivity and specificity. In ET, smell ability is impaired little if at all, and this information can be used to help differentiate ET from other types of tremor, such as tremulous Parkinson's disease or some varieties of cerebellar tremor. Olfactory dysfunction occurs to a variable degree in other degenerative disorders such as Huntington's chorea and motor neuron disease, but rarely matching the severity of Alzheimer's disease or Parkinson's disease.

The OVH for Alzheimer's disease and Parkinson's disease proposes that an initiating event may be entry of a pathogen through the nose prior to brain invasion. Although this hypothesis has largely been discounted by critics, its viability is still unclear and the possibility exists that exogenous agents are responsible for the olfactory loss and the initiation of central pathology in genetically susceptible individuals. Whether and how this occurs is largely unknown, although it clearly represents a challenging question for future research.

REFERENCES

Abele M, Riet A, Hummel T, Klockgether T, Wullner U. Olfactory dysfunction in cerebellar ataxia and multiple system atrophy. *Journal of Neurology* 2003, **250**, 1453–5.

Adler CH, Caviness JN, Sabbagh MN, Hentz JG, Evidente V and Shill H. Olfactory testing in Parkinson's disease and other movement disorders: correlation with Parkinsonian severity. *Movement Disorders*, 2005, **20**(Suppl. 10), Abs. 231.

Aggarwal NT, Bienias JL, Bennett DA *et al.* The relation of cigarette smoking to incident Alzheimer's disease in a biracial urban community population. *Neuroepidemiology*, 2006, **26**(3), 140–6.

Ahlskog JE, Waring SC, Petersen RC *et al.* Olfactory dysfunction on Guamanian ALS parkinsonism and dementia. *Neurology*, 1998, **51**, 1672–7.

Amsterdam JD, Settle RG, Doty RL, Abelman E and Winokur A. Taste and smell perception in depression. *Biological Psychiatry*, 1987, **22**(12), 1481–5.

Ansari KA and Johnson AJ. Olfactory function in patients with Parkinson's disease. *Journal of Chronic Diseases*, 1975, **28**, 493–7.

Antunes M, Bowler RM and Doty RL. San Francisco/Oakland Bay Bridge Welder Study: olfactory function. *Neurology*, 2007, **69**(12), 1278–84.

Arriagada PV, Louis DN, Hedley-Whyte ET and Hyman BT. Neurofibrillary tangles and olfactory dysgenesis. *Lancet*, 1991, **337**(8740), 559.

Ascherio A, Chen H, Weisskopf MG *et al.* Pesticide exposure and risk for Parkinson's disease. *Annals of Neurology*, 2006, **60**(2), 197–203.

Bacon AW, Bondi MW, Salmon DP and Murphy C. Very early changes in olfactory functioning due to Alzheimer's disease and the role of apolipoprotein E in olfaction. *Annals of the New York Acadamy of Sciences*, 1998, **855**, 723–31.

Baker H and Genter MB. The olfactory system and the nasal mucosa as portals of entry of viruses, drugs, and other exogenous agents into the brain. In: RL Doty, ed., *Handbook of Olfaction and Gustation.* New York, NY: Marcel Dekker, 2003, pp. 549–73.

Baker KB and Montgomery EB Jr. Performance on the PD test battery by relatives of patients with progressive supranuclear palsy. *Neurology*, 2001, **56**(1), 25–30.

Ball M J and Nuttall K. Neurofibrillary tangles granulovacuolar degeneration and neuron loss in Down's syndrome: quantitative comparison with Alzheimer's dementia. *Annals of Neurology*, 1980, **7**, 462–5.

Ballard C, Ziabreva I, Perry R *et al.* Differences in neuropathologic characteristics across the Lewy body dementia spectrum. *Neurology*, 2006, **67**(11), 1931–4.

Barnett EM, Cassell MD and Perlman S. Two neurotropic viruses, herpes simplex virus type 1 and mouse hepatitis virus, spread along different neural pathways from the main olfactory bulb. *Neuroscience*, 1993, **57**(4), 1007–25.

Barz S, Hummel T, Pauli E, Majer M, Lang CJ and Kobal G. Chemosensory event-related potentials in response to trigeminal and olfactory stimulation in Parkinson's disease. *Neurology*, 1997, **49**, 1424–31.

Bedard A and Parent A. Evidence of newly generated neurons in the human olfactory bulb. *Brain Research, Developmental Brain Research*, 2004, **151**(1–2), 159–68.

Berger PC and Vogel FS. The development of the pathologic changes of Alzheimer's disease and senile dementia in patients with Down's syndrome. *American Journal of Pathology*, 1973, **73**, 457–76.

Betarbet R, Sherer TB, MacKenzie G *et al.* Chronic systemic pesticide exposure reproduces features of Parkinson's disease. *Nature Neuroscience*, 2000, **3**, 1301–6.

Boesveldt S, Verbaan D, Knol DL, van Hilten JJ and Berendse HW. Assessment of odor identification and discrimination in Dutch Parkinson's disease patients. *Movement Disorders*, 2007, **22**(Suppl. 16), S161 (abstract).

Boeve BF, Silber MH and Parisi JE *et al.* Synucleinopathy pathology and REM sleep behavior disorder plus dementia or parkinsonism. *Neurology*, 2003, **61**(1), 40–5.

Bohnen NI, Gedela S and Kuwabara H *et al.* Selective hyposmia and nigrostriatal dopaminergic denervation in Parkinson's disease. *Journal of Neurology*, 2007, **254**(1), 84–90.

Bond JA. Bioactivation and biotransformation of xenobiotics in rat nasal tissue. In: CS Barrow, ed., *Toxicology of the Nasal Passages*. Washington, DC: Hemisphere Publishing Corporation, 1986, pp. 249–61.

Bostantjopoulou S, Katsarou Z, Papadimitriou A, Veletza V, Hatzigeorgiou G and Lees A. Clinical features of parkinsonian patients with the alpha-synuclein (G209A) mutation. *Movement Disorders*, 2001, **16**(6), 1007–13.

Bower JH, Maraganore DM, Peterson BJ, Ahlskog JE and Rocca WA. Immunologic diseases, anti-inflammatory drugs, and Parkinson disease: a case-control study. *Neurology*, 2006; **67**, 494–6.

Braak H and Braak E. Evolution of neuronal changes in the course of Alzheimer's disease. *Journal of Neural Transmission. Supplementum*, 1998, **53**, 127–40.

Braak H, Del Tredici K, Rub U, de Vos RA, Jansen Steur EN and Braak E. Staging of brain pathology related to sporadic Parkinson's disease. *Neurobiology of Aging*, 2003a, **24**, 197–211.

Braak H, Rub U, Gai WP and Del Tredici K. Idiopathic Parkinson's disease: possible routes by which vulnerable neuronal types may be subject to neuroinvasion by an unknown pathogen. *Journal of Neural Transmission*, 2003b, **110**(5), 517–36.

Braak H, Ghebremedhin E, Rüb U, Bratzke H and Del Tredici K. Stages in the development of Parkinson's disease-related pathology. *Cell Tissue Research*, 2004, **318**(1), 121–34.

Braak H, de Vos RAI, Bohl J and Del Tredici K. Gastric-synuclein immunoreactive inclusions in Meissner's and Auerbach's plexuses in cases staged for Parkinson's disease-related brain pathology. *Neuroscience Letters*, 2006, **396**, 67–72.

Brittebo EB, Eriksson VF, Bakke J and Brandt I. Toxicity of 2 6-dichlorothiobenzamide (Chlorthiamid) and 2 6-dichlorobenzamide in the olfactory nasal mucosa of mice. *Fundamental and Applied Toxicology*, 1991, **17**, 92–102.

Brousseau K and Brainerd HG. *Mongolism: A Study of the Physical and Mental Characteristics of Mongolian Imbeciles*. Baltimore, MD: Williams & Wilkins, 1928.

Busenbark KL, Huber SJ, Greer G, Pahwa R and Koller WC. Olfactory function in essential tremor. *Neurology*, 1992, **42**, 1631–2.

Buxton PH and Hayward M. Polyneuritis cranialis associated with industrial trichloroethylene exposure. *Journal of Neurology Neurosurgery and Psychiatry*, 1967, **30**, 511–18.

Bylsma FW, Moberg PJ, Doty RL and Brandt J. Odor identification in Huntington's disease patients and their offspring with and without the genetic mutation for HD. *Journal of Neuropsychiatry and Clinical Neuroscience*, 1997, **9**, 598–60.

Calderón-Garcidueñas L, Reed W, Maronpot RR *et al.* Brain inflammation and Alzheimer's-like pathology in individuals exposed to severe air pollution. *Toxicologic Pathology*, 2004, **32**, 650–8.

Calderón-Garciadueñas L, Franco-Lira M, Doty RL *et al.* Olfactory epithelium and olfactory bulb pathology in urban air pollution exposed dogs and humans: the pathological bases for olfactory deficits in exposed young healthy adults. (in press)

Charles PC, Walters E, Margolis F and Johnston RE. Mechanism of neuroinvasion of Venezuelan equine encephalitis virus in the mouse. *Virology*, 1995, **208**, 662–71.

Connelly T, Farmer JM, Lynch DR and Doty RL. Olfactory dysfunction in degenerative ataxias. *Journal of Neurology, Neurosurgery and Psychiatry*, 2003, **74**(10), 1435–7.

Crino PB, Martin JA, Hill WD, Greenberg B, Lee VM and Trojanowski JQ. Beta-amyloid peptide and amyloid precursor proteins in olfactory mucosa of patients with Alzheimer's disease Parkinson's disease and Down syndrome. *Annals of Otology, Rhinology and Laryngology*, 1995, **104**, 655–61.

Dahl AR. Possible consequences of cytochrome P-450 dependent monooxygenases in nasal tissues. In: CS Barrow, ed., *Toxicology of the Nasal Passages*. Washington, DC: Hemisphere Publishing Corporation, 1986, pp. 263–73.

Dahl AR. The effect of cytochrome P-450-dependent metabolism and other enzyme activities in olfaction. In: FL Margolis and TV Getchell, eds. *Molecular Neurobiology of the Olfactory System*. New York, NY: Plenum Press, 1988, pp. 51–70.

Daniel SE and Hawkes CH. Preliminary diagnosis of Parkinson's disease using olfactory bulb pathology. *Lancet*, 1992, **340**, 186 (letter).

Daum RF, Sekinger B, Kobal G and Lang CJ. Olfactory testing with "sniffin' sticks" for clinical diagnosis of Parkinson disease. *Nervenarzt*, 2000, **71**, 643–50.

Deeb J, Findley LJ, Shah M, Muhammed N and Hawkes CH. Smell tests compared to dopamine transporter imaging in diagnosis of idiopathic parkinson's disease: a pilot study. *Journal of Neurology Neurosurgery and Psychiatry*, 2006, **77**, 127 (P014).

Del Tredici K and Braak H. Idiopathic Parkinson's disease: staging an-synucleinopathy with a predictable pathoanatomy. In: P Kahle and C Haass, eds, *Molecular Mechanisms in Parkinson's Disease*. Georgetown, TX: Landes Bioscience, 2004, pp. 1–32.

Devanand DP, Michaels-Marston KS, Liu X *et al.* Olfactory deficits in patients with mild cognitive impairment predict Alzheimer's disease at follow-up. *American Journal of Psychiatry*, 2000, **157**, 1399–405.

Diaz-Maroto MC, Perez-Coello MS and Cabezudo MD. Headspace solid-phase microextraction analysis of volatile components of spices. *Chromatographia*, 2002, **55**, 723–8.

Ding X and Coon MJ. Immunochemical characterisation of multiple forms of cytochrome P-450 in rabbit nasal microsomes and evidence for tissue specific expression of P-450s NMa and NMb. *Cellular Pharmacology*, 1990, **37**, 489–96.

Doty RL. Olfactory dysfunction in neurodegenerative disorders. In: TV Getchell, RL Doty, LM Bartoshuk and JB Snow Jr (eds), *Smell and Taste in Health and Disease*. New York, NY: Raven Press, 1991, pp. 735–50.

Doty RL. Olfaction. *Annual Review of Psychology*, 2001, **52**, 423–52.

Doty RL. Odor perception in neurodegenerative disease. In: RL Doty, ed., *Handbook of Olfaction and Gustation* (second edition). New York, NY: Marcel Dekker, 2003a, Chapter 23.

Doty RL. Introduction and historical perspective. In: RL Doty, ed., *Handbook of Olfaction and Gustation* (second edition). New York, NY: Marcel Dekker, 2003b, pp. xv–xiv.

Doty RL. The olfactory vector hypothesis of neurodegenerative disease: is it viable? *Annals of Neurology*, 2008, **63**, 7–15.

Doty RL, Shaman P, Applebaum SL, Giberson R, Siksorski L and Rosenberg L. Smell identification ability: changes with age. *Science*, 1984, **226**(4681), 1441–3.

Doty RL, Reyes PF and Gregor T. Presence of both odor identification and detection deficits in Alzheimer's disease. *Brain Research Bulletin*, 1987, **18**, 597–600.

Doty RL, Deems DA and Stellar S. Olfactory dysfunction in parkinsonism: a general deficit unrelated to neurologic signs disease stage or disease duration. *Neurology*, 1988, **38**, 1237–44.

Doty RL, Riklan M, Deems DA, Reynolds C and Stellar S. The olfactory and cognitive deficits of Parkinson's disease: evidence for independence. *Annals of Neurology*, 1989, **25**, 166–71.

Doty RL, Perl DP, Steele JC *et al.* Odor identification deficit of the parkinsonism–dementia complex of Guam: equivalence to that of Alzheimer's disease and idiopathic Parkinson's disease. *Neurology*, 1991, **41**(Suppl. 2), 77–81.

Doty RL, Stern MB, Pfeiffer C, Gollomp SM and Hurtig HI. Bilateral olfactory dysfunction in early stage treated and untreated idiopathic Parkinson's disease. *Journal of Neurology, Neurosurgery and Psychiatry*, 1992a, **55**, 138–42.

Doty RL, Singh A, Tetrud J and Langston JW. Lack of major olfactory dysfunction in MPTP-induced parkinsonism. *Annals of Neurology*, 1992b, **32**, 87–100.

Doty RL, Golbe LI, McKeown DA, Stern MB, Lehrach CM and Crawford D. Olfactory testing differentiates between progressive supranuclear palsy and idiopathic Parkinson's Disease. *Neurology*, 1993, **43**, 962–5.

Double KL, Rowe DB, Hayes M *et al.* Identifying the pattern of olfactory deficits in Parkinson disease using the brief smell identification test. *Archives of Neurology*, 2003, **60**, 545–9.

Duda JE, Shah U, Arnold SE, Lee VM and Trojanowski JQ. The expression of alpha-beta- and gamma-synucleins in olfactory mucosa from patients with and without neurodegenerative diseases. *Experimental Neurology*, 1999, **160**, 515–22.

Duda JE, Noorigian JV, Petrovitch H, White LR and Ross WR. Pattern of Lewy body progression suggested Braak staging system is supported by analysis of a population based cohort of patients. *Movement Disorders*, 2007, **22** (Suppl. 16), LB5 (late-breaking abstract).

Duff K, McCaffrey RJ and Solomon GS. The Pocket Smell Test: successfully discriminating probable Alzheimer's dementia from vascular dementia and major depression. *Journal of Neuropsychiatry and Clinical Neurosciences*, 2002, **14**, 197–201.

Dunn LM. *Peabody Picture Vocabulary Test – Revised Manual for Forms L and M*. Circle Pines, MN: American Guidance Service, 1981.

Elbaz A, Levecque C, Clavel J *et al.* CYP2D6 polymorphism pesticide exposure and Parkinson's disease. *Annals of Neurology*, 2004, **55**(3), 430–4.

Elian M. Olfactory impairment in motor neuron disease: a pilot study. *Journal of Neurology, Neurosurgery and Psychiatry*, 1991, **54**, 927–8.

Evidente VG, Esteban RP, Hernandez JL *et al.* Smell testing is abnormal in 'Lubag' or X-linked dystonia-parkinsonism: a pilot study. *Parkinsonism and Related Disorders*, 2004, **10**(7), 407–10.

Fearnley JM and Lees AJ. Ageing and Parkinson's disease: substantia nigra regional selectivity. *Brain*, 1991, **114**(Pt 5), 2283–301.

Fernandez-Ruiz J, Diaz R, Hall-Haro C *et al*. Olfactory dysfunction in hereditary ataxia and basal ganglia disorders. *Neuroreport*, 2003, **14**, 1339–41.

Ferreira JJ, Guedes LC, Rosa MM *et al*. High prevalence of LRRK2 mutations in familial and sporadic Parkinson's disease in Portugal. *Movement Disorders*, 2007, **22**(8), 1194–201.

Ferreyra-Moyano H and Barragan E. The olfactory system and Alzheimer's disease. *International Journal of Neuroscience*, 1989, **49**(3–4), 157–97.

Flexner S and Clark PF. A note on the mode of infection in epidemic poliomyelitis. *Proceedings of the Society for Experimental Biology and Medicine*, 1912, **10**, 1–2.

Flexner S and Lewis PA. Experimental epidemic poliomyelitis in monkeys. *Journal of Experimental Medicine*, 1910, **12**, 227–55.

Galvin JE, Pollack J and Morris JC. Clinical phenotype of Parkinson disease dementia. *Neurology*, 2006, **67**(9), 1605–11.

Geser F, Wenning GK, Poewe W and McKeith I. How to diagnose dementia with Lewy bodies: state of the art. *Movement Disorders*, 2005, **20**(Suppl. 12), S11–20.

Gillner M, Brittebo EB, Brandt I, Soderkvist Appelgren L-E and Gustafsson J-A. Uptake and specific binding of 2 3 7 8-tetrachlorodibenzo-p-dioxin in the olfactory mucosa of mice and rats. *Cancer Research*, 1987, **47**, 4150–9.

Gottofrey J and Tjalve H. Axonal transport of cadmium in the olfactory nerve of the pike. *Pharmacology & Toxicology*, 1991, **69**, 242–52.

Graves AB, Bowen JD, Rajaram L *et al*. Impaired olfaction as a marker for cognitive decline: interaction with apolipoprotein E epsilon4 status. *Neurology*, 1999, **22**(3), 1480–7.

Gray JM, Young AW, Barker WA, Curtis A and Gibson D. Impaired recognition of disgust in Huntington's disease gene carriers. *Brain*, 1997, **120**(Pt 11), 2029–38.

Gresham LS, Molgaard CA and Smith RA. Induction of cytochrome P-450 enzymes via tobacco smoke: a potential mechanism for developing resistance to environmental toxins as related to parkinsonism and other neurologic diseases. *Neuroepidemiology*, 1993, **12**(2), 114–16.

Haehner A, Hummel T, Hummel C, Sommer U, Junghanns S and Reichmann H. Olfactory loss may be a first sign of idiopathic Parkinson's disease. *Movement Disorders*, 2007, **22**(6), 839–42.

Halliday G, Del Tredici K and Braak H. Critical appraisal of the Braak staging of brain pathology related to sporadic Parkinson's disease. *Journal of Neural Transmission. Supplementum*, 2006, **70**, 99–103.

Hamilton JM, Murphy C and Paulsen JS. Odor detection learning and memory in Huntington's disease. *Journal of the International Neuropsychological Society*, 1999, **5**, 609–15.

Hardy J. Expression of normal sequence pathogenic proteins for neurodegenerative disease contributes to disease risk: 'permissive templating' as a general mechanism underlying neurodegeneration. *Biochemical Society Transactions*, 2005, **33**(Pt 4), 578–81.

Harrison PJ. Neurodegeneration and the nose. *Clinical Otolaryngology and Allied Sciences*, 1990, **15**(4), 289–91.

Hawkes CH. Olfaction in neurodegenerative disorder. *Movement Disorders*, 2003, **18**, 364–72.

Hawkes CH. Parkinson's disease and aging: the same or a different process? *Journal of Neurology Neurosurgery and Psychiatry*, 2007, **78**, 206 (abstract).

Hawkes CH and Deeb J. Predicting Parkinson's disease, worthwhile but we are not there yet. *Practical Neurology*, 2006, **6**, 272–7.

Hawkes CH and Shephard BC. Olfactory impairment in Parkinson's disease: evidence of dysfunction measured by olfactory-evoked potentials and smell identification tests. *Annals of Neurology*, 1992, **32**, 248 (abstract).

Hawkes CH and Shephard BC. Selective anosmia in Parkinson's disease? *Lancet*, 1993, **341**(8842), 435–6.

Hawkes CH and Shephard BC. Olfactory evoked responses and identification tests in neurological disease. *Annals of the New York Academy of Sciences*, 1998, **855**, 608–15.

Hawkes CH, Shephard BC and Daniel SE. Olfactory dysfunction in Parkinson's disease. *Journal of Neurology Neurosurgery and Psychiatry*, 1997, **62**, 436–46.

Hawkes CH, Shephard BC, Geddes JF, Body GD and Martin JE. Olfactory disorder in motor neuron disease. *Experimental Neurology*, 1998, **50**, 248–53.

Hawkes CH, Shepherd BC and Daniel SE. Is Parkinson's disease a primary olfactory disorder? *Quarterly Journal of Medicine*, 1999, **92**, 473–80.

Hawkes CH, Fogo A and Shah M. Smell identification declines from age 36 years and mainly affects pleasant odors. *Movement Disorders*, 2005, **20**(Suppl. 10), 160 (abstract).

Hawkes CH, Del Tredici K and Braak N. Parkinson's disease: a dual-hit hypothesis. *Neuropathology and Applied Neurobiology*, 2007, **33**(6), 599–614.

Hemdal P, Corwin J and Oster H. Olfactory identification deficits in Down's syndrome and idiopathic mental retardation. *Neuropsychologia*, 1993, **31**, 977–84.

Hensiek AE, Bhatia K and Hawkes CH. Olfactory function in drug induced parkinsonism. *Journal of Neurology*, 2000, **247**(Suppl. 3), P303, III/82.

Hentschel K, Baba Y, Williams LN *et al.* Olfaction in familial Parkinsonism (FP). *Movement Disorders*, 2005, **20**(Suppl. 10), p. 175.

Hext PM and Lock EA. The accumulation and metabolism of 3-trifluoromethylpyridine by rat olfactory and hepatic tissues. *Toxicology*, 1992, **72**, 61–75.

Huisman E, Uylings HB and Hoogland PV. A 100% increase of dopaminergic cells in the olfactory bulb may explain hyposmia in Parkinson's disease. *Movement Disorders*, 2004, **19**(6), 687–92.

Iranzo A, Molinuevo JL, Santamaria J *et al.* Rapid-eye-movement sleep behavior disorder as an early marker for a neurodegenerative disorder: a descriptive study. *Lancet Neurology*, 2006, **5**(7), 572–7.

Iscan M, Reuhl K, Weiss B and Maines MD. Regional and subcellular distribution of cytochrome P-450-dependent drug metabolism in monkey brain: the olfactory bulb and the mitochondrial fraction have high levels of activity. *Biochemical and Biophysical Research Communications*, 1990, **169**(3), 858–63.

Itzhaki R and Itzhaki R. Herpes simplex virus type 1, apolipoprotein E and Alzheimer's disease. *Herpes*, 2004, **11**(Suppl. 2), 77A–82A.

Kalaitzakis ME, Graeber MB, Gentleman SM and Pearce RKB. The dorsal motor nucleus of the vagus is not an obligatory trigger site of Parkinson's disease: a critical analysis of alpha-synuclein staging. *Neuropathology and Applied Neurobiology*, 2008, **34**(3), 284–95.

Kalmey JK, Thewissen JG and Dluzen DE. Age-related size reduction of foramina in the cribriform plate. *Anatomical Record*, 1998, **251**(3), 326–9.

Kareken DA, Doty RL, Moberg PJ *et al*. Olfactory-evoked regional cerebral blood flow in Alzheimer's disease. *Neuropsychology*, 2001, **15**(1), 18–29.

Katzenschlager R, Zijlmans J, Evans A, Watt H and Lees AJ. Olfactory function distinguishes vascular parkinsonism from Parkinson's disease. *Journal of Neurology, Neurosurgery and Psychiatry*, 2004, **75**(12), 1749–52.

Katzman R. Alzheimer's disease. *New England Journal of Medicine*, 1986, **314**, 964–73.

Kaufmann H, Nahm K, Purohit D and Wolfe D. Autonomic failure as the initial presentation of Parkinson disease and dementia with Lewy bodies. *Neurology*, 2004, **63**(6), 1093–5.

Khan NL, Katzenschlager R, Watt H *et al*. Olfaction differentiates parkin disease from early-onset parkinsonism and Parkinson disease. *Neurology*, 2004, **62**(7), 1224–6.

Khan NL, Jain S, Lynch JM *et al*. Mutations in the gene LRRK2 encoding dardarin (PARK 8) cause familial Parkinson's disease: clinical, pathological, olfactory and functional imaging and genetic data. *Brain*, 2005, **128**(Pt 12), 2786–96.

Killgore WDS and McBride SH. Odor identification accuracy declines following 24 h of sleep deprivation. *Journal of Sleep Research*, 2006, **15**(2), 111–16.

Kishikawa M, Iseki M, Sakae M, Kawaguchi S and Fujii H. Early diagnosis of Alzheimer's? *Nature*, 1994, **369**(6479), 365–6.

Klimek L. Sense of smell in allergic rhinitis. *Pneumologie*, 1998, **52**, 196–202.

Kobal G and Plattig KH. Objective olfactometry: methodological annotations for recording olfactory EEG-responses from the awake human. *Elektroenzephalogr Elektromyogr Verwandte Geb*, 1978, **9**, 135–45.

Kovacs T, Cairns NJ and Lantos PL. Olfactory centres in Alzheimer's disease: olfactory bulb is involved in early Braak's stages. *Neuroreport*, 2001, **12** (12), 285–8.

Kovacs T, Papp MI, Cairns NJ, Khan MN and Lantos PL. Olfactory bulb in multiple system atrophy. *Movement Disorders*, 2003, **18**(8), 938–42.

Li AA, Mink PJ, McIntosh LJ, Teta MJ and Finley B. Evaluation of epidemiologic and animal data associating pesticides with Parkinson's disease. *Journal of Occupational and Environmental Medicine*, 2005, **47**(10), 1059–87.

Liberini P, Parola S, Spano PF and Antonini L. Olfaction in Parkinson's disease: methods of assessment and clinical relevance. *Journal of Neurology*, 2000, **247**, 88–96.

Liou HH, Tsai MC, Chen CJ *et al*. Environmental risk factors and Parkinson's disease: a case-control study in Taiwan. *Neurology*, 1997, **48**(6), 1583–8.

Louis ED and Jurewicz EC. Olfaction in essential tremor patients with and without isolated rest tremor. *Movement Disorders*, 2003, **18**(11), 1387–9.

Louis ED, Bromley SM, Jurewicz EC and Watner D. Olfactory dysfunction in essential tremor: a deficit unrelated to disease duration or severity. *Neurology*, 2002, **59**(10), 1631–3.

Louis ED, Vonsattel JP, Honig LS, Ross GW, Lyons KE and Pahwa R. Neuropathologic findings in essential tremor. *Neurology*, 2006, **66**(11), 1756–9.

Lovell MA. Jafek BW, Moran DT and Rowley JC. Biopsy of human olfactory mucosa: an instrument and a technique. *Archives of Otolaryngology*, 1982, **108**(4), 247–9.

Luzzi S, Snowden JS, Neary D, Coccia M, Provinciali L and Lambon Ralph MA. Distinct patterns of olfactory impairment in Alzheimer's disease, semantic dementia, frontotemporal dementia, and corticobasal degeneration. *Neuropsychologia*, 2007, **45**(8), 1823–31.

Mann DM. Alzheimer's disease and Down's syndrome. *Histopathology*, 1988, **13**, 125–37.

Mann DM. The pathogenesis and progression of the pathological changes of Alzheimer's disease. *Annals of Medicine*, 1989, **21**(2), 133–6.

Markopoulou K, Larsen KW and Wszolek EK *et al.* Olfactory dysfunction in familial parkinsonism. *Neurology*, 1997, **49**, 1262–7.

Marras C, Goldman S and Smith A *et al.* Smell identification ability in twin pairs discordant for Parkinson's disease. *Movement Disorders*, 2005, **20**(6), 687–93.

Masucci MG. Epstein–Barr virus oncogenesis and the ubiquitin-proteasome system. *Oncogene*, 2004, **23**, 2107–15.

McKeith IG. Consensus guidelines for the clinical and pathologic diagnosis of dementia with Lewy bodies (DLB): report of the Consortium on DLB International Workshop. *Journal of Alzheimer's Disease*, 2006, **9**(Suppl. 3), 417–23.

McKeown DA, Doty RL, Perl DP, Fryc RE, Simms I and Mester A. Olfactory function in young adolescents with Down's syndrome. *Journal of Neurology, Neurosurgery and Psychiatry*, 1996, **61**, 412–14.

McShane RH, Nagy Z, Esiri MM *et al.* Anosmia in dementia is associated with Lewy bodies rather than Alzheimer's pathology. *Journal of Neurology, Neurosurgery and Psychiatry*, 2001, **70**, 739–43.

Mesholam RI, Moberg PJ, Mahr RN and Doty RL. Olfaction in neurodegenerative disease: a meta-analysis of olfactory functioning in Alzheimer's and Parkinson's diseases. *Archives of Neurology*, 1998, **55**, 84–90.

Mitchell IJ, Heims H, Neville EA and Rickards H. Huntington's disease patients show impaired perception of disgust in the gustatory and olfactory modalities. *Journal of Neuropsychiatry and Clinical Neuroscience*, 2005, **17**(1), 119–21.

Miwa T, Watanabe A, Mitsumoto Y, Furukawa M, Fukushima N and Moriizumi T. Olfactory impairment and Parkinson's disease-like symptoms observed in the common marmoset following administration of 1-methyl-4-phenyl-1 2 3 6-tetrahydropyridine. *Acta Otolaryngologica*, 2004, **553**(Suppl.), 80–4.

Moberg PJ and Doty RL. Olfactory function in Huntington's disease patients and at-risk offspring. *International Journal of Neuroscience*, 1997, **89**, 133–9.

Moberg PJ, Pearlson GD, Speedie LJ, Lipsey JR, Strauss ME and Folstein SE. Olfactory recognition: differential impairments in early and late Huntington's and Alzheimer's disease. *Journal of Clinical and Experimental Neuropsychology*, 1987, **9**, 650–64.

Montgomery EB Jr, Baker KB, Lyons K and Koller WC. Abnormal performance on the PD test battery by asymptomatic first-degree relatives. *Neurology*, 1999, **52**, 757–62.

Montgomery EB Jr, Lyons K and Koller WC. Early detection of probable idiopathic Parkinson's disease: II. A prospective application of a diagnostic test battery. *Movement Disorders*, 2000, **15**(3), 474–8.

Morgan CD and Murphy C. Olfactory event-related potential in Alzheimer's disease. *Journal of the International Neuropsychological Society*, 2002, **8**, 753–63.

Muller A, Mungersdorf M, Reichmann H, Strehle G and Hummel T. Olfactory function in Parkinsonian syndromes. *Journal of Clinical Neuroscience*, 2002, **9**(5), 521–4.

Muller CM, de Vos RA, Maurage CA, Thal DR, Tolnay M and Braak H. Staging of sporadic Parkinson disease-related alpha-synuclein pathology: inter- and intra-rater reliability. *Journal of Neuropathology and Experimental Neurology*, 2005, **64**(7), 623–8.

Murphy C and Jinich S. Olfactory dysfunction in Down's syndrome. *Neurobiology of Aging*, 1996, **17**, 631–7.

Murphy C, Schubert CR. Cruickshanks KJ. Klein BE. Klein R and Nondahl DM. Prevalence of olfactory impairment in older adults. *Journal of the American Medical Association*, 2002, **288**(18), 2307–12.

Nee LE and Lippa CF. Inherited Alzheimer's disease PS-1 olfactory function: a 10-year follow-up study. *American Journal of Alzheimer's Disease and Other Dementias*, 2001, **16**(2), 83–4.

Nee LE, Scott J and Polinsky RJ. Olfactory dysfunction in the Shy–Drager syndrome. *Clinical Autonomic Research*, 1993, **3**(4), 281–2.

Newman R and Winans SS. An experimental study of the ventral striatum of the golden hamster. II Neuronal connections of the olfactory tubercle. *Journal of Comparative Neurology*, 1980, **191**, 193–212.

Nijjar RK and Murphy C. Olfactory impairment increases as a function of age in persons with Down syndrome. *Neurobiology of Aging*, 2002, **23**(1), 65–73.

Nordin S, Monsch AU and Murphy C. Unawareness of smell loss in normal aging and Alzheimer's disease: discrepancy between self-reported and diagnosed smell sensitivity. *Journal of Gerontology. Series B, Psychological Sciences and Social Sciences*, 1995a, **50**(4), P187–92.

Nordin S, Paulsen JS and Murphy C. Sensory- and memory-mediated olfactory dysfunction in Huntington's disease. *Journal of the International Neuropsychological Society*, 1995b, **1**, 281–90.

Nordin S, Almkvist O, Berglund B and Wahlund LO. Olfactory dysfunction for pyridine and dementia progression in Alzheimer disease. *Archives of Neurology*, 1997, **54**(8), 993–8.

Okamoto K, Hirai S, Shoji M and Takatama M. Senile changes in the human olfactory bulbs. In: T Nagatsu, ed. *Basic, Clinical, and Therapeutic Aspects of Alzheimer's and Parkinson's Diseases*. New York, NY: Plenum Press, 1990, pp. 349–52.

Olichney JM, Murphy C, Hofstetter CR *et al*. Anosmia is very common in the Lewy body variant of Alzheimer's disease. *Journal of Neurology, Neurosurgery and Psychiatry*, 2005, **76**(10), 1342–7.

Oliver C, Holland AJ. Down's syndrome and Alzheimer's disease: a review. *Psychological Medicine*, 1986, **16**, 307–22.

Oyanagi K. The nature of the parkinsonism–dementia complex and amyotrophic lateral sclerosis of Guam and magnesium deficiency. *Parkinsonism and Related Disorders*, 2005, **11**(Suppl. 1), S17–23.

Papaioannou N, Tooten PC, van Ederen AM *et al*. Immunohistochemical investigation of the brain of aged dogs. I. Detection of neurofibrillary tangles and of 4-hydroxynonenal protein, an oxidative damage product, in senile plaques. *Amyloid*, 2001, **8**(1), 11–21.

Parkkinen L, Kauppinen T, Pirttila T, Autere JM and Alafuzoff I. α-Synuclein pathology does not predict extrapyramidal symptoms or dementia. *Annals of Neurology*, 2005, **57**, 82–91.

Paulsen JS, Langbehn DR, Stout JC *et al.* Detection of Huntingdon's disease decades before diagnosis: the predict-HD study. *Journal of Neurology Neurosurgery and Psychiatry*, 2008, **79**, 874–80.

Pavese N, Gerhard A, Tai YF *et al.* Microglial activation correlates with severity in Huntington disease: a clinical and PET study. *Neurology*, 2006, **66**(11), 1638–43.

Pearce RKB, Hawkes CH and Daniel SE. The anterior olfactory nucleus in Parkinson's disease. *Movement Disorders*, 1995, **10**, 283–7.

Pearson RC, Esiri MM, Hiorns RW, Wilcock GK and Powell TP. Anatomical correlates of the distribution of the pathological changes in the neocortex in Alzheimer disease. *Proceedings of the National Academy of Science of the United States of America*, 1985, **82**(13), 4531–4.

Ponsen MM, Stoffers D, Booij J, van Eck-Smit BL, Wolters ECH and Berendse HW. Idiopathic hyposmia as a preclinical sign of Parkinson's disease. *Annals of Neurology*, 2004, **56**(2), 173–81.

Quinn NP, Rossor MN and Marsden CD. Olfactory threshold in Parkinson's disease. *Journal of Neurology, Neurosurgery and Psychiatry*, 1987, **50**, 88–9.

Rebeck GW and Hyman BT. Neuroanatomical connections and specific regional vulnerability in Alzheimer's disease. *Neurobiology and Aging*, 1993, **14**(1), 45–7.

Roberts E. Alzheimer's disease may begin in the nose and may be caused by aluminosilicates. *Neurobiology and Aging*, 1986, **7**, 561–7.

Robertson EG. An examination of the olfactory bulbs in fatal cases of poliomyelitis during the Victorial epidemic of 1937–1938. *Medical Journal of Australia*, 1940, **I**, 156–8.

Ross GW, Petrovitch H, Abbott RD *et al.* Parkinsonian signs and substantia nigra neuron density in descendents elders without PD. *Annals of Neurology*, 2004, **56**, 532–9.

Ross W, Abbott RD, Petrovitch H *et al.* Association of olfactory dysfunction with incidental Lewy bodies. *Movement Disorders*, 2006, **21**(12), 2062–7.

Ross W, Petrovitch H, Abbott RD *et al.* Association of olfactory dysfunction with risk of future Parkinson's disease. *Annals of Neurology*, 2008, **63**(2), 167–73.

Royall DR, Chiodo LK, Polk MS and Jaramillo CJ. Severe dysosmia is specifically associated with Alzheimer-like memory deficits in nondemented elderly retirees. *Neuroepidemiology*, 2002, **21**(2), 68–73.

Sabin AB. Olfactory bulbs in human poliomyelitis. *American Journal of Diseases in Children*, 1940, **60**, 1313–18.

Sabin AB and Olitsky PK. Influence of pathway of infection on pathology of olfactory bulbs in experimental poliomyelitis. *Proceedings of the Society for Experimental Biology and Medicine*, 1936, **35**, 300–1.

Sajjadian A, Doty RL, Gutnick D, Chirurgi RJ, Sivak M and Perl D. Olfactory dysfunction in amyotrophic lateral sclerosis. *Neurodegeneration*, 1994, **3**, 153–7.

Schiffman SS, Graham BG, Sattely-Miller EA, Zervakis J and Welsh-Bohmer K. Taste, smell and neuropsychological performance of individuals at familial risk for Alzheimer's disease. *Neurobiology and Aging*, 2002, **23**, 397–404.

Schlitt M, Chronister RB and Whitley RJ. Pathogenesis and pathophysiology of viral infections of the central nervous system. In: WM Scheld, RJ Whitley and DT Durack, eds, *Infections of the Central Nervous System.* New York, NY: Raven Press, 1991, pp. 7–18.

Schultz EW and Gebhardt, LR. Prevention of intranasally inoculated poliomyelitis in monkeys by previous intranasal irrigation with chemical agents. *Proceedings of the Society for Experimental Biology and Medicine,* 1936, **34**, 133–5.

Schultz, EW and Gebhardt LR. Zinc sulfate prophylaxis in poliomyelitis. *Journal of the American Medical Association,* 1937, **108**, 2182–4.

Schwartz BS, Doty RL, Monroe C, Frye R and Barker S. Olfactory function in chemical workers exposed to acrylate and methacrylates vapors. *American Journal of Public Health,* 1989, **79**(5), 613–18.

Schwartz BS, Ford DP, Bolla KI, Agnew J, Rothman N and Bleecker ML. Solvent-associated decrements in olfactory function in paint manufacturing workers. *American Journal of Industrial Medicine,* 1990, **18**(6), 697–706.

Semchuk KM, Love EJ and Lee RG. Parkinson's disease and exposure to agricultural work and pesticide chemicals. *Neurology,* 1992, **42**(7), 1328–35.

Shackelford J and Pagano JS. Targeting of host-cell ubiquitin pathways by viruses. *Essays in Biochemistry,* 2005, **41**, 139–54.

Shah M, Findley LJ, Muhammed N and Hawkes CH. Olfaction is normal in essential tremor and can be used to distinguish it from Parkinson's disease. *Movement Disorders,* 2005, **20**(Suppl. 10), 563 (abstract).

Shah M, Deeb J, Fernando M *et al.* Abnormality of taste and smell in Parkinson's disease. *Parkinsonism and Related Disorders,* 2008, July 5, (Epub ahead of print).

Sherer TB, Betarbet R, Testa CM *et al.* Mechanism of toxicity in rotenone models of Parkinson's disease. *Journal of Neuroscience,* 2003, **23**, 10, 756–64.

Shipley MT. Transport of molecules from nose to brain: transneuronal anterograde and retrograde labelling in the rat olfactory system by wheatgerm agglutin–horseradish peroxidase applied to the nasal epithelium. *Brain Research Bulletin,* 1985, **15**, 129–42.

Siderowf A, Newberg A and Chou KL *et al.* (^{99m}Tc)TRODAT-1 SPECT imaging correlates with odor identification in early Parkinson disease. *Neurology,* 2005, **64**(10), 1716–20.

Sienkiewicz-Jarosz H, Scinska A, Kuran W *et al.* Taste responses in patients with Parkinson's disease. *Journal of Neurology, Neurosurgery and Psychiatry,* 2005, **76**(1), 40–6.

Silveira-Moriyama L, Williams D, Katzenschlager R and Lees AJ. Pizza, mint, and licorice: smell testing in Parkinson's disease in a UK population. *Movement Disorders,* 2005, **20**(Suppl. 10), P471 (abstract).

Silveira-Moriyama L, Guedes L, Kingsbury A *et al.* Olfaction in dardarin/LRRK2 associated Parkinsonism. *Movement Disorders,* 2007, **22**(Suppl. 16), S258.

Singleton A, Gwinn-Hardy K, Sharabi Y *et al.* Association between cardiac denervation and parkinsonism caused by alpha-synuclein gene triplication. *Brain,* 2004, **127** (Pt 4), 768–72.

Smith CAD, Gough AC, Leigh PN *et al.* Debrisoquine hydroxylase gene polymorphism and susceptibility to Parkinson' disease. *Lancet,* 1992, **339**, 1375–7.

Smith DH, Uryu K, Saatman KE, Trojanowski JQ and McIntosh, TK. Protein accumulation in traumatic brain injury. *Neuromolecular Medicine*, 2003, **4**, 59–72.

Smutzer GS, Doty RL, Arnold SE and Trojanowski JQ. Olfactory system neuropathology in Alzheimer's disease. Parkinson's disease and schizophrenia. In: RL Doty, ed., *Handbook of Olfaction and Gustation* (second edition). New York, NY: Marcel Dekker, 2003, Chapter 24.

Sobel N, Thomason ME, Stappen I *et al.* An impairment in sniffing contributes to the olfactory impairment in Parkinson's disease. *Proceedings of the National Academy of Science of the United States of America*, 2001, **98**, 4154–9.

Sommer U, Hummel T, Cormann K *et al.* Detection of presymptomatic Parkinson's disease: combining smell tests transcranial sonography and SPECT. *Movement Disorders*, 2004, **19**(10), 1196–202.

Spiegel J, Hellwig D, Mollers MO *et al.* Transcranial sonography and [^{123I}]FP-CIT SPECT disclose complementary aspects of Parkinson's disease. *Brain*, 2006, **129**(Pt 5), 1188–93.

Stern MB, Doty RL, Dotti M *et al.* Olfactory function in Parkinson's disease subtypes. *Neurology*, 1994, **44**, 266–8.

Stiasny-Kolster K, Doerr Y, Moller JC *et al.* Combination of 'idiopathic' REM sleep behavior disorder and olfactory dysfunction as possible indicator for alpha-synucleinopathy demonstrated by dopamine transporter FP-CIT-SPECT. *Brain*, 2005, **128**(Pt 1), 126–37.

Swan GE and Carmelli D. Impaired olfaction predicts cognitive decline in nondemented older adults. *Neuroepidemiology*, 2002, **21**(2), 58–67.

Tabert MH, Liu X, Doty RL *et al.* A 10-item smell identification scale related to risk for Alzheimer's disease. *Annals of Neurology*, 2005, **58**(1), 155–60.

Talamo BR, Rudel R, Kosik KS *et al.* Pathological changes in olfactory neurons in patients with Alzheimer's disease. *Nature*, 1989, **23**, 337(6209), 736.

Tanner CM, Goldman SM, Aston DA *et al.* Smoking and Parkinson's disease in twins. *Neurology*, 2002, **58**(4), 581–8.

Tisdall FF, Brown A, Defries RD, Ross MA and Sellers AH. Nasal spraying as preventive of poliomyelitis. *Canadian Public Health Journal*, 1937, **28**, 431–4.

Tissingh G, Berendse HW, Bergmans P *et al.* Loss of olfaction in de novo and treated Parkinson's disease: possible implications for early diagnosis. *Movement Disorders*, 2001, **16**(1), 41–6.

Tjalve H and Henriksson J. Uptake of metals in the brain via olfactory pathways. *Neurotoxicology*, 1999, **20**, 181–95.

Tjalve H, Henriksson J, Tallkvist, J, Larsson BS and Lindquist NG. Uptake of manganese and cadmium from the nasal mucosa into the central nervous system via olfactory pathways in rats. *Pharmacology & Toxicology*, 1996, **79**, 347–56.

Tomlinson AH and Esiri MM. Herpes simplex encephalitis: immuno-histological demonstration of spread of virus via olfactory pathways in mice. *Journal of Neurological Science*, 1983, **60**, 473–84.

Trojanowski JQ, Newman PD, Hill WD and Lee VM. Human olfactory epithelium in normal aging Alzheimer's disease and other neurodegenerative disorders. *Journal of Comparative Neurology*, 1991, **310**, 365–76.

Tsuboi Y, Wszolek ZK, Graff-Radford NR, Cookson N and Dickson DW. Tau pathology in the olfactory bulb correlates with Braak stage Lewy body pathology and apolipoprotein epsilon4. *Neuropathology and Applied Neurobiology*, 2003, **29**(5), 503–10.

Tyas SL, Manfreda J, Strain LA and Montgomery PR. Risk factors for Alzheimer's disease: a population-based, longitudinal study in Manitoba, Canada. *International Journal of Epidemiology*, 2001, **30**, 590–7.

Tzen KY, Lu CS, Yen TC, Wey SP and Ting G. Differential diagnosis of Parkinson's disease and vascular parkinsonism by (^{99m})Tc-TRODAT-1. *Journal of Nuclear Medicine*, 2001, **42**(3), 408–13.

Uchida K, Kihara N, Hashimoto K, Nakayama H and Yamaguchi RT. Age-related histological changes in the canine substantia nigra. *Journal of Veterinary Medicine and Science*, 2003, **65**(2), 179–85.

Vogt BA, Van Hoesen GW and Vogt LJ. Laminar distribution of neuron degeneration in posterior cingulate cortex in Alzheimer's disease. *Acta Neuropathologica*, 1990, **80**(6), 581–9.

Wakabayashi K, Takahashi H, Ohama E and Ikuta F. Parkinson's disease: an immunohistochemical study of Lewy body-containing neurons in the enteric nervous system. *Acta Neuropathologica*, 1990, **79**, 581–3.

Warner MD, Peabody CA and Berger PA. Olfactory deficits and Down's syndrome. *Biological Psychiatry*, 1988, **23**, 836–9.

Wenning GK, Shephard B, Magalhaes M, Hawkes CH and Quinn NP. Olfactory function in multiple system atrophy. *Neurodegeneration*, 1993, **2**, 169–71.

Wenning GK, Shephard B, Hawkes CH, Petruckevitch A, Lees A and Quinn N. Olfactory function in typical parkinsonian syndromes. *Acta Neurologica Scandinavica*, 1995a, **91**, 247–50.

Wenning GK, Shephard BC, Hawkes CH, Lees A and Quinn N. Olfactory function in progressive supranuclear palsy and corticobasal degeneration. *Journal of Neurology, Neurosurgery and Psychiatry*, 1995b, **57**, 251–2.

Westervelt HJ, Carvalho J and Duff K. Presentation of Alzheimer's disease in patients with and without olfactory deficits. *Archives of Clinical Neuropsychology*, 2007, **22**(1), 117–22.

Wetter S and Murphy C. Individuals with Down's syndrome demonstrate abnormal olfactory event-related potentials. *Clinical Neurophysiology*, 1999, **110**(9), 1563–9.

Wetter S and Murphy C. Apolipoprotein E epsilon4 positive individuals demonstrate delayed olfactory event-related potentials. *Neurobiology and Aging*, 2001, **22**, 439–47.

Wetter S, Peavy G, Jacobson M, Hamilton J, Salmon D and Murphy C. Olfactory and auditory event-related potentials in Huntington's disease. *Neuropsychology*, 2005, **19**(4), 428–36.

Williams DR, de Silva R, Paviour DC *et al.* Characteristics of two distinct clinical phenotypes in pathologically proven progressive supranuclear palsy: Richardson's syndrome and PSP-parkinsonism. *Brain*, 2005, **128**(Pt 6), 1247–58.

Wilson RS, Arnold SE, Schneider JA, Tang Y and Bennett DA. The relation of cerebral Alzheimer's disease pathology to odor identification in old age. *Journal of Neurology, Neurosurgery and Psychiatry*, 2007a, **78**(1), 30–5.

Wilson RS, Schneider JA, Arnold SE, Tang Y, Boyle PA and Bennett DA. Olfactory identification and incidence of mild cognitive impairment in older age. *Archives of General Psychiatry*, 2007b, **64**, 802–8.

Wisniewski KE, Wisniewski HM, and Wen GY. Occurrence of neuropathological changes and dementia of Alzheimer's disease in Down's syndrome. *Annals of Neurology*, 1985, **17**, 278–82.

Witt M, Gudziol V, Haehner A, Reichmann H and Hummel T. Nasal mucosa in patients with Parkinson's disease. *Chemical Senses*, 2006, **31**(5), 479–93 (abstract 106).

Wright J. *A History of Laryngology and Rhinology*. Philadelphia, PA: Lea & Febiger, 1914.

Yahr MD, Orosz D and Purohit DP. Co-occurrence of essential tremor and Parkinson's disease: clinical study of a large kindred with autopsy findings. *Parkinsonism and Related Disorders*, 2003, **9**(4), 225–31.

Yamada M, Onodera M, Mizuno Y and Mochizuki H. Neurogenesis in olfactory bulb identified by retroviral labeling in normal and MPTP-treated adult mice. *Neuroscience*, 2004, **124**(1), 173–81.

Yamagishi M, Ishizuka Y and Seki K. Pathology of olfactory mucosa in patients with Alzheimer's disease. *Annals of Otology, Rhinology and Laryngology*, 1994, **103**, 421–7.

Youngentoub SL, Schwob JE, Saha S, Manglapus G and Jubelt B. Functional consequences following infection of the olfactory system by intranasal infusion of the olfactory bulb line variant (OBLV) of mouse hepatitis strain JHM. *Chemical Senses*, 2001, **26**(8), 953–63.

Yousem DM, Oguz KK and Li C. Imaging of the olfactory system. *Seminars in Ultrasound CT and MR*, 2001, **22**(6), 456–72.

Zijlmans JC, Thijssen HO, Vogels OJ *et al.* MRI in patients with suspected vascular parkinsonism. *Neurology*, 1995, **45**(12), 2183–8.

Zucco GM and Negrin NS. Olfactory deficits in Down subjects: a link with Alzheimer disease. *Perception and Motor Skills*, 1994, **78**(2), 627–31.

5

Investigation, treatment, and general management of olfactory disease

Investigation of smell loss

In common with most medical disorders, a careful history is critical to establish probable cause and direct subsequent elements of the evaluation and examination. Most people complaining of taste loss will, in fact, have olfactory loss. Before administering either taste or smell tests, it is useful to ask the patient the following questions: Do you experience the sweetness of sugar on breakfast cereal or when added to coffee or tea? Do you experience the saltiness of potato chips or saltiness when salt is added to your food from a salt-shaker? Do you experience the sour taste of grapefruit or lemon juice? Can you detect the bitterness in tonic water (quinine)? If a patient reports "yes" to these questions the patient's primary problem is highly likely to be olfactory and smell testing should be initiated. This reflects the fact that such questions have a high negative predictive value, i.e., they are sensitive in detecting people who have no taste problem. However, such questions are not very sensitive in detecting people who have a true taste problem, i.e., they have low positive predictive value (Sorter et al., 2008). Therefore, when true taste deficits are suspected, they must be verified by quantitative taste tests.

Validated olfactory tests are now widely available for assessing olfactory function in the clinic, as described in detail in Chapter 2. For screening purposes of suspected olfactory defects there has to be a compromise between the time required for the test, its reliability, and its validity. In general, the reliability of a test is proportional to the number of items of the test or the time required for its administration (Doty et al., 1995); lengthy tests, such as some threshold tests, are usually impractical for outpatient screening. Since many olfactory tests correlate relatively well with one another (e.g., tests of odor identification, detection, and discrimination) (Doty et al., 1994), simple tests of odor identification with forced-choice responses are generally preferred. Although brief (e.g., three-item) odor identification tests may be sensitive to total anosmia (Jackman & Doty, 2005), their sensitivity and specificity in detecting various degrees of microsmia or hyposmia are compromised. Longer screening procedures, such as the 12-item "Sniffin' Sticks" and the 12-item "Brief Smell Identification Test" (B-SIT), are more sensitive and specific, although these tests still have limited ability to differentiate between categories of dysfunction and cannot detect malingering with reliability. Hence, whenever possible, longer tests should be employed. Procedures amenable to self-administration should still be administered by an examiner to patients with disability, such as those with poor eyesight or movement disorder, in order to ensure the validity of the testing.

Once it is clear that an olfactory deficit is present, the next step is to decide whether the defect is conductive, sensorineural, or both. Exclusion of sinonasal disease is done best by nasal endoscopy, which will overlook only about 10 percent of nasal pathologies. The presence of local nasal disease may also be detected by acoustic rhinometry, rhinomanometry, ciliary motility, and skin tests, although microinflammation within the olfactory epithelium cannot be determined by endoscopy or such testing. If there is still doubt, a short course of systemic steroids will usually clarify if there is an inflammatory problem. If this is the case, then at least some smell function will return briefly. Additionally, a high-resolution computed tomography (CT) scan of the nose and paranasal sinuses may be of value. In general, for the investigation of smell problems, ear, nose, and throat (ENT) surgeons prefer CT scanning (which is better for local nasal problems), whereas neurologists prefer magnetic resonance imaging (MRI), as it delineates better the olfactory path both peripherally and centrally. MRI yields good images of the nose and sinuses, as well as the brain itself, and provides acceptable definition of bone structure; however, MRI sometimes overemphasizes the magnitude of sinus disease.

For evaluation of suspected central causes of anosmia there is a choice of CT, MRI, and single-photon emission computed tomography (SPECT). MRI has particular value for determining the integrity of the olfactory bulbs and tracts, and special imaging with multiple cuts through the cribriform plate region can usually establish whether these structures are grossly abnormal. Functional MRI (fMRI) and positron emission tomography (PET), which are detailed in Chapter 3, still belong to the domain of research. If the patient describes an olfactory aura, then epilepsy needs to be considered. Here electroencephalography (EEG) and MRI brain scan are the preliminary investigations of choice. If mass lesions are excluded, an MRI epilepsy protocol may then be required, with high-resolution coronal slices through the medial temporal area.

Treatment

Therapy directed to the underlying cause is the obvious treatment for local nasal inflammatory disease and tumor, whether growing in the nose, sinuses, or intracranially. Any process that is obstructing the flow of air to the olfactory mucosa should be corrected, either with surgery, steroids, or anti-inflammatory sprays. Surgery for polyps is usually indicated only for large medically refractory polyps or where there is diagnostic uncertainty. Predictably, steroids are used for granulomata affecting the nose, such as Wegener granulomatosis or sarcoidosis. Wegener granulomatosis usually needs more vigorous immunosuppression than steroids alone can provide, e.g., cylcophosphamide, azathioprine, or methotrexate, although some report that sulphonamides such as cotrimoxazole may be just as effective (Stegeman et al., 1996). If hyposmia is associated with nasal polyps, steroids may be of value because of their anti-inflammatory and anti-edema effects. They are more beneficial when given systemically than topically. Although a short course of systemic steroids may improve smell function, subsequent topical management of the nasal inflammation often fails. The efficacy of steroid sprays or drops can be enhanced by administering them with the head in the inverted position, where the bridge of the nose is perpendicular to the floor (e.g., Moffett's position), thereby allowing the steroid to enter the olfactory meatus.

Unconfirmed reports suggest that vitamin A might aid recovery in chronic nasal sinus disease (Steck-Scott et al., 2004). Use of this vitamin has been suggested frequently for treatment of olfactory problems (e.g., Duncan & Briggs, 1962), but in the absence of vitamin A deficiency such therapy is unlikely to be effective. The original idea that vitamin A would be helpful stemmed from the now outdated concept that pigmentation within the olfactory neuroepithelium is an important element of olfactory transduction (Briggs & Duncan, 1961). Nevertheless, bioactive vitamin A derivatives (retinoids) play an important role in the survival of mature olfactory neurons (Hagglund et al., 2006). Other agents, such as zinc and α-lipoic acid, an over-the-counter antioxidant, have been reported to be of value in mitigating smell loss (Hummel et al., 2002; Schechter et al., 1972). Unfortunately these investigations lacked appropriate controls and when double-blind studies have been performed, i.e., in the case of zinc and vitamin A, such efficacy has not been supported (Henkin et al., 1976; Lill et al., 2006). Despite this, zinc repletion in people with zinc deficiencies and chemosensory disturbance secondary to renal or liver disease can help taste dysfunction (e.g., Mahajan et al., 1980; Weisman et al., 1979).

For the patient who has become hyposmic from head injury, steroids are tried often, but there are no large randomized trials to validate their use. Many clinicians give prednisolone in high doses for the first few weeks and with a taper for the following three weeks. The rationale is that scarring around the cribriform plate area may impede the growth of regenerating centripetal olfactory neurons and, if the scarred tissue can be softened, then connection with the bulb might be reestablished (Jafek et al., 1989). More likely, any beneficial effect results from reduction of local nasal edema and any long-term benefit on olfaction is dubious.

Hyperosmia

Treatment of hyperosmia is not easy. Anecdotally, the only compounds that seem to be of benefit are the anti-epileptic preparations which are given on the assumption that there is increased firing activity possibly with ephaptic

---

Case report 5.1: A 23-year-old housewife with hyperosmia after minor head injury

This lady was involved in a rear-end collision while stationary in her car at a traffic light. She was in the driver's seat, the seat belt was applied correctly, and there were head restraints, but the airbag did not inflate. The impact caused her to bang her head on the sun visor, resulting in a laceration of the forehead. There was no alteration of consciousness. Over the next few days she became headachy and noticed hypersensitivity to smells, particularly perfume and deodorants. She had experienced a similar degree of hyperosmia during the early months of pregnancy and consulted her GP on two occasions, each time thinking she might be pregnant again but the appropriate urine tests were negative. When examined five months after the accident she was still complaining of hyperosmia, but no abnormality of the nose or sinuses was detected. A basic taste identification test was normal and she scored 37/40 (normal) on the University of Pennsylvania Smell Identification Test (UPSIT). After the test she remarked, "I hope I never have to do this test again as I feel very sick now." An MRI brain scan showed no sinonasal disease and gradient-echo sequences did not disclose any areas of petechial hemorrhage.

Comment: The initial injury was clearly trivial, but it is likely there was minor injury to the olfactory tracts from shearing forces at the time of accident. The proximity of hyperosmia to the time of accident gives credulity to her story, and so does her initial belief that she might have been pregnant. Another possibility would be triggering of migraine by the head trauma and the associated hyperosmia that is occasionally experienced by migraineurs. She gave no history of migraine or prior hyperosmia apart from that reporting during early pregnancy. No treatment was requested by the patient. As mentioned in Chapter 3 the existence of true hyperosmia is doubted and many apparent cases reflect hyperreactivity rather than increased power of detection. Her UPSIT score was unremarkable and no threshold test data were available to confirm her complaint of hypersensitivity. There is little available guidance on the prognosis for hyperosmia but most cases tend to resolve gradually over the course of several years.

(short-circuiting) transmission somewhere along the olfactory pathway. The selection of medication is a matter of personal choice but many use carbamazepine (Tegretol®), sodium valproate (Epilim®, Depakene®), gabapentin (Neurontin®), or pregabalin (Lyrica®). With all these medications it is important to start at a low dose then build up to the maximum tolerable. On basic principles an antidepressant might help, whether used alone or in conjunction with an anticonvulsant.

On the industrial front there are a large number of olfactory toxins that may cause damage, as listed in Chapter 3 (Table 3.4). Unquestionably there is an association between many of those listed, but several reports are anecdotal or based on small numbers from financially motivated individuals. Some odor symptoms concerning pollutants are primarily the result of sensory properties of the pollutants themselves which should resolve spontaneously once the individual is removed from the workplace. People exposed to pollutants may be receiving or have taken medication that, by itself, can affect smell sense or they may suffer coexisting disease known to alter olfaction. Note should be made of the compound alleged to have caused the olfactory defect and whether several substances were involved simultaneously. For most compounds there is a published threshold limit value (TLV) that gives an idea of maximum safe exposure levels and from this the magnitude of exposure may be estimated. This is of most relevance in cases of acute exposure, but for chronic exposure there may be individual susceptibility. The duration of exposure, latency of onset to first symptoms, their progression, and presence of dysosmia need to be recorded as well as the quality of ventilation, efficiency of filtration, and whether one or more workers had comparable symptoms at the same time.

Medicolegal aspects

Head injury is a common cause of anosmia, as described already. It should be recalled that severe trauma can lead to damage of the frontal and temporal poles, both of which are areas concerned with olfactory function. Thus, damage to the temporal pole may injure the amygdala or piriform nucleus, both of which are primary olfactory regions; frontal pole injury may involve the orbitofrontal cortex, which is an association area for smell (and taste). Anosmia commonly develops from mild trauma in the absence of skull fracture and possibly after whiplash injury (Kramer, 1983). Medical experts working for insurance companies, who deal with head-injured patients, often forget to ask about smell impairment, and if any tests are done they are usually inadequate. If injury directly involves the face there may be conductive anosmia from fracture of nasal bones, displacement of the septum, or

---

Case report 5.2: A 56-year-old heavy goods vehicle driver and amateur chef with posttraumatic anosmia

In November 2002 this man was hit just above the left eyebrow by a piece of protruding scaffolding. There was no laceration or impairment of consciousness. Later that day he noted lack of smell when using deodorant, and during the evening when eating a curry dish, there was no smell from the food although it tasted spicy. On the following day he experienced a peculiar burning odor, described as an "acid-sharp burning" sensation which persisted for one week. It sometimes woke him from sleep. A further week later, the smell sense disappeared completely. He specifically mentioned lack of odor from onions, ammonia, or bleach; all food tasted bland. When interviewed two years after the accident he reported no improvement in the sense of smell and no recurrence of parosmia. One of his hobbies was to cook meals for friends each week. Following the accident, it became difficult to mix sauces by their smell or taste and he resorted to cooking simpler dishes. He took the precaution of installing smoke and gas detectors throughout the house and a special malodor detector for the fridge. General neurological examination was unremarkable; likewise a brief identification test to five tastants was normal. His score on the UPSIT was within the anosmic (but not malingering) range at 16/40.

Comment: The most reasonable explanation is posttraumatic anosmia resulting from a relatively minor blow to the head. It is now accepted that even minor blows to the head may damage the sense of smell. The history is convincing because of the immediate appearance of smell loss and association with transient parosmia. The UPSIT scores are within the anosmic range and show no sign of malingering (range usually 0–5). His test scores and medical history are convincing and would strongly support his claim for anosmia and disruption of his main hobby as an amateur chef. Assuming the smell loss to be complete, the likelihood of recovery of useful smell function is poor.

---

nasal congestion from blood and debris, etc. Smell dysfunction due to this type of injury may resolve after surgical correction and resolution of edema, so further testing is desirable, say, 6–12 months after the trauma. Such patients may demonstrate unilateral anosmia over the initial months, but it can be persistent and will be overlooked if the nostrils are not tested independently. It is not sufficient just to ask a head-injured (or indeed any) patient about their smell perception. By analogy with cognitively normal patients with Parkinson's disease, only about 40 percent will be aware

Case report 5.3: A 56-year-old manual laborer and amateur archer with microsmia and probable Parkinson's disease after head trauma

This manual laborer, who was a keen amateur archer, became involved in an accident at work in April 2005. He slipped on a wet floor surface, striking the left side of his head on a metal girder. He was concussed but did not lose consciousness. There was blood oozing from the left ear and subsequent examination revealed a perforation injury of the tympanic membrane. Two weeks later he became aware of shaking of the left hand. During archery practice, he found it difficult to operate the bow and maintain the arrow steady because of tremulous movement. He was referred for a neurological opinion one year after the accident.

Examination revealed an intermittent rest tremor without any increase of tone. MRI brain scan was normal but the dopamine transporter imaging (DATScan) showed bilateral reduction of transporter uptake in the putamen on both sides. The UPSIT score was 26/40, which is within the microsmic range for a male of 56 years. The Mini-Mental State Examination (MMSE) score was normal at 28/30 and so were tests of taste threshold.

Comment: This man had good evidence on neurological examination, smell testing, and DATScan of tremulous Parkinson's disease, probably of the classical variety. The UPSIT score was within a range suggestive of considerable, but not total, loss of function, and there was no evidence of malingering or amplification of symptoms. The medicolegal question posed was whether the accident could have caused a tremor which emerged after just two weeks. There is a large and confusing literature on posttraumatic Parkinson's disease without any clear consensus, apart from those rare instances of parkinsonism resulting from repeated blows to the head, as in boxing. The latent period of two weeks from accident to tremor is far too short for the development of classical Parkinson's disease. Furthermore, an injury to the left skull, if it caused tremor at all, would be more likely to do so on the right side of the body unless there was a contre-coup effect, which would be unusual for subcortical structures. The most reasonable explanation is that the subject was in the early stages of Parkinson's disease at the time of accident and that the injury unmasked latent Parkinson's disease. The abnormal smell tests are compatible with a diagnosis of Parkinson's disease. A normal UPSIT score would have been more in keeping with a parkinsonian syndrome (e.g., progressive supranuclear palsy, corticobasal degeneration, vascular parkinsonism) or essential tremor. If the smell defect is secondary to Parkinson's disease, it will be permanent.

of a defect (Hawkes *et al.*, 1997) and if there is cognitive impairment, which is often the case where there has been brain injury, the figure is higher still. Although practical brief olfactory tests are available for preliminary vetting in outpatient practice (see Chapter 2 and the beginning of this chapter), more comprehensive assessment is necessary to detect malingerers reliably. Assuming a deficit does not relate to malingering, then further evaluation or repeated measurement would be appropriate at, say, yearly intervals, although the prognosis for recovery is poor overall and depends upon the patient's age and severity of initial loss (London *et al.*, 2008) (see Table 3.2, Chapter 3).

During the recovery phase a number of patients complain of distorted smell perception so that everyday odors taste bland or unpleasant (parosmia). Such distortions usually dissipate over time, although in rare instances they can be chronic, as described in Chapter 3. Treatment is problematic but antiepileptic or antidepressant medication could be tried in the first instance, as described above, for the management of hyperosmia.

According to guidance given by Sumner (1976) the law courts will wish to satisfy themselves on several counts:

- That trauma or industrial exposure can produce anosmia itself – a now incontrovertible fact.
- That there was no evidence of anosmia before the episode.
- That local causes of anosmia have been excluded.
- That there is no sign of amplification of symptoms or frank malingering.
- That the prognosis for recovery is based on reasoned assessment.

It is sometimes difficult to know when to finalize a claim for anosmia as there is prospect for recovery after a prolonged period. In broad terms, an interval not exceeding three years from the date of injury would be reasonable. If the sense of smell has not recovered by then it is likely to be permanent. An exception appears to be parosmia, the prevalence of which in one series decreased from 41.1 percent to 15.4 percent over eight years posttrauma (Doty *et al.*, 1997). Few people are willing to wait that long and serial assessment at yearly intervals may be helpful in determining the point at which no further improvement has taken place.

Detection of malingering and patients with nonorganic psychiatric disorders

"Malingering" is defined as the intentional production of false or grossly exaggerated physical or psychological symptoms that is motivated by some external incentive (e.g., financial gain). For example, on forced-choice tests, the known correct answer may be deliberately deselected, giving an abnormallylow score. Those with non-organic disorders variously termed "functional" or "hysterical" may also score badly on tests, but in our experience such patients are extremely rare. At one extreme would be a patient with true hysteria, where there may be no deliberate deception but the patient has assumed the features of disease – so-called "conversion hysteria." Between true hysteria and malingering are those subjects who, because of various stressors (anxiety, depression, etc.), score badly. This may be unintentional but nonetheless extremely difficult to quantify.

Traditionally it has been assumed that malingering can be detected reliably by having a patient inhale a strong trigeminal stimulant, such as ammonia, and asking whether a smell is perceived. If denial occurs, the assumption is made that malingering is present. Unfortunately, this procedure is unreliable, since ammonia usually produces reflex coughing, secretion from nasal membranes, or other rejection reactions which the patient obviously cannot deny. Furthermore, trigeminal thresholds vary considerably; some may experience little reaction to the ammonia and truthfully report perceiving no sensations. Indeed, anosmia is often associated with heightened trigeminal thresholds (Gudziol *et al.*, 2001). The clever malingerer may be smart enough to report the irritant effect, so the accuracy of the procedure is questionable and, in the authors' view, this test should not be employed.

The results of longer forced-choice tests, including identification and detection threshold measures, can be examined for improbable responses that usually signify malingering. On the UPSIT, for example, malingerers typically score between 0/40 and 5/40 (see Chapter 2, Figure 2.4). The binomial probability of achieving a score of say, 1/40 on this four-alternative forced-choice test by a true anosmic is 0.000134 (Doty *et al.*, 1995). To achieve such a low score, the patient must first identify the odor and then avoid the correct answer. In general, if a patient scores within the probable malingering region on the UPSIT, the test should be repeated to confirm the apparent avoidance of correct responses. Multiplication of the two probabilities is then used to establish the statistical likelihood of malingering. Some malingerers may repetitively provide the same response to every test item (e.g., always indicate the first response item in each set of four response alternatives on the UPSIT), but this is also true for some anosmia sufferers, and in both cases the test score would not fall in the probable malingering range. Hence, such responses do not definitively establish malingering. Some true anosmics scratch the UPSIT pad so hard that they abrade the strip down to its cardboard backing (Doty *et al.*, 1998) – a feature not seen in malingering.

The olfactory event-related potential (OERP) is of potential value in detecting a malingerer as long as the technical difficulties can be overcome, the patient cooperates with the examiner (e.g., does not exhibit significant body movements), and the subject is not unduly stressed by the obvious importance and complexity of the procedure. In theory, olfactory agnosia in such cases cannot be ruled out – so that a patient with a temporal lobe defect could have difficulty naming odors in the presence of a normal OERP. Brain imaging by MRI, CT, or SPECT may show posttraumatic change in a relevant area, e.g., temporal lobes, insular, or orbitofrontal cortices. The gradient echo MRI sequence is particularly useful in revealing petechial areas of hemorrhage, which can persist for several years after injury and may be invisible on conventional MRI. There may be atrophy of the olfactory bulb (Yousem *et al.*, 1999), a point of relevance where there is a suspicion of amplification or malingering. Even with this procedure, there are added difficulties as there are no large healthy control measurements that take into account the effect of age and sex, and it is unknown whether the olfactory bulbs regress in size in a uniform manner over time among different individuals. Nonetheless, there is growing evidence of strong associations between MRI-determined olfactory bulb volumes and olfactory function in both normal individuals and in persons with olfactory deficits. For example, a –0.86 correlation was noted by Turetsky *et al.* (2000) between MRI-determined olfactory volumes and detection thresholds for phenyl ethyl alcohol in a group of 22 healthy subjects. Theoretically, malingering might be detected by fMRI or PET studies using olfactory stimuli, but such measures may not be reliable and activity could be present in primary olfactory areas but not in tertiary ones, making it possible that the subject is genuinely unaware of odors. All this assumes, as noted above, that a malingerer will cooperate with a complex test – which is unlikely.

Some patients with genuine smell impairment but preserved taste may deliberately avoid correct answers on forced choice *taste* tests. This pattern reflects a naïve attempt to embellish the "taste loss" which, in reality, stems from lack of retronasal stimulation of the olfactory receptors. Such behavior usually confirms a normal ability to taste.

Several cognitive tests are used by neuropsychologists on which amnesic patients perform well, yet malingerers fail to do so. One example is the Rey's Memory Test, also known as Rey's 3×5 test, and the Rey 15-item memory test (Rey, 1964). The rationale behind this is that malingerers typically fail at a memory task that all but the most retarded or severely brain-damaged people perform easily. This is a highly specialized area of evaluation for which the reader should consult elsewhere (e.g., Hall & Pritchard, 1996).

Case report 5.4: An 18-year-old office worker with probable malingering

This lady reported having lost her sense of taste and smell in an accident in which she fell from the back of a pickup truck, hitting her head on the ground. She suffered concussion and amnesia for the entire event. A CT brain scan revealed a transverse fracture of the left temporal bone predominantly through the mastoid portion. She experienced transient decrease in hearing on the left, as well as mild positional vertigo. She was referred for assessment by her lawyer three years after the accident, when she was 21 years of age. According to the patient records, she had previously reported to an otolaryngologist (who was following up her case) that her sense of smell was improving. Upon testing, the UPSIT score was 1, which fell within the probable malingering range of the test. The UPSIT was repeated, giving a score of 3, a value that similarly fell within the probable malingering range. On a two-alternative forced-choice odor detection threshold test, in which a blank and an odor were presented in random fashion, the patient performed correctly on only 24 of the 96 trials (25 percent). On a forced-choice regional taste test, in which six trials each of sweet-, sour-, bitter- and salty-tasting substances are presented to four regions of the tongue (six trials × four tastants × four tongue regions = 96 trials), this patient missed 79/96 trials, i.e., she only provided correct responses on 17/96 trials (18 percent). On this test, a forced-choice response is also required to four response alternatives (sweet, sour, bitter, and salty).

Comment: This lady most likely suffered transient loss of smell from head trauma, but had subsequently improved and was malingering for litigation purposes. A true anosmia sufferer would, on average, answer correctly one-quarter of the UPSIT items, or have a predicted average score of 10. There is a sampling distribution around this value, but the binomial probability of achieving a score of 1 out of 40 on this four-alternative forced-choice test by an anosmic is 0.000 134. On the second administration, she scored 3 out of 40, which has a binomial probability of occurrence of 0.003 67. The combined probability of her being a true anosmic, based on these test responses alone, is $0.000\,134 \times 0.003\,67 = 3.70^{-8}$. On the olfactory threshold test, the binomial probability of missing 72 out of 96 trials by chance is <0.000 001. Her taste tests also suggested she was deliberately avoiding correct responses. For example, on a test in which 25 percent of 96 trials would be expected on the basis of random responding (i.e., 24), she detected correctly only 17. The probability of performing this badly and not avoiding the correct responses would be less than 1 in 1000. OERPs were not done but they should be normal in this case.

Case report 5.5: A 57-year-old housewife with smell and taste impairment related to fungal sinus infection

This lady, who had a degree in psychology, suffered recurrent urinary tract infection for several years and was placed on a long-term antibiotic, nitro-furantoin (Furadantin®, Macrodantin®, Macrobid®). This worked well, but after three years' use she developed chronic active hepatitis, a recognized complication of long-term use of this drug. This was treated by long-term steroids, but after two months' use of these she developed progressive blurring of vision and a lower altitudinal field defect in the left eye. Investigation showed a fungal infection (aspergillus) in the sphenoid and ethmoid sinuses. Treatment with an antifungal drug, amphotericin B (Fungilin®; Fungisome®) and spheno-ethmoidotomy resulted in improved vision. Two weeks after surgery, she returned home and noticed for the first time that the sense of smell was impaired. Sweet food and chocolates appeared to taste normal, but there was no sensation from flowers or shrubs and she lost all interest in cooking. There was some odorous sensation if she held garlic close to the nose. Formerly, she was able to tell if her urine was infected by its abnormal odor, but this became impossible. On one occasion, her husband came home to find the house full of gas. A writ had been served on her primary care physicians for failing to monitor liver function whilst taking long-term nitrofurantoin and the subsequent development of chronic active hepatitis and complications of steroid use.

Detailed evaluation was performed about three years after surgery at the request of her solicitor. The electrical taste threshold over the tongue tip using a Rion electrogustometer was elevated significantly at 64 μA (normal below 25 μA). The UPSIT was 12/40, which is well within the anosmic range. She became tearful and distressed throughout this test, commenting that everything smelt the same. Evaluation with the Smell Threshold Test (phenyl ethyl alcohol) using the single staircase method was also abnormal, being above −2.00 log vol/vol in light mineral oil (normal would be in the range of −6.0 to −5.0). OERPs showed a normal latency to H_2S of 412 ms, recorded from Pz.

Comment: Several interesting points are raised by this case. Most likely, long-term steroid exposure caused the fungal infection in the sinuses. Such infection could easily have impaired the sense of smell but so could the decompressive surgery and use of the antifungal agent, amphotericin B. On questioning she affirmed that smell impairment was first noticed only on arriving home after she would have completed 16 days of amphotericin therapy. She did not think it occurred immediately after surgery.

The first question is whether the smell loss was genuine. The history alone is convincing in many respects; her inability to detect the smell of

Case report 5.5: (cont.)

infected urine and of the house filled with gas unknown to her. Her score on UPSIT was at chance level, and the smell threshold value was elevated markedly, in keeping with a diagnosis of anosmia. Although no problem with taste was declared, the electrogustometer suggested partial impairment. Despite the fact that this patient had a degree in psychology and therefore might have sufficient knowledge to fabricate some of her symptoms, there was no evidence that this occurred. It is of interest, however, that the OERP, which could have been a deciding "objective" test, was within normal limits. The final advice offered was that the anosmia was in fact genuine and the delay in reporting a problem related to general malaise in hospital where she was recovering from major surgery. It was considered that, when she had fully recuperated from inpatient treatment, she would have been better placed to detect other less severe problems. It was advised that the normal OERP may have been a technical issue caused by inadvertent stimulation of healthy nasal trigeminal afferent fibers. The cause of anosmia was thought to be a mixture of fungal infection, possibly sinus surgery, and exposure to a drug (amphotericin B) known to produce anosmia. Amphotericin B probably caused the mild impairment of taste as well. Useful recovery of smell sense in someone with such severe loss is unlikely to occur three years after the initiating event. This case was eventually settled in the claimant's favor, out of court.

General advice and vocational issues

The medicolegal and indeed everyday clinical importance of anosmia or hyposmia in part relate to occupation. A wine taster or chef may well be unemployable if there is even the smallest reduction in olfactory identification or threshold and their potential for legitimate financial compensation is high. This contrasts with the unskilled laborer who would be entitled to less. In general a plaintiff's former employment should be allowed to continue unless a good sense of smell is essential or the person had to work alone in a potentially dangerous environment. A retired person would command less financial reward, but the dangers in everyday life must not be underestimated, nor the lack of enjoyment of food or drink and the overall reduction in the quality of life.

Disability awards and compensations are provided in the USA under the 1963 amendment to the Workman's Compensation Law. Where a diminution of future earning power is apparent, the Veterans Administration awards a 10 percent disability for total anosmia. In general, there is considerable interstate variability in workman compensation payment and the results of private individual settlements are hardly ever made public. Up to a 5 percent compensation for anosmia is suggested by the 6th edition of the American Medical Association *Guides to the Evaluation of Permanent Impairment*:

Only rarely does complete loss of the closely related senses of olfaction and taste seriously affect an individual's performance of the usual activities of daily living. For this reason, a 1% to 5% impairment of the whole person is suggested for use in cases involving partial or complete bilateral loss of either sense due to peripheral lesions. (Anderson & Cocchiarella, 1995)

This is surprising, given that anosmia or dysosmia disqualifies applicants for service in the US Armed Forces, including the Coast Guard, and can be a basis for discharge or retirement (Air Force Instructions 2006). Private accident insurance policies in the UK recompense their clients by less than 10 percent of that awarded for parallel cases in the USA. In the UK an average level of compensation for non-vocational smell disorder is £12 000 for partial loss of smell and £18 000 for complete loss.

   Anosmic patients, and even those experiencing natural decline of smell function through aging, should be given guidance on simple precautions. A significant number of elderly people die from gas poisoning each year (Chalke & Dewhurst, 1956) and presumably if they were properly advised this tragedy would be less. Consumption of infected food probably causes minor ailments in the elderly and, on occasion, food poisoning. Nutritional problems and weight loss in the aged may relate to decreased smell function, as food loses its appeal. Indeed, it is suspected that the frequent finding of weight loss in patients with advanced Parkinson's disease relates to hyposmia, which as mentioned in Chapter 4, affects at least 80–90 percent of these individuals (Hawkes *et al.*, 1997). A smoke detector is essential for the kitchen and in every room where there is the potential for fire. It is preferable to have a detector in all bedrooms, particularly in those belonging to smokers. An electric cooker is preferable to one operated by gas. If the household has a gas supply, patients should purchase a detector for this as well. Propane, butane, and petroleum spirit (gasoline) are heavier than air and because of this detectors for them should be placed near the ground. Natural gas and smoke are lighter than air so the detectors for this need to be situated near the ceiling or top of the stairwell. An anosmic person may have difficulty appreciating spoiled food, which can be hazardous to eat even if kept in the refrigerator. Such people should be encouraged to discard leftover food and ideally ask someone with normal smell sense to check all food before consumption. Finally, advice – ideally from a dietician – should be given on how to enhance the appeal of food with artificial flavorings, without inducing weight gain.

An often underappreciated fact is that simply quantifying the degree of olfactory loss and ruling out serious causes is extremely beneficial for the psychological well-being of a patient, whether or not treatment is possible. Helping the patient place into perspective the magnitude of his or her loss is very therapeutic, and in some cases mitigates depression and other symptoms produced by fear or by uncaring medical providers. Many patients feel alienated and are unaware that others suffer the same problems. Meeting other patients with similar problems in a waiting room, for example, has proven in our experience to be most helpful, since patients become directly aware they are not alone in terms of their malady. It can be pointed out to half of older persons that their olfactory test scores actually are above the 50th percentile relative to individuals of their age and sex. This patient then leaves with the understanding that whilst loss has occurred, he or she is still "hanging in there" and is outperforming the majority of his or her peers.

Importantly, patients who fear safety issues, such as inability to detect leaking natural gas and fire, can be counseled about smoke and gas detectors, as well as changing gas appliances to electrical ones when economically possible. Psychological strategies to aid patients in dealing with their disability are beyond the scope of this book, but have been described in detail elsewhere (Tennen *et al.*, 1991).

Summary

Treatment of olfactory disorder is directed to the underlying disease and assisting patients to cope with their problem from the psychological perspective. Steroids, zinc supplements, and various antioxidants are tried extensively but their value is dubious. Steroids are beneficial only for local nasal conditions, particularly where there is conductive anosmia from polyps or hay fever. Some benefit may accrue from nasal operations that facilitate sinus drainage and reduce infection, although topical steroids are usually required to minimize local inflammation. Where compensation is pursued the patient is best directed to a unit specializing in assessment of olfactory medicolegal problems. It is important to help sufferers cope psychologically with their problem and put their deficit in perspective, as well as provide them with general advice about their occupation, safety in the home, and how food may be made more palatable.

REFERENCES

Air Force Instructions 48–123. Accession, retention and administration. *Medication Examination and Standards*, **2**, 5 June 2006.

Anderson GBJ and Cocchiarella L. *Guides to the Evaluation of Permanent Impairment*, 6th edn. Chicago, IL: American Medical Association Press, 1995.

Briggs MH and Duncan RB. Odor receptors. *Nature*, 1961, **91**, 1310–11.

Chalke HD and Dewhurst JR. Loss of smell in old people. *Public Health*, 1956, **72**, 223.

Doty RL, Smith R, McKeown DA and Raj J. Tests of human olfactory function: principal components analysis suggests that most measure a common source of variance. *Perception and Psychophysics*, 1994, **56**(6), 701–7.

Doty RL, McKeown DA, Lee WW and Shaman P. A study of the test–retest reliability of ten olfactory tests. *Chemical Senses*, 1995, **20**(6), 645–56.

Doty RL, Yousem DM, Pham LT, Kreshak AA, Geckle R and Lee WW. Olfactory dysfunction in patients with head trauma. *Archives of Neurology*, 1997, **54**(9), 1131–40.

Doty RL, Genow A and Hummel T. Scratch density differentiates microsmic from normosmic and anosmic subjects on the University of Pennsylvania Smell Identification Test. *Perceptual and Motor Skills*, 1998, **86**, 211–16.

Duncan RB and Briggs MH. Treatment of uncomplicated anosmia by vitamin A. *Archives of Otolaryngology*, 1962, **75**, 116–24.

Gudziol H, Schubert M and Hummel T. Decreased trigeminal sensitivity in anosmia. *Journal for Oto-Rhino-Laryngology and its Related Specialties*, 2001, **63**(2), 72–5.

Hagglund M, Berghard A, Strotmann J and Bohm S. Retinoic acid receptor-dependent survival of olfactory sensory neurons in postnasal and adult mice. *Journal of Neuroscience*, 2006, **26**, 3281–91.

Hall HV and Pritchard DA. *Detecting Malingering and Deception*. Delray Beach, FL: St. Lucie Press, 1996.

Hawkes CH, Shephard BC and Daniel SE. Olfactory dysfunction in Parkinson's disease. *Journal of Neurology, Neurosurgery and Psychiatry*, 1997, **62**, 436–46.

Henkin RI, Schechter PJ, Friedewald WT *et al.* A double-blind study of the effects of zinc sulfate on taste and smell dysfunction. *American Journal of Medical Science*, 1976, **272**, 167–74.

Hummel T, Heilmann S and Huttenbriuk KB. Lipoic acid in the treatment of smell dysfunction following viral infection of the upper respiratory tract. *Laryngoscope*, 2002, **112**, 2076–80.

Jackman AH and Doty RL. Utility of a three-item smell identification test in detecting olfactory dysfunction. *Laryngoscope*, 2005, **115**(12), 2209–12.

Jafek BW, Eller PM, Esses BA and Moran DT. Post-traumatic anosmia. Ultrastructural correlates. *Archives of Neurology*, 1989, **46**(3), 300–4.

Kramer G. Diagnosis of neurologic disorders after whiplash injuries of the cervical spine. *Deutsche Medizinische Wochenschrift*, 1983, **108**(15), 586–8.

Lill K, Reden J, Muller A, Zahnert T and Hummel T. Olfactory function in patients with post-infectious and post-traumatic smell disorders before and after treatment with vitamin A: a double-blind, placebo-controlled, randomized clinical trial. *Chemical Senses*, 2006, **31**(5), Abstract A33.

London B, Nabet B, Fisher AR, White B, Sammel MD and Doty RL Predictors of prognosis in patients with olfactory disturbance. *Annals of Neurology*, 2008, **63**(2), 159–66.

Mahajan SK, Prasad AS, Briggs WA *et al*. Improvement in uremic hypogeusia by zinc: a double-blind study. *American Journal of Clinical Nutrition*, 1980, **33**, 1517–21.

Rey A. *L'Examen Clinique en Psychologie*. Paris: Presses Universitaires de France, 1964.

Schechter PJ, Friedewald WT, Bronzert DA *et al*. Idiopathic hypogeusia: a description of the syndrome and a single blind study with zinc sulfate. *International Review of Neurobiology*, 1972, **1**(Suppl.), 125–40.

Sorter A, Kim J, Jackman A, Tourbier I, Kaul A and Doty RL. Accuracy of self-report in detecting taste dysfunction. *Laryngoscope*, 2008, **118**, 611–17.

Steck-Scott S, Forman MR, Sowell A *et al*. Carotenoids, vitamin A and risk of adenomatous polyp recurrence in the polyp prevention trial. *International Journal of Cancer*, 2004, **112**(2), 295–305.

Stegeman CA, Cohen Tervaert JW, de Jong PE and Kallenberg CG. Trimethoprim–sulfamethoxazole (co-trimoxazole) for the prevention of relapses of Wegener's granulomatosis. Dutch Co-Trimoxazole Wegener Study Group. *New England Journal of Medicine*, 1996, **335**, 16–20.

Sumner D. Disturbances of the senses of smell and taste after head injuries. In: PJ Vinken and GW Bruyn, eds., *Handbook of Clinical Neurology*. Amsterdam: Elsevier Press, 1976, pp. 1–25.

Tennen H, Affleck G and Mendola R. Coping with smell and taste disorders. In: TV Getchell, RL Doty, LM Bartoshuk and JB Snow Jr., eds., *Smell and Taste in Health and Disease*. New York, NY: Raven Press, 1991, pp. 787–802.

Turetsky BI, Moberg PJ, Yousem DM, Doty RL, Arnold SE and Gur RE. Reduced olfactory bulb volume in patients with schizophrenia. *American Journal of Psychiatry*, 2000, **157**, 828–30.

Weisman K, Christensen E and Dreyer V. Zinc supplementation in alcoholic cirrhosis: a double-blind clinical trial. *Acta Medica Scandinavica*, 1979, **205**, 361–6.

Yousem DM, Geckle RJ, Bilker WB, Kroger H and Doty RL. Posttraumatic smell loss: relationship of psychophysical tests and volumes of the olfactory bulbs and tracts and the temporal lobes. *Academic Radiology*, 1999, **6**(5), 264–72.

Index

Note: page numbers in *italics* refer to figures and tables.